QP   Morehouse
301   Physiology of exercise
M65
1976

               Date Due   108571

APR 2 3 1984		
JAN 2 5 1988		
DEC 0 8 1989		
JAN 0 2 1990	MAY 2 1 1998	
MAY 1 1 1992	SEP 1 4 1999	
JUL 1 6 1992	MAR 2 8 2005	
NOV 4 1992	APR 1 8 2005	
	MAY 1 0 2005	
MAR 2 2 1995		
	OCT 2 0 2008	

D1165270

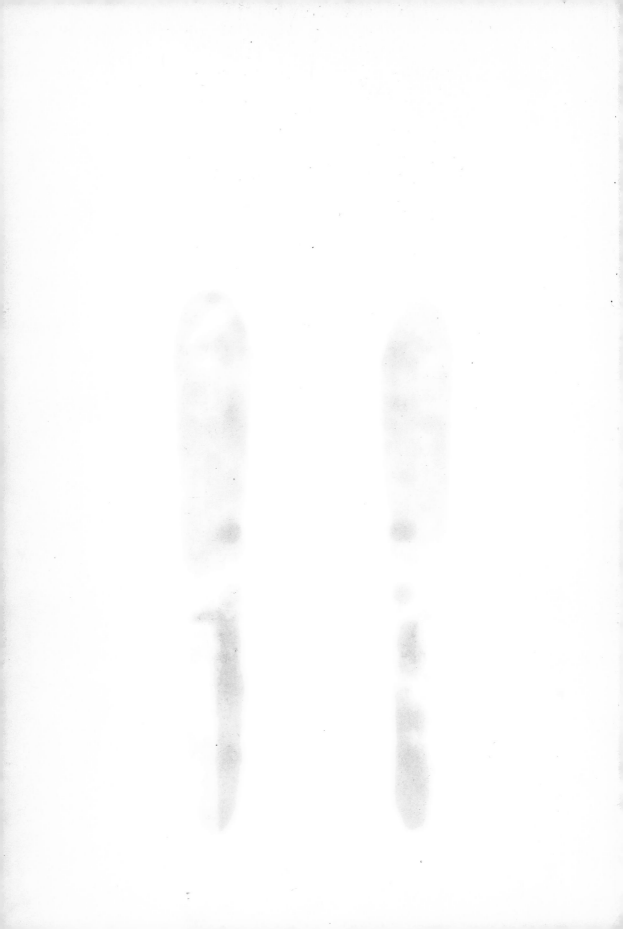

PHYSIOLOGY OF EXERCISE

PHYSIOLOGY OF EXERCISE

LAURENCE E. MOREHOUSE, Ph.D.

Professor of Kinesiology, University of
California at Los Angeles, Los Angeles, Calif.

AUGUSTUS T. MILLER, Jr., M.D., Ph.D.

Professor of Physiology, University of
North Carolina Medical School, Chapel Hill, N.C.

Seventh edition

with 33 illustrations

Saint Louis

The C. V. Mosby Company

1976

SEVENTH EDITION

Copyright © 1976 by The C. V. Mosby Company

All rights reserved. No part of this book may be reproduced
in any manner without written permission of the publisher.

Previous editions copyrighted 1948, 1953, 1959, 1963, 1967, 1971

Printed in the United States of America

Distributed in Great Britain by Henry Kimpton, London

Library of Congress Cataloging in Publication Data

Morehouse, Laurence Englemohr, 1913-
    Physiology of exercise.

    Bibliography: p.
    Includes index.
    1. Exercise—Physiological effect. I. Miller,
Augustus Taylor, 1910-   joint author. II. Title.
[DNLM: 1. Exertion. WE103 M838p]
QP301.M65 1976   612'.76   75-22186
ISBN 0-8016-3485-7

VH/VH/VH   9   8   7   6   5   4   3   2   1

FOREWORD*

Physical exercise is an activity in which every human being engages, to one degree or another, during the course of his life. It is of the utmost importance to know the physiological mechanisms that sustain and act as the basis of every body response to exercise. Accordingly, there is a definite need for textbooks that will give the nonspecialized professional the fundamentals of exercise physiology in clear, everyday language.

In the course of physical exertion a number of coordinated and compensatory adjustments take place throughout the body which involve metabolic functions and the nervous, muscular, circulatory, and respiratory systems. Important roles are played by environmental conditions, stress, training, and fatigue.

The tendency to exercise and to move rhythmically is inborn. Exercise improves muscle tone and creates a sense of well-being. These factors, among several others, characterize the importance of exercise.

Besides creating pleasure, exercise helps to sustain agility and alertness and it exerts a deep social and psychological influence; the lack of it can cause obesity and degenerative metabolic diseases. In short, exercise favors both psychic and physical health. However, excesses in physical exertion are harmful and must be carefully avoided.

At present, knowledge about physiology is progressing at a steady pace. Some old creeds and formerly held beliefs must be corrected or perfected, if not entirely renewed; therefore, a textbook on the influence of physiology on human exercise must be clear, modern, fundamental, stimulating, and as simple as possible.

*From the Spanish edition, translated by A. Leveroni and M. Martini.

v

Drs. Morehouse and Miller's book complies with every one of these requirements and may be recommended as a good modern textbook. It covers all the basic topics and fundamental ideas that lead to a complete understanding and thorough knowledge of this branch of science.

Bernardo A. Houssay
Nobel Laureate in Physiology
Buenos Aires

PREFACE

The scientific study of exercise physiology is becoming increasingly important with the growing realization of the relation of exercise to health. Field and laboratory observations on exercising human subjects are being supplemented with physiologic and biochemical studies on laboratory animals, with the result that many of the phenomena associated with acute and chronic exercise can now be explained at basic cellular and molecular levels. For this reason, a new chapter has been added to this edition entitled "The Production of Energy by Cells." The assistance of V. Reggie Edgerton in the preparation of this new chapter is gratefully acknowledged.

Other new chapters in this edition reflect the extension of exercise physiology studies beyond the fields of physical education and athletics, especially into therapeutic areas including sports medicine and cardiac rehabilitation. These other new chapters are entitled: "Muscular Performance," "Maximal Effort and Fatigue," "Nutrition and Ergogenic Aids," "Body Structure," "Muscular Development," "Circulorespiratory Development," "Exercise in Relation to Obesity and Diabetes," "Motor Rehabilitation," and "Exercise and Heart Disease."

Exercise physiology is emerging as an independent discipline with its unique problems and its own methods of study. For the student whose major is exercise physiology, this text is an introductory survey of this branch of knowledge.

The *Laboratory Manual for Physiology of Exercise*, by L. E. Morehouse, published by The C. V. Mosby Company, 1972, is available for students of exercise physiology. References to this manual in this text are cited as *Laboratory Manual*.

Comments from our readers will be received with appreciation.

Laurence E. Morehouse
Augustus T. Miller, Jr.

CONTENTS

PART SEVEN

Therapeutic exercise

PART EIGHT

Age and sex factors

PART ONE

CELLULAR DYNAMICS OF EXERCISE

1 THE PRODUCTION OF ENERGY BY CELLS

Exercise requires the contraction of skeletal muscles, and muscle contraction requires energy. The purpose of this chapter is to explain the manner in which all cells, including muscle cells (fibers), obtain the energy needed for their various activities. For many students this chapter will be a perhaps unnecessary review, but for others it may be helpful in understanding some aspects of exercise physiology to be discussed in later chapters.

For many years students were taught that the energy required by the body is derived from the oxidation of foodstuffs (carbohydrates, fats, and proteins). As we shall see, this is true only in a limited sense. Actually, the immediate source of energy for the activities of cells is the compound ATP (adenosinetriphosphate), which is formed mostly in the mitochondria (small structures or "organelles" about the size of bacteria, which are present in large numbers in the cytoplasm of the cell). An "average" cell (e.g., liver) may contain about 1,000 mitochondria, each of which contains all the machinery required for the production of ATP. Mitochondria occupy almost half the volume of the average cardiac muscle cell and a considerable part of the volume of skeletal muscle cells.

When the cells require energy, they obtain it by splitting stored ATP molecules, a process that results in the liberation of energy, together with the formation of a simpler compound, ADP (adenosinediphosphate), and inorganic phosphate. The reaction may be written $ATP \rightleftharpoons ADP + Pi +$ energy. Energy is often expressed in terms of calories; the splitting of 1 mol of ATP liberates about 7,000 calories of energy (the exact amount depends on conditions in the cell, discussion

3

of which is beyond the scope of this book). The manner in which the energy liberated by the splitting of ATP is utilized varies in different types of cells; the situation in muscle cells will be discussed in Chapter 2.

Our present concern is with the chemical reactions that result in the formation of ATP, so that the ATP stores are maintained at an adequate level, available for instant use when needed. This is where the "oxidation" of foodstuffs enters the picture. Biological oxidations usually involve the removal of hydrogen (or electrons), rather than the addition of oxygen, such as occurs when wood is burned; however, the terms oxidation and dehydrogenation are often used interchangeably in textbooks. Before proceeding to a more detailed discussion of the reactions involved in the formation of ATP, one additional point should be mentioned: ATP can be formed during both aerobic and anaerobic metabolism, that is, in the presence or absence of oxygen. The characteristics of these two types of metabolism will now be discussed.

AEROBIC AND ANAEROBIC METABOLISM

Both aerobic and anaerobic metabolism involve oxidations; the two types of metabolism differ in a number of ways but most basically in the nature of the hydrogen acceptor in each type. In chemical reactions, the oxidation of one compound must always be accompanied by the reduction of another compound. Since in biological reactions oxidations usually involve the removal of hydrogen or electrons, the compound being oxidized is called the hydrogen (or electron) *donor,* and the compound being reduced is the hydrogen (or electron) *acceptor.* As an example, let AH_2 represent a compound that is being oxidized:

$$AH_2 + \tfrac{1}{2}O_2 \rightarrow A + H_2O$$

In this reaction AH_2 is the hydrogen *donor* and O_2 is the hydrogen *acceptor.* This is an example of an oxidation that does actually involve oxygen. Consider, on the other hand, the following reaction:

$$NADH_2 + \text{pyruvic acid} \rightleftharpoons NAD^+ + \text{lactic acid}$$

($NADH_2$ and NAD^+ are the reduced and oxidized forms, respectively, of one of the common coenzymes—nicotinamide adenine dinucleotide; NAD was called DPN in the older literature—for diphosphopyridine nucleotide.) Here $NADH_2$ is oxidized to NAD^+ by the removal of hydrogen; pyruvic acid acts as the hydrogen acceptor, thereby undergoing reduction to lactic acid. In some of the cytochrome reactions in the mitochondria, oxidation consists of the removal of electrons from a reduced cytochrome (electron donor) and their acceptance by the next cytochrome in the chain (electron acceptor) or by *molecular oxygen* in the case of the last member of the chain. Thus, we may say that aerobic and anaerobic metabolism differ essentially in the nature of the *final hydrogen (or electron) acceptor;* this is oxygen in aerobic metabolism, but some other compound in anaerobic metabolism. Other important differences between aerobic and anaerobic metabolism will be pointed out in succeeding sections of this chapter.

AEROBIC FORMATION OF ATP

The aerobic formation of ATP involves two sets of reactions: the Krebs cycle (also called the citric acid or TCA cycle), and the respiratory chain (also called the electron transport chain or ETC). Both sets of reactions occur exclusively in the mitochondria.

The Krebs cycle is a cycle of chemical reactions into which simple compounds derived from the foodstuffs are fed at several points (Fig. 1). At four points in the cycle, oxidation (removal of hydrogen) occurs; the resulting hydrogen is then passed down the respiratory chain to oxygen, the final hydrogen acceptor (Fig. 2). The Krebs cycle itself produces no energy, only hydrogen for the respiratory chain. However, as hydrogen (or electrons) is passed stepwise down the respiratory chain (in which each compound in the chain successively reduces the

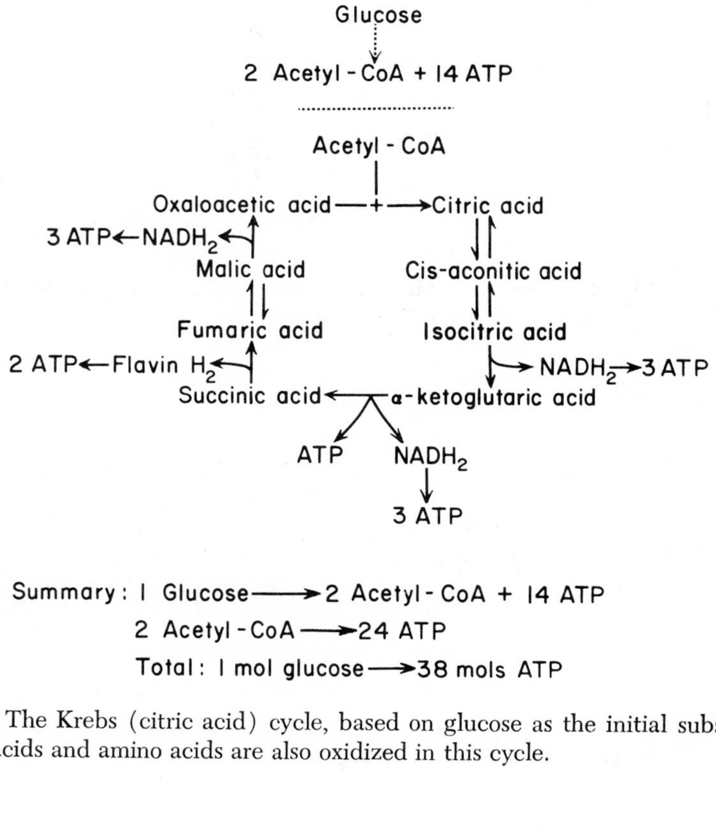

Glucose

2 Acetyl - CoA + 14 ATP

. . . .

Acetyl - CoA

Oxaloacetic acid —+—→ Citric acid

3 ATP←NADH$_2$←

Malic acid   Cis-aconitic acid

Fumaric acid   Isocitric acid

2 ATP←Flavin H$_2$←   NADH$_2$→3 ATP

Succinic acid←   α-ketoglutaric acid

ATP   NADH$_2$

3 ATP

Summary: 1 Glucose———→2 Acetyl-CoA + 14 ATP

2 Acetyl-CoA——→24 ATP

Total: 1 mol glucose——→38 mols ATP

Fig. 1. The Krebs (citric acid) cycle, based on glucose as the initial substrate. Fatty acids and amino acids are also oxidized in this cycle.

5

compound below it), a molecule of ATP is formed at three points (only at these three points is the free energy change great enough to form a molecule of ATP). It is generally believed that the enzymes involved in the Krebs cycle are located in the interior or *matrix* of the mitochondrion (Fig. 3), while the components of the respiratory chain are attached in sequential order to the cristae of the inner mitochondrial membrane (Fig.

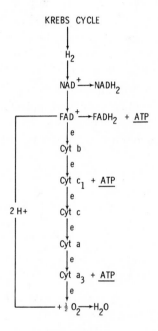

Fig. 2. The mitochondrial respiratory chain (electron transport chain), showing the sites at which ATP is formed.

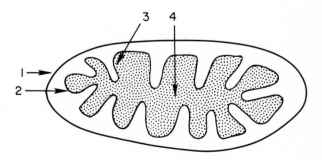

Fig. 3. Schematic cross section of a mitochondrion. *1*, Outer membrane; *2*, inner membrane; *3*, infolding of inner membrane to form a crista; *4*, matrix.

3). We may summarize by saying that the function of the Krebs cycle is to provide hydrogen for transport down the respiratory chain to oxygen, and that ATP is formed during this transport by a process known as oxidative phosphorylation. The details of this process are still poorly understood.

When oxygen is available, derivatives of the three foodstuffs (carbohydrates, fats, and proteins) are fed into the Krebs cycle and hence ultimately contribute to the formation of ATP. When oxygen is not available, the Krebs cycle and respiratory chain are nonfunctional, and ATP can be formed only by anaerobic metabolism, to be discussed in the next section.

ANAEROBIC FORMATION OF ATP

When oxygen is not available, carbohydrate is the only one of the three foodstuffs that can be used in the formation of ATP. This involves the process known as glycolysis (which takes place in the cytoplasm of the cell), in which glucose or glycogen is converted, through a series of reactions, to the three-carbon compound pyruvic acid (Fig. 4). Glycolysis, to this point, is common to both aerobic and anaerobic metabolism of carbohydrates. When oxygen is available, the pyruvic acid is converted to acetic acid which, after further modification, enters the Krebs cycle and is metabolized as described in the preceding section. However, when oxygen is not available the pyruvic acid is reduced to lactic acid, which is a metabolic dead end and hence accumulates in the cells and diffuses into the blood. It is for this reason that blood lactic acid concentration serves as an indicator of anaerobic metabolism in exercise.

The formation of lactic acid from pyruvic acid under anaerobic conditions does not produce energy. What, then, is its purpose? If we examine the chain of reactions involved in glycolysis (Fig. 4), we note that one reaction involves an oxidation: the conversion of glyceraldehyde-3-phosphate to 1, 3-diphosphoglyceric acid, and that this is made possible by the simultaneous reduction of NAD^+ to $NADH_2$. The supply of NAD^+ in the cytoplasm is limited, and it would soon be exhausted if there were no mechanism to restore it; in this case, glycolysis would come to a standstill. Fortunately, this does not occur, since $NADH_2$ can be reoxidized to NAD^+ coupled with the reduction of pyruvic acid to lactic acid. Thus the "purpose" of lactic acid formation under anaerobic conditions is the restoration of the NAD^+ required for glycolysis. In the pathway of glycolysis from glucose to pyruvic acid, two molecules of ATP are used and four are produced; the net result is that the anaerobic metabolism of one molecule of glucose yields two molecules of ATP. Under aerobic conditions, the metabolism of one molecule of glucose via

7

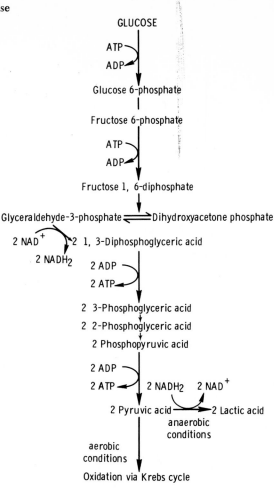

Fig. 4. Glycolysis.

the Krebs cycle and respiratory chain yields thirty-eight molecules of ATP. The end products, carbon dioxide and water, are also readily disposable while the lactic acid formed in anaerobic metabolism is not, and causes a metabolic acidosis. A final advantage of aerobic metabolism is that it can utilize all three of the major foodstuffs (carbohydrates, fats, and proteins), while anaerobic metabolism can utilize only carbohydrates. The sole virtue of anaerobic metabolism is that it does not require oxygen. The importance of this fact will become clear in subsequent chapters.

THE SHUTTLE SYSTEMS

In the metabolism of glucose or glycogen to the stage of pyruvic acid, NAD^+ is reduced to $NADH_2$, and this NAD^+ must eventually be

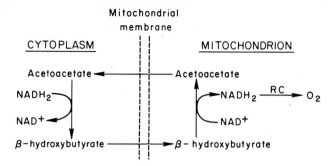

Fig. 5. Acetoacetate-β-hydroxybutyrate shuttle system for transferring reducing equivalents from cytoplasm to mitochondria, coupled with reoxidation of cytoplasmic NADH$_2$ derived from glycolysis. This is merely one example of many such shuttle systems.

restored if the process of glycolysis is to continue. We have just seen that, when oxygen is not available, this is accomplished by coupling the oxidation of NADH$_2$ to NAD$^+$ with the reduction of pyruvic acid to lactic acid. When oxygen *is* available, the NAD$^+$ is restored in an entirely different manner without the formation of lactic acid. This is accomplished by the mitochondria, but it must be done indirectly because NADH$_2$ cannot penetrate into the mitochondria.[2] It has been suggested that a device known as a *shuttle* brings this about,[1] as shown in Fig. 5. The oxidation of NADH$_2$ formed in glycolysis is coupled with the reduction of one of a number of compounds in the cytoplasm which *can* penetrate into the mitochondria. This reduced compound diffuses into the mitochondria where it is reoxidized by reacting with NAD$^+$ in the respiratory chain. The resulting NADH$_2$ is oxidized in the usual manner by passing its hydrogen down the respiratory chain to oxygen. In the meantime, the acetoacetate formed in the mitochondria diffuses back into the cytoplasm to perpetuate the shuttle. The acetoacetate-β-hydroxybutyrate system is only one of a number of similar shuttle systems. It is of interest that many types of cancer cells appear to lack these shuttle systems, and as a result they form lactic acid even when oxygen is abundant and the Krebs cycle is operating. This is known as aerobic glycolysis.

CREATINE PHOSPHATE

Certain organs (primarily brain, heart, and skeletal muscle) contain, in addition to ATP, another high-energy compound called creatine phosphate (CP). Unlike ATP, CP is apparently not involved directly as a source of energy for cell activities. Instead, it helps to maintain an ade-

9

quate concentration of ATP when the latter is being utilized:

$$ATP \longrightarrow ADP + Pi + energy$$
$$CP + ADP \xrightarrow{CPK} ATP + C$$

(CPK is an enzyme, creatine phosphokinase)

Ultimately, the creatine thus formed is rephosphorylated to CP by ATP. What is gained by this elaborate device? One gain may be an additional store of high-energy compounds that would be useful in sudden spurts of intense activity. It would seem, however, that this could be accomplished simply by maintaining a larger store of ATP (since the mitochondria are normally working far below their maximal capacity). It is possible that CP may participate in a *shuttle system* for transferring the energy of ATP from the mitochondria, where it is formed, to the cytoplasm, where it is used (such as in muscle contraction). Such an arrangement would be beneficial because the mitochondrial membrane is not freely permeable to ATP. According to this scheme, as ATP is used for activities in the cytoplasm (involving, for example, the contraction of muscle) it is immediately restored by CP. The resulting creatine diffuses to the surface of the mitochondrion; in the wall of the mitochondrion there is a bound form of the enzyme creatine phosphokinase which transfers a high-energy phosphate group across the membrane from mitochondrial ATP to cytoplasmic creatine. This restores the cytoplasmic creatine phosphate and makes it available once more for maintaining a high concentration of ATP in the cytoplasm, where it is needed for various cell activities. The ADP formed in the mitochondrion in this reaction is promptly rephosphorylated in the usual way by the respiratory chain. The net result is that energy formed in the mitochondria is rapidly made available to the cytoplasm, where it is needed for the performance of work. This hypothesis is consistent with the fact that creatine phosphate occurs in high concentration in only three organs, and that these are organs with a high energy requirement, either constantly (brain, heart) or occasionally (skeletal muscle). There are also other "carriers" in the mitochondrial membrane that facilitate the transfer of ATP from the mitochondria to the cytoplasm.[2]

REGULATION OF THE ENERGY METABOLISM OF CELLS

The preceding sections have described the reactions that produce energy for the cell. It remains to be seen how the *rate* of energy formation is adapted to the changing energy needs of the cell. A rapidly contracting skeletal muscle cell, for example, may require 100 times as much energy as a resting cell. In the following discussion we shall assume that all the

10

compounds and enzymes required for energy formation are present, just as an automobile has all the essentials for traveling faster at the whim of the driver. When the activity of a cell is increased, the extra energy required is supplied by the breakdown of ATP to ADP + Pi + energy. The increase in the concentration of ADP stimulates the rate of oxygen consumption by the mitochondria, and this in turn results in the formation of more ATP by oxidative phosphorylation in the mitochondrial respiratory chain. The extra hydrogen for passage down the respiratory chain is provided by an increased rate of the reactions in the Krebs cycle (mass action effect).

The rate of glycolysis is also increased in times of increased energy need, to provide the extra pyruvic acid to channel into the Krebs cycle. This regulation is a little more complex than that controlling energy formation in the mitochondria. There are several rate-limiting enzymes in glycolysis, the most important of which is phosphofructokinase (PFK). Anything that stimulates this enzyme will increase the rate of glycolysis, and anything that inhibits it will slow the rate of glycolysis. PFK is stimulated by several factors, including a *decrease* in ATP and citric acid (one of the intermediates in the Krebs cycle), and an *increase* in ADP and inorganic phosphate. Thus the very change associated with increased breakdown of ATP will increase the rate of glycolysis and hence provide more fuel for the Krebs cycle and the ultimate formation of ATP.

The regulation of the rate of energy metabolism in the cells provides an excellent example of biological regulation by *negative feedback;* we shall encounter many other examples in our study of the physiology of exercise.

SUMMARY

The energy for muscle contraction is obtained from the breakdown of the high-energy compound, ATP. The ATP is then restored by new formation in the mitochondria, when oxygen is present (aerobic metabolism). This involves successive "oxidation" (removal of hydrogen) of compounds derived from carbohydrates, fats, and proteins, which takes place in the Krebs cycle. The hydrogen thus removed is passed down the respiratory chain to oxygen, and during this passage of hydrogen ATP is formed. When oxygen is not available, the formation of ATP occurs anaerobically by the process of glycolysis. This utilizes only carbohydrate and results in the formation of lactic acid.

Aerobic metabolism yields thirty-eight molecules of ATP per molecule of glucose, while anaerobic metabolism yields only two molecules of ATP per molecule of glucose.

References

1. Boxer, G. E., and Devlin, T. M.: Pathways of intracellular hydrogen transport, Science 134:1495-1501, 1961.
2. Lehninger, A. L.: Biochemistry, New York, 1970, Worth Publishers, pp. 400-408.

Suggested readings

Bergström, J.: Local changes of ATP and phosphorylcreatine in human muscle tissue in connection with exercise, Circulat. Res. Suppl. 1 to volumes 20 and 21:I-91—I-98, 1967. (The first studies on ATP and creatine phosphate changes in human muscle during exercise.)

Cain, D. F., and Davies, R. E.: Breakdown of adenosine triphosphate during a single contraction of working muscle, Biochem. Biophys. Res. Communications 8:361-366, 1962. (This is a classic paper—the first to demonstrate that ATP is the immediate source of energy for muscle contraction.)

Gollnick, P. D., and King, D. W.: Energy release in the muscle cell, Med. Sci. Sports 1:23-31, 1969. (A good review.)

PART TWO

THE NATURE
OF NEUROMUSCULAR
ACTIVITY

2 CONCEPTS OF MUSCULAR CONTRACTIONS

All movements of the human body are caused by contraction, or shortening of the skeletal muscles. They are referred to as skeletal muscles because they attach to a skeletal system. Other types of muscle tissue in the body are cardiac muscle and smooth muscle, also frequently called involuntary muscle because of a lack of voluntary control of contraction. Smooth muscles control the degree of vasodilatation or vasoconstriction in blood vessels, and in the gastrointestinal tract they regulate by rhythmic contractions of the gut wall the advancement of ingested material through the stomach and intestines.

Skeletal muscles cause body movement by a shortening or pulling action of muscle on its bony attachment. A flowing or smooth efficient movement depends on the proper sequence of recruitment of specific motor units (motoneuron together with the muscle fibers that it activates). Some variables that must be controlled in order to produce the desired movement are the proper selection of the number and kind of motoneurons, as well as the pattern of stimulation of each motoneuron.

MORPHOLOGICAL FEATURES OF SKELETAL MUSCLE

All muscles are divided into bundles or fascicles; several hundred muscle fibers may make up a bundle, and hundreds of bundles may make up a single muscle. Although some connective tissue surrounds and separates bundles and fibers (Fig. 6), even more encases whole muscles. Blood vessels and nerves travel throughout the muscles within the connective tissue components. Skeletal muscle also contains a sensory system, muscle spindles, which senses variables such as muscle tension. This information is transmitted to the central nervous system, providing a

15

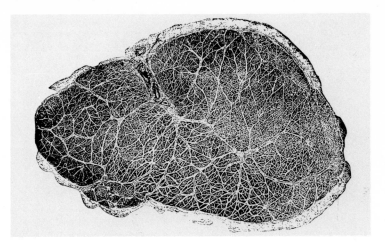

Fig. 6. Cross section through a human sartorius muscle, showing the subdivision into bundles of various sizes by connective tissues. ($\times 4$) (Photograph by Müller, from Heidenhain. In Bloom, W., and Fawcett, D. W.: A textbook of histology, ed. 8, Philadelphia, 1962, W. B. Saunders Co.)

means of making appropriate modifications for performing a given movement.

A skeletal muscle fiber or cell is unique in several respects. Unlike most cells, it is very long and cylindrical in shape. It is also unique in that it has many nuclei. These spindle-shaped nuclei are located in the periphery of muscle fibers just underneath the cell membrane (sarcolemma), which surrounds the muscle fiber. The fluid component of the muscle fiber is referred to as sarcoplasm. Within the sarcoplasm there are a number of proteins which are related to glycolysis, as discussed in Chapter 1. The contractile elements of the muscle fiber make up the myofibrillar proteins. Less than two-tenths of the muscle by weight consists of proteins. The proteins are generally classified as sarcoplasmic proteins, myofibrillar proteins, and particulate or connective tissue proteins. Of the total proteins in muscle, myofibrillar proteins make up more than 60%. Sarcoplasmic proteins make up about 30% while the remainder of the protein is associated with connective tissue and other particulate structures such as the mitochondria.

MICROSCOPIC ASPECTS OF MUSCLE FIBERS

Each muscle fiber is composed of functional units referred to as sarcomeres. It is the presence of these functional units which gives the muscle fiber its striated appearance when viewed under the microscope. Consequently, skeletal muscle is also referred to as striated muscle. These striations are caused by a repetitive and specific organization of the myo-

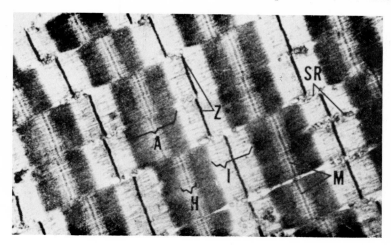

Fig. 7. Low-power electron micrograph of section of rabbit psoas muscle. The pattern of A, I, Z, and H bands may be seen much more clearly than in light microscope photographs, and the longitudinal filaments that make up the contractile material are also visible. SR = Sarcoplasmic reticulum. ($\times24,350$) (From Huxley, H. E.: Muscle cells. In Brachet, J., and Mirsky, A. E., editors: The cell, vol. 4, New York, 1960, Academic Press, Inc.)

fibrillar proteins, actin (thin), myosin (thick), and regulatory proteins within each sarcomere, as demonstrated in Fig. 7. The Z-line is a line of demarcation for each sarcomere and is located in the middle of each I-band. A darker A-band is found in the middle of each sarcomere, but within each A-band there is a centrally located, somewhat lighter zone called the H-band. The portion of the A-band which consists of myosin filaments only makes up the H-band, whereas the remainder of the A-band has both myosin and actin filaments overlapping. A further point of distinction in the center of each sarcomere is a thin line caused by localization of M-protein. The function of the M-protein is apparently to maintain a somewhat constant structural relationship between the thick and thin filaments. Note that the thin actin filaments extend from the Z-line into the A-band. Located with a regular periodicity in the actin filament are two proteins called tropomyosin and troponin, which are very important in the regulation of muscular contraction.

Muscle fibers are also divided longitudinally into subunits called myofibrils. A network of longitudinally oriented sac-like membranes with varying shapes called the sarcoplasmic reticulum partially separates myofibrils (Fig. 7). Mitochondria are also located between myofibrils.

The sarcolemma which surrounds the muscle fiber is continuous with a separate set of membranes which are transversely oriented tubular

17

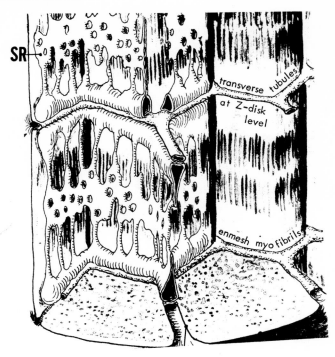

Fig. 8. Intracellular tubules may be responsible for the transportal (tranverse tubules) or storage (sarcoplasmic reticulum) of calcium, the element necessary for muscle contraction. (From Elias, H., and Pauly, J.: Human microanatomy, Philadelphia, 1966, F. A. Davis Co., p. 71.)

membranes that extend and branch throughout the cross section of the muscle fiber at strategic points (junction of the A- and I-bands) within each sarcomere. These transverse tubules (t-tubules) are in apposition but not continuous with the sarcoplasmic reticulum. The sarcoplasmic reticulum has a special ability to store and release calcium ions very efficiently.

Another important organelle within the muscle fiber is the mitochondrion. The role of the mitochondrion in ATP production is discussed in Chapter 1. Oxidative metabolism occurs in the mitochondrion; this is the organelle in which oxygen is actually utilized in the body.

Other subcellular structures that are important to the proper function of the muscle are the glycogen granules, which can be seen with the electron microscope. Ribosomes are also found in muscle fibers. Ribosomes play a key role in synthesis of proteins, a phenomenon particularly important in adaptation to chronic exercise. Myoglobin, associated with the membranes of the sarcoplasmic reticulum, is similar to hemoglobin in structure and function. It assists in maintaining an adequate oxygen concentration within the muscle fiber so that the mitochondria can function optimally. Also located in the sarcoplasm are those enzymes associated with the utilization of glycogen and glucose (glycolysis).

MUSCLE FUNCTION

A muscle contracts when the nervous system transmits an impulse to a motoneuron located in the ventral horn of the spinal cord, down the axon of the motoneuron to the nerve-muscle junction (NMJ), and down the length of the muscle fiber (Fig. 9). A single motoneuron usually innervates several hundred muscle fibers but this ranges from less than ten to more than a thousand. A motoneuron plus all of the muscle fibers it innervates is called a motor unit. It is the true functional unit of the neuromuscular system.

The arrival of the electrical impulse at the terminal ending of the axon (NMJ), which is located about halfway between the ends of each fiber, initiates the release of the neurotransmitter acetylcholine (ACh) in finite packets called quanta. The ACh diffuses across a narrow gap from the presynaptic membrane (nerve terminal) to the postsynaptic membrane (sarcolemma) of the muscle fiber. The ACh initiates a disturbance in the sarcolemma permeability (depolarization or reversal of a potential difference across the membrane), and an impulse is produced which travels down the sarcolemma toward both ends of the muscle fiber. The membrane is stabilized quickly after each impulse because an enzyme, acetylcholinesterase, destroys the ACh, deactivating its depolarizing effect. With prolonged stimulation, the number of vesicles available, for release of ACh from the presynaptic terminals can be markedly reduced.

The impulse transmitted down the length of a muscle fiber by the sarcolemma is also transmitted intracellularly via the t-tubules described earlier. This event assures that all myofibrils throughout the fiber will be activated essentially simultaneously. The t-tubule impulse in some way signals the sarcoplasmic reticulum to release calcium. The calcium binds with the regulatory protein troponin, which is located on the thin helical filaments as shown in Fig. 10. The binding of calcium to troponin abolishes the inhibition of the interaction of the actin and myosin filaments exerted by the troponin-tropomyosin complex. Once the inhibition is abolished, the heads of the myosin molecules activated by the release of energy from ATP go through a conformational change as they interact with actin in such a way as to exert pulling forces between actin and myosin. In each sarcomere, the forces pull the actin toward the center of each sarcomere, thus narrowing the H-band as the sarcomeres and therefore the whole muscle contract.

The process is reversed during relaxation. Withdrawal of the stimulus

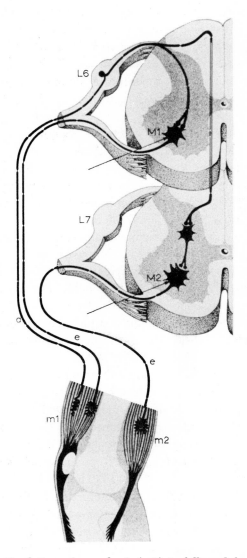

Fig. 9. Cortical stimulation of muscle 1 *(m1)* is followed by receptor (spindle) stimulation, which enters the spinal cord at *L6* and branches. One branch stimulates α-motoneuron, *M1*, to add another motor unit to the muscle contracting while the other branch indirectly stimulates *M2* in order to inhibit the antagonistic muscle *(m2)*. (From Schadé, J. B., and Ford, D. H.: Basic neurology, ed. 2, New York, 1973, Elsevier Scientific Publishing Co., p. 151.)

permits the sarcoplasmic reticulum to withdraw the calcium from the sarcoplasm, thereby permitting troponin to inhibit actin-myosin interaction again.

With this background of fundamental information about muscle contraction, several physiological properties of muscles should be considered. For example, the amount of tension that a muscle can exert is of obvious importance in physical performances. According to the all-or-none principle of muscular contraction, when a muscle fiber is stimulated as described above, it produces the maximal tension or none at all. As we shall see, this principle does not hold true for a whole muscle. Obviously, we have the ability to exert whole muscle contractions of varying strengths and speeds. Graded tensions within a single motor unit can occur by varying the frequency at which a muscle is stimulated: the higher the frequency, the greater the tension and also the greater the rate at which tension can be developed. Graded tensions of a whole muscle can also be achieved by varying the number of motor units involved.

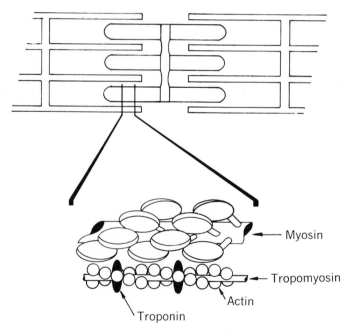

Fig. 10. A sarcomere drawn to scale. Note the relative length and thickness of the thin and thick filaments. The division in the center of the sarcomere is the M-substance. A small section of the thick and thin filament is enlarged in the lower half of the figure. Note the relative size and number of myosin heads compared to the thin filament consisting of two chains of actin molecules wound around the tropomyosin protein. Also note the periodicity of the troponin protein located on the thin filament.

Another important property of skeletal muscle with regard to physical performance is endurance, that is, the ability of the neuromuscular system to perform continuously and repetitively. Endurance of the neuromuscular system is closely related to several muscle properties. Mitochondrial concentration is related to the ability of a muscle to maintain tension when it is repetitively stimulated. It is also known that the point of exhaustion in humans working at a rate which is less than two-thirds of the maximal rate at which they can absorb oxygen is related to the point at which glycogen is essentially depleted from the skeletal muscles involved. Consequently, those muscles which have the most numerous mitochondria and the most glycogen have the greatest endurance, assuming other factors are the same. However, there are many other properties that are related to the muscle fiber's endurance. For example, we know that the myoglobin concentration and the vascularity of the muscle, as well as the concentration of creatine phosphate, are also important factors in the endurance capacity of a given muscle.

MUSCLE FIBER TYPES

It is generally recognized now that muscle fibers vary markedly in their capacity to produce tension, in the rate at which they can develop the tension, and in the length of time the tension can be maintained. Most of this variability in the strength, speed, and endurance of contraction can be explained by the presence of different muscle fiber types.

The speed at which a muscle contracts and relaxes is closely related to the rate at which the muscle can hydrolyze ATP; this is dependent on the activity of the enzyme myofibrillar adenosine triphosphatase (ATPase). Myofibrillar ATPase is also closely related to the amount of the sarcoplasmic reticulum within that muscle fiber.

Muscle tension is also closely related to the ATPase activity. However, specific properties that might be responsible for the greater tension achieved by one muscle fiber than by another are not always immediately apparent. The amount of myofibrillar protein per cross sectional area or the muscle fiber size would seem to be important. In terms of the whole muscle, the number of muscle fibers, and from the motor unit standpoint, the number of muscle fibers per motor unit, would also be related to the amount of tension that can be produced.

Endurance of a muscle is directly related to the mitochondrial content, the glycogen concentration and the vascularity, as well as the myoglobin concentration. In general, the muscle fibers that have the most numerous mitochondria also have the greatest endurance, because they are more lavishly supplied with blood via a more extensive vascular system.

By the consideration of each of these properties, speed, tension, and

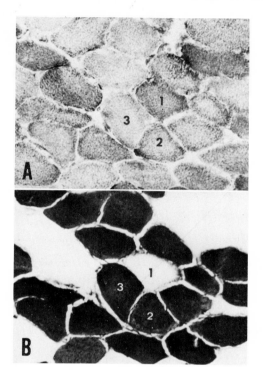

Fig. 11. Cross section of a guinea pig gastrocnemius muscle. The intensity of the staining represents the oxidative capacity of the fiber. **A,** Exercise of an endurance type results in an increase in the darker staining fibers. *1,* Slow twitch, high-oxidative fiber; *2,* fast twitch, high-oxidative fiber; and *3,* fast twitch, low-oxidative fiber. **B,** A histochemical stain (myosin ATPase) that indicates the contractile speed of a fiber (dark, fast; light, slow).

endurance, a logical classification scheme for muscle fiber types can be derived. Common classification systems that are used in reference to human muscle divide fibers into fast and slow twitch populations. These populations can be further considered in terms of their endurance capacity; that is, a muscle fiber may be fast twitch and have either a high or a low oxidative capacity. To state it in another way, a fast twitch muscle may be relatively fatigue-resistant or very fatiguable. All fast twitch fibers have a relatively higher glycolytic capacity than do slow twitch fibers. Slow twitch muscle fibers generally vary less than fast twitch in their oxidative capacity and all are relatively fatigue-resistant. These muscle fibers are often referred to as slow twitch oxidative fibers. Although the tension property of the muscle fiber is not incorporated in the various nomenclatures commonly used, tension capacity is closely related to these classification schemes. For example, muscle fibers which

23

contract at a faster rate generally produce more tension than do muscle fibers that contract more slowly. However, the endurance capacity of a muscle fiber is not so closely related to its tension properties.

Fiber types, as might be expected, seem to be very specialized in their ability to produce specific types of movements. Perhaps one of the most important properties is the tension capacity. It appears that fast twitch fibers can produce a significantly greater peak tension than slow twitch fibers. Differences in speed of shortening have advantages as well. For example, a disproportionate number of fast twitch fibers may be involved in movements that are reflexly activated. On the other hand, sustained isometric contractions producing light forces can probably be performed more efficiently by slow twitch fibers that are fatigue-resistant.

SITE OF FATIGUE

Numerous experiments have been performed which identify the primary site of fatigue of the neuromuscular system. However almost as many sites of fatigue have been identified as experiments have been performed. Various experiments have demonstrated that fatigue can occur within the spinal synapses, at the neuromuscular junction, and at the actual site of excitation-contraction coupling within the muscle. It is important to realize that these different findings are not necessarily contradictory. Under a given set of circumstances fatigue may be identified at any one of several points within the link. In short, there is excellent evidence that neuromuscular fatigue has both a neural and a muscular component. The weakest link at one time may not be the weakest at another time in the same individual. And of course, one must also consider the nature of the specific type of neuromuscular overload; that is, whether it is a highly repetitive, low resistance movement, low repetitive, high resistance, or some variation of these extremes.

EFFECTS OF TRAINING ON MUSCLE

More is known about endurance training than any other type of training. This is due in part to the fact that laboratory animals are easier to train in endurance type programs. The adaptations in response to endurance identified thus far are essentially those that one might predict from the previous discussion of the properties of different types of motor units. In general, it has been shown that with daily training in an exercise that involves highly repetitive and low resistance contractions, the mitochondrial number and size increase as do the enzymes associated with oxidative metabolism. Endurance training also results in elevated glycogen stores in the muscles and increased vascularity around individual muscle fibers, with the vascularity increasing the most around those muscle fibers which are utilized most extensively. Endurance training results in little or no alteration in the maximal capacity of skeletal muscle to produce tension. However, because of the endurance-related changes just noted, a maximal or near maximal tension can be maintained over a longer period of time with repetitive work. The question of alteration in speed of muscle contraction has been considered by numerous investigators, but the evidence is conflicting. Current information suggests that a training program lasting up to 6 months does not significantly affect muscle speed as reflected in the proportion of slow and fast twitch muscle fibers. However, training can affect the rate at which the whole muscle contracts by having a selective effect on specific types of muscle fiber populations. For example, during continuous work of sufficient intensity the first fibers that fatigue will usually be fast twitch fibers. As a result, the ability of the muscle to develop tension at a maximal rate would be affected in a fatigued state. If high tension, low resistance type muscle fibers become fatigued, tension will be markedly affected because of the difference in the relatively high tension output of the fast fibers versus the low tension capacity of the slow fibers. Since endurance training increases the oxidative capacity, exercise can cause a change in fiber types in terms of their metabolism. Muscle fibers that were fast twitch but had low oxidative capacity before training may become fast twitch with a higher oxidative capacity after training.

High resistance, low repetition exercise over a period of weeks causes skeletal muscle to enlarge. The enlargement is caused by an increase in size of muscle fibers, or muscle hypertrophy. Hyperplasia or an increase in number of muscle fibers after overload training, although sometimes claimed to occur, has not been demonstrated conclusively. A detailed review of the growth of muscle fibers with exercise has been published.[1] In essence an increase in the numbers of nuclei of muscles occurs with overload but the nuclei are those of cells other than muscle fibers, for example, endothelial cells of capillaries and fibroblasts that produce components of connective tissue.

Another adaptation to endurance training occurs at the neuromuscular junction. It has been demonstrated that cholinesterase activity increases with endurance training. Cholinesterase is the enzyme which is responsible for the degradation of the acetylcholine that is released by each nerve impulse from the nerve terminals, thereby preventing prolonged contractions. The advantage of this adaptation is not immediately apparent but does indicate that adaptation of the neuromuscular system is not confined to the muscle tissue itself. There is also some evidence that the length of the terminal nerves which make contact with the muscle fibers at the neuromuscular junction is increased with neuromuscular overload. These changes may be quite significant in light of the reported drop in electrical activity of muscles after prolonged intensive exercise. The decrease in electrical activity may be caused by a diminution of proper function of the neuromuscular junction so that the impulses do not reach the muscle fiber.

Reference

1. Edgerton, V. R.: Exercise and the growth and development of muscle tissue. In Rarick, G. L., editor: Physical activity; human growth and development, New York, 1973, Academic Press, Inc.

Suggested readings

Baldwin, K., and others: Substrate depletion in different types of muscle and in liver during prolonged running, J. Physiol. 225:1045, 1973.

Barnard, R. J., Edgerton, V. R., and Peter, J. B.: Effect of exercise on skeletal muscle. I, Biochemical and histochemical properties. II, Contractile properties, J. Appl. Physiol. 28: 762, 1970.

Burke, R., and Edgerton, V. R.: Motor unit properties and selective involvement in movement, Exercise Sports Sci. Rev. 3:31, 1975.

Holloszy, J. O.: Biochemical adaptations in muscle; effects of exercise on mitochondrial oxygen uptake and respiratory enzymes activity in skeletal muscle, J. Biol. Chem. 242:2278, 1967.

Murray, J. M., and Weber, A.: The cooperative action of muscle proteins, Sci. Am. 230:58, 1974.

Saltin, B.: Metabolic fundamentals in exercise, Med. Sci. Sports 5:137, 1973.

3 THE CHARACTERISTICS OF MUSCLE CONTRACTION

Skeletal muscles normally contract only when they are stimulated by nerve impulses coming from the brain or spinal cord. This stimulus-response mechanism is highly complex and is more easily understood after a consideration of the simpler response of an isolated muscle to direct electrical stimulation.

MUSCLE TWITCH

If a single shock is applied to the muscle, the response is a single contraction and relaxation, known as a muscle *twitch*. Although some simple reflexes such as the knee jerk may be single twitches, most muscular activity involves a more prolonged type of contraction known as a *tetanus*, which is described later.

The total duration of a single twitch varies greatly in different types of muscle. For example, the extraocular muscles that move the eyeball are extremely rapid (twitch duration = 7.5 milliseconds = 0.0075 second), while at the other extreme, the soleus muscle in the lower leg has a very long twitch duration (94 to 120 milliseconds).

SUMMATION OF CONTRACTIONS—TETANUS

When a muscle is stimulated twice in such rapid succession that the second stimulus falls during the response to the first, the tension developed in the second twitch is greater than that in the first twitch. This may be explained as follows: A certain amount of time is required for the muscle to undergo maximal shortening because of the structural rearrangements that must take place in each fiber. When a single twitch is of such short duration that these changes cannot be completed during the period of excitation of the muscle, maximal shortening cannot occur. If, however, two or more contractions occur in rapid succession, these

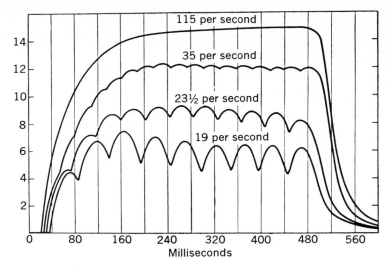

Fig. 12. The development of tetanus by increasing rates of stimulation. Complete tetanus, represented by the top curve, was obtained with a stimulation rate of 115 per second; the tension developed was more than three times that of a single twitch. (From Amberson, W. R., and Smith, D. C.: Outline of physiology, Baltimore, 1939, The Williams & Wilkins Co.)

structural changes may go to completion and greater tension is developed. If the muscle is stimulated with a series of rapidly repeated shocks, there is not sufficient time for relaxation between successive contractions, and the result is a steady, prolonged contraction known as a *tetanus*. Most muscle contractions in the body are of this type. The tension developed during tetanus may be 3 or 4 times that of a single twitch. If the rate of stimulation is not rapid enough to produce complete tetanus, there may be partial relaxation between contractions. The result is a jerky type of contraction known as incomplete tetanus (Fig. 12).

CONTRACTION OF MUSCLES IN THE BODY

Motor neurons in the central nervous system. The impulses that give rise to muscle contractions normally arise in nerve cells (neurons) in the central nervous system. In the case of voluntary movements these neurons are located in the brain; in many types of reflex movements they are located in the spinal cord (the details are considered in Chapter 4). In the present discussion, for simplicity, we shall consider only the motor neurons in the spinal cord whose nerve fibers pass directly to the muscles of the extremities. These motor neurons are located in the ventral horn (or gray matter) of the spinal cord, and each motor neuron sends a single fiber, by way of the ventral root of the spinal cord and the motor nerve, to the muscle that it innervates. When the nerve fiber reaches its muscle, it breaks up into several hundred branches and each branch supplies a single muscle fiber. The motor neuron, its fiber and branches, and the muscle fibers supplied by its branches constitute the basic unit of neuromuscular activity, the *motor unit.* The fibers of a single muscle may participate in several hundred motor units; the collection of motor neurons that supplies a single muscle is called the *motor pool* of that muscle.

The nerve impulse. The signal that originates in a motor neuron and travels along a nerve fiber is called a nerve impulse.

The membrane surrounding the neuron and its processes is polarized, that is, it possesses an electrical charge; the outer surface of the membrane is positive and the inner surface negative. This results from certain properties of the membrane itself. Sodium ions, which are abundant in the blood and extracellular fluid, diffuse through the membrane of the neuron rather slowly and are promptly pumped out again by the so-called sodium pump. This is an energy-requiring process. The major positive ion (cation) inside the neuron is potassium. Potassium ions tend to leak out of the neuron, but they are restrained from leaving it completely because they are attracted by the negatively charged protein anions, which are too large to diffuse out of the neuron. Since sodium is effectively excluded from the neuron by the sodium pump, the slight net passive movement of potassium ions from inside to outside leaves the interior of the neuron relatively negative with respect to its outer surface. This difference in potential, amounting to about 70 millivolts, is referred to as the resting membrane potential, and the nerve impulse is essentially a transient reversal of the polarity of the membrane.

When a nerve fiber is excited, either by an electrical stimulus in the laboratory or by a nerve impulse in the body, there is a sudden increase in the permeability of the membrane to sodium ions. The inrush of positive ions momentarily reverses the polarity of the membrane, causing a local electrical current to flow between this region of the membrane and the adjacent region, which is still normally polarized. This results in reversal of the polarity at this site, setting up another local current flow. The series of local current flows is propagated down the nerve fiber as the nerve impulse or nerve action potential. The reversal of polarity at any one site on the membrane is of very brief duration; the sodium ions are pumped out again very quickly and the normal polarity is reestablished. The nerve fiber is now ready to conduct another nerve impulse.

TRANSMISSION OF EXCITATION FROM NERVE TO MUSCLE

The transmission of excitation from one neuron to another across a synapse and from a nerve fiber to a muscle fiber across a neuromuscular junction involves a common mechanism. In each case, the prejunctional nerve endings contain minute vesicles filled with a chemical transmitter substance, acetylcholine. The arrival of a nerve impulse causes the rupture of some of these vesicles and release of the acetylcholine, which diffuses across the gap and stimulates the postjunctional membrane of the nerve cell or muscle fiber. The result is a wave of excitation that is conducted along the membrane of the nerve or muscle fiber, as described in the previous section.

THE MUSCLE ACTION POTENTIAL

The membrane of the individual muscle fiber is polarized in the same manner as the membrane of the nerve fiber, and the wave of excitation that spreads along the muscle fiber membrane has the same characteristics as the nerve impulse. In the region of the Z line of the muscle fiber, the excitation is transmitted to a system of membranes called the transverse tubules, which penetrate into the muscle fiber. The excitation spreads from the transverse tubules to another system of membranes, called the sarcoplasmic reticulum. This causes a release of calcium ions, which initiates the contraction of the muscle fiber, as described in Chapter 2.

The waves of excitation that spread along the muscle fibers and cause them to contract can be recorded by sensitive electrodes inserted into the muscle. The resulting record, the electromyogram (or EMG), is often used in both physiological research and clinical testing to reveal the pattern of excitation of skeletal muscle fibers, just as the electrocardiogram is used for analyzing the excitation of cardiac muscle.

ALL-OR-NONE NATURE OF ACTION POTENTIALS

Any stimulus that is strong enough to cause a contraction of a muscle fiber will cause a maximal contraction—a further increase in the strength of the stimulus will elicit no increase in the force of contraction. It must be emphasized that the all-or-none law assumes that all conditions other than stimulus strength remain constant. We have seen, for example, that the force of contraction of a muscle fiber can be increased by an increase in the *frequency* of stimulation (summation of contractions) and decreased by fatigue.

The all-or-none law also applies to the action potentials of nerve and muscle fibers; that is, any stimulus that is strong enough to produce reversal of the polarity of the membrane produces a maximal reversal, which is always of the same magnitude if other conditions remain constant. As a matter of fact, the all-or-none nature of the muscle action potential is the basis of the all-or-none contraction of the muscle fiber. The contractile elements in the muscle fiber can be made to contract with greater force if a powerful electrical stimulation is applied directly to the muscle; this is, of course, an artificial situation which does not occur in ordinary muscular activity.

The motor unit, rather than the individual muscle fiber, is the basic unit of neuromuscular activity, and it obeys the all-or-none law. This means that if a motor neuron in the spinal cord or brain stem sends an impulse to a skeletal muscle, all the muscle fibers making up the motor unit contract in an all-or-none manner.

GRADING OF THE STRENGTH OF MUSCLE CONTRACTIONS

It is a matter of common experience that the strength of a muscle contraction is adjusted in accordance with the force required to perform the muscular act. The lifting of a heavy weight requires a more powerful muscle contraction than does the lifting of a light weight. If muscle contractions were always of maximal strength, they would be very wasteful of energy in most of the activities of daily life. The manner in which the nervous system determines the strength of contraction that is adequate will be discussed later. At this time we are concerned rather with the manner in which this adjustment is carried out in the muscle. Two basic mechanisms are involved: (1) variation in the number of muscle fibers that contract and (2) variation in the frequency with which the muscle fibers contract. These two mechanisms will be considered.

Each motor nerve cell in the spinal cord sends a single nerve fiber to its muscle. Within the muscle the nerve fiber breaks up into branches, each of which supplies a single muscle fiber. In this way a single nerve cell controls the contraction of about 100 to 150 muscle fibers. The nerve cell, its nerve fiber, and the group of muscle fibers supplied by the terminal branches of the nerve fiber constitute a *motor unit*. When the nerve cell discharges an impulse, all the muscle fibers in that motor unit contract. The average skeletal muscle may have about 300 motor units, which means that a group of 300 nerve cells in the spinal cord controls the contraction of the muscle. Theoretically a contraction of the muscle could involve any number of motor units between 1 and 300. On this basis a contraction involving 200 motor units would be twice as strong as a contraction involving only 100 motor units. This is the first and probably the more important mechanism for grading the strength of a muscle contraction.

The second basic mechanism that determines the strength of a muscle contraction is the frequency of stimulation of the muscle. A muscle de-

31

velops greater tension when the rate of stimulation is great enough to produce complete tetanus. At lower frequencies of stimulation there is partial relaxation between contractions, and the tension developed is less. On the average, the tension developed in tetanus is about 4 times that of a single twitch. Incomplete tetanus has the advantage of requiring less energy expenditure than does complete tetanus so that the requirements of a weak contraction may be met by incomplete tetanus in a fraction of the total number of motor units. The jerky type of contraction obtained with incomplete tetanus in the laboratory does not normally occur in the intact organism because the different motor units are not all active at the same time. At any one time some units are active, while others are not, so that the average tension does not fluctuate.

The operation of these two basic mechanisms may be illustrated by the following example. In lifting a 100-pound weight all 300 motor units might be active, each exerting 4 units of tension in complete tetanus and requiring 100 nerve impulses per second along each motor nerve fiber. The total tension would be $300 \times 4 = 1,200$ units. In lifting a 25-pound weight perhaps only 150 motor units are active, each unit exerting 2 units of tension because of lower frequency of stimulation, and requiring 50 nerve impulses per second. The total tension in this case would be $150 \times 2 = 300$ units.

ISOTONIC AND ISOMETRIC CONTRACTIONS

If the load against which a muscle contracts is not too great, the muscle undergoes shortening and a movement occurs; this type of contraction is called isotonic. This word literally means constant tension, and it is a misnomer since the tension *does* change during the shortening. It is, however, useful in distinguishing this type of contraction from one in which the load opposing the muscle is too great to permit shortening of the muscle. This is called an isometric contraction, and its only effect is to exert a force. In an isometric contraction, no work (in the classic physical sense of $W = F \times D$) is done, and all the energy of contraction is dissipated as heat. (See *Laboratory Manual,* Chapter 3, for further types of applications of muscular force.)

FACTORS INFLUENCING MUSCLE CONTRACTION

It was mentioned previously that a muscle can exert greater tension during a tetanus than during a single twitch because of the summation of contractions; thus the *frequency* of stimulation is one factor that determines the force of contraction. Within limits, increasing the *intensity* of the stimulus also increases the force of contraction. Since experiments on single muscle fibers have shown that a fiber contracts maximally in response to any stimulus that is strong enough to excite (all-or-none law), the increasing force of contraction of a whole muscle in response to increasing stimulus strength must result from the progressive stimulation of more fibers. When the stimulus strength is adequate to excite all the fibers in a muscle, no further increase in tension follows increased intensity of the stimulus. Under special experimental conditions it can be shown that the all-or-none law applies not to the contractile elements in the muscle fiber (they contract more forcefully in response to stronger stimuli) but rather to the intensity of the excitation transmitted along the fiber membrane in response to the usual type of stimulation. Since muscle fibers in the intact body are always stimulated by an excitation wave conducted along the fiber membrane, they obey the all-or-none law.

The force exerted by a contracting muscle is influenced by the *resistance* against which the muscle shortens and by the *velocity* of the shortening. In an isolated muscle the velocity of shortening is greatest when there is no resistance, and it diminishes progressively with increasing load or resistance. The interrelations of load, velocity of shortening, and efficiency of work in the intact body are discussed in Chapter 10.

Contractile fatigue. When an excised muscle is stimulated repeatedly at a frequency of about once per second, the height of each contraction eventually begins to decrease. Not only is the amount of shortening diminished but also the relaxation becomes slower and incomplete (contracture). Finally the muscle fails to respond even to the strongest stimulation; that is, its irritability is completely lost. This diminished capacity for response that results from previous activity is called *fatigue.*

If a fatigued excised muscle is cut across and the cut surface tested with litmus paper, it is found that the interior of the muscle is acid. Since the normal muscle gives an alkaline reaction with litmus, it is apparent that fatigue is associated with an accumulation of acid. Chemical analysis reveals that the amount of glycogen (energy-yielding carbohydrate) is less in the fatigued muscle than in the normal muscle. These experiments suggest that fatigue may be caused by the accumulation of acid waste products that decrease the irritability of the muscle or by exhaustion of stored fuel supplies. The accumulation of acid waste products (largely lactic acid) in the excised muscle is due in large part to the absence of a normal circulation of blood. As a result the amount of oxygen supplied to the muscle is not sufficient to prevent the formation of lactic acid, nor can it be removed from the muscle by diffusion into the circulating blood. Conditions are, of course, different in the case of muscles in the body. The fuel is constantly being replenished by way of the circulation, and the oxygen supply may be adequate to provide most, if not all, of the energy required without the formation of lactic acid. Any lactic acid that is formed diffuses from the muscle to the blood; it is then transported to the liver and other organs for disposal.

Site of fatigue. When muscles tire during exercise (for example, weight lifting), the defect might be in the muscles themselves or in the nervous system. The classic view has placed the principal blame on the neuromuscular junction or the nervous system because of experiments of the following type:

1. If a frog muscle is stimulated repeatedly via its motor nerve until it fails to contract and the stimulus is then applied directly to the muscle, a contraction results.

2. If voluntary muscle contractions are carried to the point of fatigue and the motor nerve is then stimulated by electrodes placed on the skin just over the site of entrance of the nerve into the muscle, contractions of the muscle may be obtained.

Other experiments have produced evidence favoring the view that the site of fatigue is in the muscle itself, not in the nervous system or in the transmission of the stimulus from the nerve to the muscle.[5,6] The impairment of muscle function in fatigue may result in part either from the decreased rate of formation and release of the transmitter substance acetylcholine at the neuromuscular junction or from desensitization of cholinergic receptors in end-plate membranes of the muscle fibers. These would result in failure of some of the impulses arriving over the motor nerves to stimulate the muscle fibers, and would increase the impairment caused by fatigue of the muscle itself.[8] As suggested in Chapter 2, fatigue can occur at any one of several points within the neuromuscular system, and the site may depend on the type of overload.

MUSCULAR PAIN, SORENESS, AND STIFFNESS

During and following strenuous muscular exercise, particularly in untrained subjects, there may be muscle pain, soreness, and stiffness.

Muscle pain commonly occurs during or shortly after exercise, whereas soreness and stiffness usually appear some hours later. It is well known that when muscles are forced to work without adequate blood supply (for example, rapid flexion and extension of the fingers with the circulation occluded by a blood pressure cuff) severe pain results. The inadequate blood flow results in failure of complete removal of the products of muscle metabolism, and it is probable that the pain of strenuous exercise is the result of an outward passage of potassium across the muscle cell membrane into the tissue spaces. It may also be caused by the accumulation of lactic acid that irritates the pain nerve endings located in the muscles. When the exercise ceases, the pain disappears as the lactic acid diffuses from the muscles to the bloodstream.

Fluid collects in muscles during activity, and a number of hours may be required for its reabsorption into the bloodstream. The resulting swelling of the muscle causes it to become shorter and thicker and more resistant to stretching. This gives rise to a sensation of stiffness when the muscle is stretched during the contraction of antagonistic muscles.

The cause of muscle soreness is not completely understood. Two types have been postulated: (1) general soreness resulting from the presence of diffusible metabolic waste products, which usually disappears within 3 or 4 hours after the cessation of exercise and (2) localized soreness or *lameness* that appears 8 to 24 hours after exercise and may persist for several days. The second type of soreness is probably caused by the rupture of muscle fibers, or of the sarcolemma, which transmits the contraction to the tendon. Greater muscle soreness is more likely to occur after vigorous eccentric (lengthening) contraction in which there is an external force against the muscle, than after concentric (shortening) contraction in which the muscle fibers are controlling the movement. The less frequently used fibers and the sarcolemma covering them are probably more susceptible to strain than are the fibers more frequently used in ordinary contractions. The generalized type of soreness is alleviated by immediate cold applications followed by light work that hastens the circulatory removal of the metabolic waste products, while the localized lameness, which is caused by actual injury, needs rest with heat and only enough exercise to prevent the formation of adhesions between the injured muscle fibers.

Cramps or spasms are spontaneous, enduring, and sometimes painful muscular contractions. They are most common in weight-bearing muscles, such as those of the foot, calf, leg, and hip. They can occur with or without warning or obvious cause. They may occur during sleep or after vigorous contraction of fresh muscle, slight contraction of a tired muscle, or intensive exercise. Cramps may result from a blow or strain, but they often occur without apparent provocation.

During a muscle cramp nearly all motor units are in continuous action. There is no single explanation that can account for all cases. In some a reduction in salt in the body through sweating may have increased the susceptibility of a muscle to cramp due to a disturbance in fluid and electrolyte balance. In others there may have been an impairment of blood flow. Another possibility is a localized shortage or lack of cholinesterase, which allows a persistent contraction until acetylcholine is broken down by the cholinesterase.

Cramps are relieved by stretching the muscle slightly and putting firm pressure on it through a gentle kneading action. Those with a tendency toward cramps may reduce the incidence by warming up (p. 236) before vigorous exercise and by ingesting salt and water before and after prolonged exercise (p. 209).

MUSCLE STRENGTH

The maximal tension that an isolated muscle can exert is influenced by a number of factors, including the size of the muscle (especially its cross section area), the arrangement of the fibers in the muscle, the velocity of contraction, the presence or absence of fatigue, and the nutritional state. The situation is even more complex in the case of intact muscles in the body; this is discussed in detail in Chapter 5.

THE EFFECTS OF TRAINING ON MUSCLE

It is a matter of common knowledge that muscles increase in size as a result of certain types of training. Since muscle fibers do not undergo cell division (except during fetal development) the increase in muscle size resulting from training must be due to an increase in the size of the individual muscle fibers (that is, it represents hypertrophy rather than hyperplasia).[2] Dynamic exercises have other effects (including improved neuromuscular coordination and increased muscle circulation because of proliferation of muscle capillaries), which will be discussed in Chapter 19.

Strenuous training (treadmill exercise) has striking effects on the capacity of the muscles for forming ATP.[1,3,4] In rats subjected to strenuous exercise, the mitochondria in muscle cells increase in both number and size and some of the oxidative enzymes are present in greater amounts. As a result, the muscles of the trained individual are able to remove more of the oxygen from the blood that supplies them during exercise. It has been claimed that the increased capacity of trained subjects to utilize oxygen may be due as much to this factor as to their increased ability to transport oxygen to their muscles. The cellular changes resulting from training will be discussed at greater length in Chapter 19.

References

1. Barnard, R. J., Edgerton, V. R., and Peter, J. B.: Effect of exercise on skeletal muscle. I, Biochemical and histochemical properties. II, Contractile properties, J. Appl. Physiol. **28:** 762, 1970.
2. Etemadi, A. A., and Hosseimi, F.: Frequency and size of muscle fibers in athletic body build, Anat. Rec. **162:**269, 1968.
3. Gollnick, P. D., and King, D. W.: Effect of exercise and training on mitochondria of rat skeletal muscle, Am. J. Physiol. **216:**1502, 1969.
4. Holloszy, J. O.: Biochemical adaptations in muscle; effects of exercise on mitochondrial oxygen uptake and respiratory enzymes activity in skeletal muscle, J. Biol. Chem. **242:**2278, 1967.
5. Kugelberg, E., and Edström, L.: Differential histochemical effects of muscle contractions on phosphorylase and glycogen in various types of fibers; relation to fatigue, J. Neurol. Neurosurg. Psychiat. **31:**415, 1968.
6. Merton, P. A.: Problems of muscular fatigue, Brit. Med. Bull. **12:**219, 1956.
7. Norris, F. H., Jr., Gasteiger, E. L., and Chatfield, P. O.: An electromyographic study of induced and spontaneous muscle cramps, Electroenceph. Clin. Neurophysiol. 9:139, 1957.

8. Porter, C. W., and others: Types and locations of cholinergic receptor-like molecules in muscle fibers, Nature **241**:3, 1973.

Suggested readings

Henneman, E.: Peripheral mechanisms involved in the control of muscle. In Mountcastle, V. B., editor: Medical physiology, ed. 12, Vol. 2, St. Louis, 1968, The C. V. Mosby Co., pp. 1697-1706.

Vander, A. J., Sherman, J. H., and Luciano, D. S.: Human physiology, ed. 2, New York, 1975, McGraw-Hill Book Co., pp. 189-225.

4 NERVOUS CONTROL OF MUSCULAR ACTIVITY

One of the distinguishing features of a good athlete is the skill with which he executes complex muscular movements. This is largely a matter of the central nervous system; in a very literal sense the muscles are the servants of the brain. The development of motor skills of various types, one of the major objectives of physical education, consists primarily of improvement in the speed and accuracy with which the nervous system coordinates activity.

The central nervous system is made up of two types of cells—neurons and glia. The neurons (nerve cells) have as their most obvious functions the receipt of messages (nerve impulses) from other neurons and the transmission of these messages to still other neurons or to muscle or gland cells. The glia, long regarded as functionally inert supporting cells, are now believed to have complex metabolic functions of their own, but the details are beyond the scope of this book. Neurons have other activities in addition to the transmission of nerve impulses, such as the storage and retrieval of memory traces and the processes involved in abstract reasoning; these are poorly understood and will not be discussed.

A neuron has a cell body, which contains the nucleus and a number of branching processes extending from the cell body. These are of two types: the dendrites, which receive incoming nerve impulses, and the single axon, which transmits the nerve impulse to the next cell in the chain. Excitation is transmitted from one neuron to another across a junctional structure, the synapse, and from a motor nerve fiber to a skeletal muscle fiber across another type of junctional structure, the motor end-plate. A single neuron usually receives excitation from numerous other neurons and, through the terminal branches of its axon, it in turn excites more than one neuron downstream. In like manner, a single nerve fiber (axon) from a motor nerve cell in the brain stem or spinal cord breaks up into many branches when it reaches a skeletal muscle, and each branch supplies a single muscle fiber. A motor neuron and the group of muscle fibers supplied by the terminal branches of its axon constitute a *motor unit,* which is the functional unit of neuromuscular activity.

CONTROL OF THE ACTIVITIES OF THE MOTOR NEURONS

A convenient way to begin our consideration of the control of movements and posture is to analyze the influences that act on the motor neurons in the spinal cord. These are the neurons that discharge impulses by way of the motor nerve to a skeletal muscle and cause that muscle to contract. They are large cells and are called alpha neurons, to distinguish them from the smaller gamma neurons, to be discussed later. Each alpha motor neuron receives afferent impulses from many sources; it has been estimated that a single alpha neuron may receive about 15,000 synaptic endings, which converge onto it from many sources.[2] Some of these synapses excite the motor neuron, while others inhibit it; thus the final result is a balance between opposing influences. We may divide the afferent influences that act on the alpha motor neuron into two general categories—those which originate in the muscle innervated by that neuron and those which originate from other sources, including higher brain centers. The first of these is exemplified by the stretch reflex, and the second by the mechanisms responsible for voluntary movements.

The stretch reflex. Embedded within skeletal muscles are groups of modified muscle fibers called spindle fibers. Afferent nerve endings are wrapped around the central portions of these specialized muscle fibers; the whole is enclosed within a fibrous capsule and is called a *muscle spindle*. The muscle spindles are arranged in such a manner that stretching the whole muscle pulls on the spindle fibers. This stimulates their receptor nerve endings, and afferent impulses are sent back to the alpha motor neurons which innervate the same muscle; neurons are excited, and the muscle which they supply contracts. This is the stretch reflex; it is an important element in the maintenance of posture, as we shall see later. On the other hand, contraction of a muscle relaxes the tension on the muscle spindles and inhibits the stretch reflex.

The situation is actually somewhat more complicated. Some of the endings of the afferent fibers from the muscle spindles synapse on the motor neurons of the antagonistic muscles (which would oppose the reflex response) and inhibit them. A common example of a stretch reflex is the knee jerk. Tapping the tendon of the knee extensor muscles causes them to contract, while at the same time the flexors of the knee joint are inhibited and thus do not oppose the jerk. This relaxation of antagonistic muscles that would otherwise oppose a contraction is called reciprocal inhibition. A third group of fibers from the muscle spindles terminates on the motor neurons that supply synergistic muscles whose contraction assists the reflex contraction, and a fourth group of afferent fibers synapses on neurons whose fibers convey information about muscle length to areas of the brain concerned with the coordination of muscle movements.

In summary, when a muscle is stretched, the muscle spindle receptors are stimulated and afferent impulses are transmitted to the spinal cord, where they: (1) stimulate the alpha motor neurons supplying the same muscle, causing it to contract; (2) stimulate the alpha motor neurons supplying synergistic muscles whose contraction aids the reflex contraction; (3) inhibit the motor neurons of antagonistic muscles; and (4) stimulate neurons that transmit information about muscle length to coordinating centers in the brain.

Golgi tendon organs. The muscle spindles are not the only sensory receptors in skeletal muscles. A second set of receptors, the Golgi tendon organs, are stimulated by the stretch generated by the shortening of a muscle when it contracts, and the impulses transmitted to the spinal cord exert an inhibitory influence on the motor neurons of the contracting muscle and an excitatory influence on the motor neurons of the antagonistic muscles. In addition, impulses from the Golgi tendon organs supply the motor control systems with continuous information about the degree of tension generated in the muscle, and thus inform them whether or not the flow of impulses from the motor areas of the brain is causing the muscles to exert sufficient tension to perform the task required. Some of the Golgi tendon organs respond only to great muscle tension and may serve to protect the muscle from damage from excessive tension by restraining the contraction.

The gamma loop. The large alpha motor neurons innervate the ordinary skeletal muscle fibers, while the smaller gamma neurons innervate the fibers in the muscle spindles. The contraction of the muscle spindle fibers brought about by impulses from the gamma neurons stimulates the muscle spindle receptors, and the impulses thus generated pass back into the spinal cord; here they stimulate the alpha motor neurons and thus increase the tension in their corresponding muscle. This pathway from gamma motor neurons and their efferent fibers to the muscle spindle and back to the spinal cord over the muscle spindle afferents is the gamma loop. The gamma motor neurons receive most of their afferent input from motor centers in the brain, unlike the alpha motor neurons which receive afferent input both from higher brain cells and from the muscle which they innervate. What is the function of this gamma loop system? We are not certain. One suggestion is that it causes continuous tension to be exerted on the spindle stretch receptors by contraction of the spindle fibers. If the spindle fibers were allowed to relax during contraction of the muscle, the stretch receptors would stop firing and information about muscle length would be lost. A second function may be to reinforce the inhibition of antagonistic muscles and the stimulation of synergistic muscles during a contraction. At any rate, both the alpha and gamma systems appear to be essential for optimal coordination of movement.

BASIC TYPES OF MUSCULAR ACTIVITY

Muscle contractions normally accomplish one of two things—they maintain a posture or they cause movement. *Posture*, in the physiological sense, means a certain orientation of the body in space (for example, standing) or of parts of the body in relation to other parts (for example, arms outstretched). Frequently the posture opposes the force of gravity (as in standing) and involves the mechanisms for maintaining balance and for restoring balance if it has been disturbed. *Movements*, on the other hand, either change the position of the body in space or of parts of the body in relation to other parts. Movements may be either reflex or volitional. A *reflex* is an invariable response to a definite stimulus affecting a sensory receptor. Many acts that are often referred to as reflexes because they do not require attention (for example, walking) are actually very complex acts involving many of the higher brain centers. Reflexes do not have to be learned; they are inborn. The acquired or conditioned reflexes described by Pavlov are in a sense an exception to this statement. They consist essentially in retraining a reflex so that it is elicited by a different stimulus, but once established it resembles the usual type of reflex in being an automatic and predictable response to a specific stimulus.

POSTURE AND BALANCE

One of the basic elements in posture is the *stretch reflex;* it is important in the maintenance of posture and balance and is best developed in the extensor muscles, which are ordinarily involved in maintaining a posture against the force of gravity. (For this reason they are often called the antigravity muscles.) For example, in order for the body to be held erect, the tendency for the weight of the body to cause flexion at the hip and knee must be counteracted. If the knees begin to buckle under the influence of gravity, the extensor muscles acting across the knee joint are stretched, and their muscle spindles are stimulated. The resulting reflex contraction of the extensor muscles then straightens the knee joint and preserves the upright posture.

Although the basic element in posture is reflex in nature, the participation of higher centers in the brain is necessary, as indicated by the fact that loss of consciousness abolishes the ability to stand erect.

Another group of postural reactions that is of paramount importance in sports is concerned with the maintenance of equilibrium or balance. In complex motor skill activities it is essential that the body be in the correct posture for the performance of the necessary movements. A boxer who is staggered by a blow or a football player who stumbles while running "automatically" makes compensatory movements that tend to restore the normal erect posture. Such movements are not "thought out"; they can occur in experimental animals in the absence of the cerebral cortex so that they must be considered to be complex reflex patterns.

There are three major sources of sensory impulses that initiate these reflex movements: (1) visual stimulation, (2) proprioceptors in the inner ear (the semicircular canals and the otolith organs), and (3) stretch receptors in the neck muscles. The example of the football player who stumbles and begins to fall may clarify the operation of the mechanisms of balance. The abnormal *position* of the head in space results in altered stimulation of nerve endings in the retina of the eye and in the otolith organs of the inner ear. There follows a reflex contraction of the neck muscles that restores the head to its normal position in space. Some of the neck muscles are stretched by this movement of the head, and the resulting stretch reflex causes reflex movements of the arms, trunk, and legs that serve to restore the rest of the body to its normal position. The abnormal *movement* of the head during falling and also during the performance of gymnastic maneuvers such as turning somersaults or cartwheels causes stimulation of receptors in the semicircular canals of the inner ear which produce the same types of corrective movements as those just described. The maintenance of posture and the corrective movements that restore balance involve the activities of a large portion of the skeletal musculature and many parts of the central nervous system. Every movement starts from a posture and ends in a posture, but during the execution of the movement the postural contractions are altered or abolished. This implies an accurate coordination between postural contractions and phasic contractions (those that produce movements).

REFLEX AND VOLITIONAL (VOLUNTARY) MOVEMENTS

A reflex is a relatively simple, unlearned motor response to a particular sensory stimulus. The structural basis of a reflex is the reflex arc, which consists of a sensory receptor, a sensory nerve fiber that passes to the spinal cord or brain stem, a synapse between the sensory nerve fiber and a motor neuron, a motor nerve fiber that conducts the excitation to the muscle, and the muscle itself. There may be one or more interneurons interposed between the sensory fiber and the motor neuron. An important feature of reflex activity is that stimulation of a particular muscle (the agonist) is associated with inhibition of the antagonistic muscle (reciprocal inhibition). This prevents the stretch reflex in the antagonist from interfering with the contraction of the agonist.

The character of the reflex response to stimulation of any particular area of the body surface is determined largely by the type of receptor stimulated. Thus, painful stimulation of the sole of the foot causes flexion of the leg that withdraws the foot from contact with the injurious agent. On the other hand, gentle pressure applied to the same point elicits extension of the leg because of stimulation of pressure receptors just under the skin. This "extensor thrust" reflex is an integral part of the whole reflex mechanism of walking and is normally operative on contact of the sole of the foot with the ground.

All reflexes are not of this simple type. Some involve higher brain centers (for example, the instantaneous turning of the head toward the source of a sudden, loud noise). Despite their greater complexity of nervous pathways, however, the general principles are the same as for the simpler types; a reflex is an invariable, predictable response to stimulation of a particular type of receptor, and the response appears to be a useful act related to the nature of the stimulus.

Volitional movements are initiated by impulses that are discharged from certain areas of the cerebral cortex. Cortical (volitional) activity differs from reflex activity in several respects, one of the most important of which is that, unlike spinal activity, it is unpredictable. This results from the fact that it is determined not only by the nature of the immediate stimulus (if any) but also by the stored memories of past experiences.

The nerve impulses that bring about volitional movements originate in nerve cells located in certain areas of the cerebral cortex. The impulses pass down in the corticospinal tract, most of the fibers crossing to the opposite side in the medulla so that the left cerebral cortex controls the movements of muscles on the right side of the body and vice versa. The muscles of the face, however, receive fibers from both sides of the cerebral cortex. The location of the cortical areas that control muscular movements has been investigated by several methods. The cortex may be stimulated systematically by applying electrodes to various regions and observing the muscular movements that result. Much information has also been obtained by a study of the impairment of movements that follows destruction of various areas of the cortex. Both methods have been used to study cortical representation of motor activity in experimental animals and in man. The results have sometimes been conflicting and are often difficult to interpret. It is not possible to duplicate precisely the natural processes of cortical activity by artificial methods of stimulation, and the results of localized destruction of cortical areas are often surprisingly slight because of the multiple representation of a single function in various areas of the cortex and in subcortical structures. For these reasons it is dangerous to be dogmatic about the details of the cortical control of muscular activity, and much of the presentation that follows must be considered to be a tentative summary of current opinions.

If the surface of the cerebral cortex is explored by stimulating electrodes, muscular movements are evoked by the stimulation of many areas—in fact from a large portion of the cortex. However, finely coordinated movements are obtained most readily by the stimulation of a strip of frontal lobe cortex lying just anterior to the central fissure, and this region has been designated the *motor area*. As shown in Fig. 13, the muscles for each portion of the body have separate representations in the motor area. The size of the cortical area that controls the activity of a given group of muscles is determined not by the size of the muscle group but rather by the complexity of its activity. For example, the cortical area that controls the movements of the fingers is much larger than the cortical area for the entire mus-

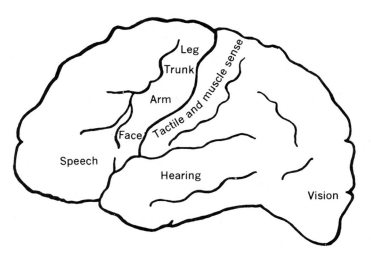

Fig. 13. Diagram of the locations of cortical areas. Areas labeled leg, trunk, arm, and face are the areas controlling contractions of the muscles of those parts of the body. (From Hamilton, W. F.: Textbook of human physiology, Philadelphia, 1949, F. A. Davis Co.)

culature of the trunk. This suggests that one of the prerequisites for finely coordinated movements is their control by a large number of cortical neurons.

Electrical stimulation of the motor cortex characteristically evokes movements, not contractions of single muscles, and this fact has led to the concept that the "cortex thinks in terms of movements, not of muscles." On the other hand, there is good evidence that the neurons that ultimately control the contraction of a given muscle are grouped closely together in the cortex, although the zones for closely related muscles may overlap to some extent. It appears that while the cortex may think in terms of movements this is not due to the arrangement of neurons in the motor area in discrete groups representing movements but rather to the multiple interconnections between neurons in the "motor area" and those in other cortical areas. The sensory areas of the cortex also play a role in the control of motor activity by interconnections with the motor areas so that movements are adjusted in accord with sensory information from the muscles and joints. We have no answer to one of the most basic problems in physical education and athletics—how do we *learn* a motor skill (as opposed to coordinating an already learned skill)? The easy answers of the past have largely been discredited, and we are now in a position of being almost completely ignorant of the physiological basis of the learning and memory of the complex skills involved in sports.

Although the motor area of the cerebral cortex initiates the muscle contractions that make up skilled activities and ensures that they are performed in proper sequence, other portions of the nervous system are required to adjust the strength, duration, and range of movements of muscles. The *cerebellum,* through its connections with the motor areas of the cortex on the one hand and with the proprioceptors of the muscles and joints on the other, is the key structure in this coordination. As a muscle begins to contract, its muscle spindles and tendon organs are stimulated, and some of the impulses are transmitted up the spinal cord to the cerebellum. In this way the cerebellum is kept constantly informed of the strength of muscle contractions and of the range of movement at the joints. Through its connections with the motor areas of the cortex, it is then able to increase or decrease cortical motor activity and therefore to adjust the strength, duration, and range of movements of muscles to the requirements of the act.

Adjustment of the range or extent of movement necessary to accomplish a given act is largely a matter of experience. We learn to correlate our visual impressions of the necessary range of movement with the corresponding proprioceptive information from the muscle spindles so that eventually we are able to make this adjustment in the

45

absence of visual stimulation. For example, in learning to type we must guide the movement of our fingers to the appropriate keys by sight. With practice, proprioceptive impulses are sufficient to guide our movements. If the cerebellum is injured, proprioceptive information is faulty, and our tendency is to overreach or underreach the keys; constant visual guidance then becomes necessary.

There is evidence that the sensory receptors in the muscles and joints may suffer fatigue during exhausting exercise. This may partially account for the faulty neuromuscular coordination that is often associated with extreme fatigue.

References

1. Asanuma, H.: Cerebral cortical control of movement, Physiologist **16:** 143, 1973.

2. Vander, A. J., Sherman, J. H., and Luciano, D. S.: Human physiology, ed. 2, New York, 1975, McGraw-Hill Book Co., chapters 16 and 17.

5 MUSCULAR PERFORMANCE

CLASSIFICATION OF MUSCULAR ACTIVITY

Muscles act in teams during movement of the body. The direction of movement of any part is the result of a difference in tension of the muscles on either side of the joint that is moved. When the arm is flexed, tension exerted by the contraction of the biceps is greater than that exerted by the triceps. Muscles arranged to act against each other on opposite sides of a joint are known as *antagonistic muscles*. Muscles working in mutual assistance to move a joint in one direction are known as *synergic muscles*. The biceps and the brachialis help each other in flexing the elbow and are examples of synergic muscles.

Rapid, rhythmic activity is accomplished by an alternation of contraction and relaxation of the antagonistic flexors and extensors of the joints in motion. Such freedom and speed of motion are allowed by a reflex reduction in tension of the muscles that are lengthening at the same time; the tension is increased in the muscles that are shortening. This reflex reduction in tension of the muscles that are lengthening during rapid, light movement is brought about involuntarily by a reduction of the motor discharges from the central nervous system. This kind of coordination has its center in the spinal cord and is called *reciprocal innervation of antagonistic muscles*.

Unresisted shortening of a muscle, as in the rapid, light, rhythmic activity just described, is called *concentric contraction*. In slow, heavy work and in a controlled motion, such as steering an automobile, tension of antagonistic muscles during lengthening is called *eccentric contraction*. The synchronous tension of antagonistic muscles is called *cocontraction*. Both concentric and eccentric contractions are called *dynamic contractions* because the increased muscular tonus results in a change in length. Such development of tension without change in length, such as that occurring in antagonistic muscles during static contraction, is known as *isometric contraction*.

It is practically impossible to hold the body still. Voluntary efforts to hold still by contracting groups of antagonistic muscles against each other, a fixation movement, never fully succeed, and the distal portion of the segment is observed to move to and fro. This movement is known as *tremor* and is caused by the unsteady muscle response caused by the synchronous nature of the volleys of nerve impulses stimulating the antagonistic muscles. An increase in muscular tension during fixation will increase tremor. Relaxation of tension will reduce tremor.

In a *slow tension movement* the antagonistic muscle groups are continuously in cocontraction, which serves to fix the joints involved in the action and to aid in accurate positioning. As slow tension movement continues, the body part moves in the direction of the group of muscles exerting the stronger pull, and there is a continual readjustment of tension of the groups of antagonistic muscles. A *rapid tension movement* such as shaking or tapping is one in which there is tension in all antagonistic muscles during the motion. Rapid tension movement is initiated by a sudden concentric contraction. There follows a contraction of the antagonists that stops the motion and reverses it. This is repeated and an oscillatory motion is set up. The maximal rate of tapping is limited by the rate of the tremor because it is not possible to modify the course of a movement except at the termination of each oscillation of the tremor. Thus, if the rate of the tremor is 10 per second, the tapping rate cannot exceed that value.

The *rapid ballistic* movement is one that is begun by a concentric contraction and proceeds unhindered by eccentric contraction of antagonists until near the end of the movement. If cocontraction of the antagonist becomes progressively intense toward the end of the movement, serving to arrest the motion, the movement is said to be *oscillatory*.

ANALYSIS OF MUSCULAR ACTION

The action of muscles during movement can be studied by simultaneous recordings of action currents occurring in the muscles under investigation. Electrical activity occurring when muscles contract is detected either by a needle thrust into the muscle or by an electrode placed on the skin over the muscle and is conducted through a cable to an electromyograph, which amplifies the current and records changes as muscular tension is altered during activity. A sample electromyogram (record of action current alterations during activity) is presented in Fig. 14. Using this technique, analysis of golf, tennis, weight lifting, and performance during acceleration in aircraft has been accomplished. Multiple, simultaneous electromyographic records of muscular activity of aircraft

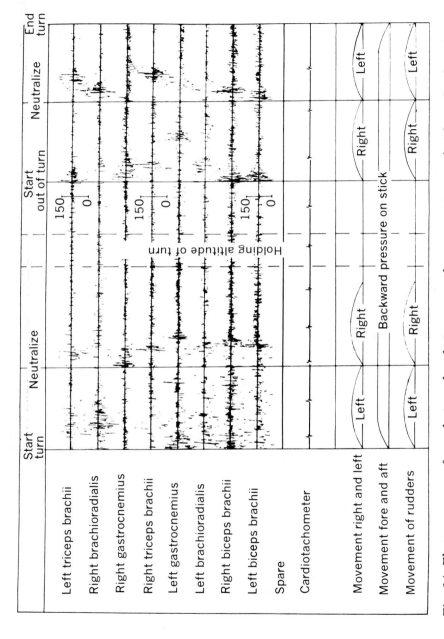

Fig. 14. Electromyogram of muscle interplay during a control movement in aircraft. The scale of 0-150 is an arbitrary calibration of amplitude of muscular activity. (From Wells, J. G.: Physical condition as a factor in pilot performance, unpublished doctoral dissertation.)

49

pilots and changes in economy of effort, coordination, and accuracy of movement were made during each hour of a simulated 7-hour flight. Poor performers were characterized by wasteful muscular activity, using forceful motions when only light ones were required. Muscular coordination during flight tasks was not observed to be affected by either a month of frequent and regular vigorous muscular exercise or a month in a hospital bed. The accuracy of muscular movements of subjects, both after bed rest and after normal duty, was observed to deteriorate during the latter portion of the long-range flight, but these errors in control were not gross enough to affect the scores of flight performance. Subjects whose physical condition was improved by exercise were able to make accurate muscular adjustments throughout the 7-hour flights.

The multiple electromyographic technique may possibly be employed as an objective measure of skill. Any muscular activity in excess of a minimum requirement for performance of standardized tasks would represent a measure of wasted effort. Performances accomplished with the least waste of effort would represent the highest standard of skill. Effects of training, drugs, fatigue, and other conditions upon skill could thus be quantitated by this method.

Procedures for recording electromyograms are found in Chapter 4 of the *Laboratory Manual*.

VOLUNTARY CONTROL OF MOVEMENT

Volition controls the whole movement, not the action of single muscles. Any movement, whether it is striking, jumping, lifting, pulling, throwing, or falling, requires a concentration on the movement and demands a disregard of the muscle action. The golf instructor who points out how the muscles should be acting during the swing of the club will soon have his pupil in the state of the centipede who "was happy quite, until a frog in fun said, 'Pray, which leg comes after which?' This wrought her up to such a pitch, she lay distracted in the ditch considering how to run." This condition is termed *paralysis by analysis*.

MECHANICAL EFFICIENCY

Human body designed for speed. The human body is designed for speed rather than for overcoming great loads. In most of the levers of the body the distance between the fulcrum and the point of application of power, the power arm, is relatively shorter than the distance between the fulcrum and the center of the weight, the weight arm. This is unlike most man-made mechanical levers in which the power arm is relatively long and the weight arm short so that great loads may be overcome by the application of a small force. The source of power in the body is placed at a great mechanical disadvantage, and extraordinarily strong forces must be applied through the short power arms and through the short distances. The muscles that are the source of power must be strong and efficient in order to work effectively at such mechanical disadvantage.

Factors affecting mechanical efficiency. In general the mechanical efficiency of muscular movements is affected by the following mechanical conditions: (1) the length of the power arm, (2) the length of the weight arm, (3) the load and the speed of movement of the load, (4) momentum, (5) the angle of the pull by the muscle as affected by the attachment to the lever, (6) the stretched condition of the pulling muscle, and (7) the action of synergic and antagonistic muscles.

Length of the power arm. A *long* power arm in comparison with the length of the weight arm gives the lever a mechanical advantage that enables heavy loads to be lifted. A *short* power arm results in a mechanical disadvantage in lifting heavy loads but imparts speed to the movement if the muscular power is sufficient. The calcaneus presents a long power arm that enables a person to rise on his toes while carrying a heavy weight. The olecranon is a short power arm that allows great speed in throwing.

Length of the weight arm. A *long* weight arm is a disadvantage in lifting heavy loads but is an advantage in movements of speed and in imparting momentum to light objects A *short* weight arm in relation to the power arm gives the lever a mechanical advantage in lifting loads.

Load and speed of movement of the load. The closer a load is placed to the fulcrum, the greater is the mechanical advantage. The further a light object is held from the fulcrum, the greater is the advantage for speed. A lightweight ball is thrown with the arm extended, whereas the heavy shot is put from close to the shoulder.

The magnitude of the load determines the speed at which the lever can be moved. The heavier the load, the slower is the movement. In the case of heavy loads the amount determines the distance through which a load can be lifted. The importance of the most effective application of muscular power and mechanical efficiency becomes greater as the load to be lifted becomes heavier. A load that is difficult to lift by the use of inefficient movements becomes less difficult if efficient mechanical principles are applied. Heavy loads are best moved by the arm through a flexion of approximately 150 to 160 degrees or through an extension from approximately 45 to 90 degrees.

The speed of the movement of the load affects the maximum load that can be moved. Heavy loads can only be lifted slowly. If a fast movement is required, the weight must be light. A heavy weight can be moved faster if it is held closer to the fulcrum (for example, the shot put).

51

Momentum. Momentum affects the amount of power that must be applied in moving a load. A greater amount of power must be applied to overcome the inertia of a stationary object than to maintain the speed of a moving object. Likewise, a greater amount of power is needed to stop a moving object quickly than to stop it by gradually reducing the speed. A greater momentum can be imparted to a movable object if the weight arm is lengthened. Less power is necessary to change the direction of a moving object if the object is kept moving than if the object is brought to a stop before it is moved in the new direction. The turn in swimming is a continuous motion through a short circle, not an abrupt reversal of the direction of movement.

Angle of pull. A pull at right angle to the lever gives the maximum mechanical efficiency. The greater the deviation from the right angle, the less efficient is the angle of pull. In a flexion of a fully extended arm most of the force is wasted by pulling the radius and ulna against the humerus.

If the pull of a muscle is not directly away from its point of insertion, additional muscles must be called into activity in order to hold the lever in the desired position during the movement. Most arm movements in swimming, for example, are angular and require the contraction of synergic muscles.

Stretched condition of the pulling muscle. One of the general properties of all types of muscle is that the force developed during contraction is greater if the muscle is under stretch at the time of contraction. In the case of skeletal muscle, the optimal degree of stretching corresponds roughly to the natural or resting length of the muscle in the body (that is, the muscle must be stretched about 25% to bridge the distance between its origin and its insertion).

Action of synergic and antagonistic muscles. The reciprocal action of synergic and antagonistic muscles increases the steadiness and accuracy of a movement. The greater the number of muscles engaged in a movement, the more accurate and graceful is the movement. The more complete the relaxation of the antagonistic muscles, the more rapid and powerful is the movement. The more angular the direction of pull, the greater is the importance of the action of the synergic muscles in controlling the direction of the movement.

Motion economy. There is a best way to perform any task, and it is the job of the coach in athletics and the time-and-motion specialist in industry to find it. A few of the principles that have been found to be of importance in improving performance are as follows:

1. Momentum should be employed to overcome resistance.
2. Momentum should be reduced to a minimum if it must be overcome by muscular effort.

3. Continuous curved motions require less effort than straight-line motions involving sudden and sharp changes in direction.
4. Movements in which the muscles initiating movement are unopposed, allowing free and smooth motion, are faster, easier, and more accurate than restricted or controlled movements.
5. Work arranged to permit an easy and natural rhythm is conducive to smooth and automatic performance.
6. Hesitation or the temporary and often minute cessation from motion should be eliminated from the performance.

Textbooks with a more detailed discussion of body movement in relation to the perfomance of work and sport are listed at the end of this chapter. Methods of describing and analyzing human movement are presented in Chapter 6 of the *Laboratory Manual*.

FACTORS DETERMINING THE STRENGTH OF MUSCLE

If all other factors were equal, the absolute strength of muscle would be roughly proportional to its cross-section area. Absolute values vary from muscle to muscle, and calculations of the strength of muscle tissue per square centimeter of cross section range from 3.6 to 10 kilograms. Fluctuations within these values among persons are unrelated to age from 13 to 48 years (see Chapter 26).

Two muscles having the same area may differ in strength simply because of the difference in the amounts of *fat tissue* that they contain. Fat not only lacks contractile power but it also acts as a friction brake, limiting the rate and extent of shortening of the muscle fibers.

Arrangement of muscle fibers. The arrangement of muscle fibers determines the force of the shortening action. Muscles whose fibers run parallel to the long axis of the muscle are not as powerful as those whose fibers are placed at an oblique angle.

Fatigue. Fatigue reduces the excitability, power, and extent of contraction of muscle. Unless the stimulus is great, fatigue reduces the number of fibers that respond in repeated muscular contractions. Such reduction in the number of contractile elements reduces the power of contractions. The range of each contraction is also diminished by fatigue because of the reduction in the number of fibers stimulated and because of the reduction in the amount of shortening of each fiber (see Chapter 12).

Temperature. Muscular contraction is most rapid and most powerful when the temperature of the muscle fibers is slightly higher than the normal body temperature. In this slightly warmed condition the muscle viscosity is lowered, the chemical reactions of contraction and recovery are more rapid, and circulation is improved. The heat of muscular contractions thus tends to improve the condition of the muscles for further work. Elevations of 8° to 10° F. in skin temperature have been observed in the vicinity of exercised muscle. Excessively high body temperatures overcome the capacity of the body for circulatory adjustments and may also destroy the tissue proteins. Temperatures below the normal body temperature elevate the irritability threshold and increase the viscosity, making the muscles sluggish and stiff and therefore weak (see Chapter 16).

Stores of energy foodstuffs. If stores of energy foodstuffs, such as muscle glycogen, are diminished by starvation or prolonged work without adequate feeding, the elements essential for contraction are consumed in the metabolic processes and contractile tissue atrophies. The decline in strength during weight loss is negligible until starvation is well advanced. Rats may lose as much as 38% of their normal body weight before marked decrements occur in muscle strength. Shortly after this point, however, when the body weight loss is over 40%, death occurs (see Chapters 1 and 13).

State of training. The state of training plays a potent role in the contractile power of muscular tissue. In a muscle weakened by disuse, gain in strength due to an exercise regimen commonly exceeds 50% within the first 2 weeks. Where this gain comes from is discussed in Chapter 19.

Ability to recover from work. An additional factor affecting the strength of muscle is its ability to recover from a bout of work. This is dependent upon the supply of oxygen to the muscle tissue, the rate of removal of carbon dioxide and other wastes, the provision of energy foodstuffs, and the replacement of minerals and other elements lost during muscular work. The circulation must be adequate to carry these materials to and from the working muscles. The greater the flow of blood through a muscle during contraction and relaxation, the more rapid is the recovery. Short, frequent rest pauses result in greater efficiency in muscular work than do prolonged, infrequent rests and are equally important in preventing loss of efficiency in skilled performance. Even after an elbow flexor muscle had been allowed to work to exhaustion, 69% of its strength was regained after 30 seconds. After a rest of 2.5 minutes only 13% more was regained, and after 7.5 minutes an additional 18% was regained. After a long rest of 42.5 minutes a total of 95% of its original strength was regained—only 26% more than after a 30-second rest.

FACTORS DETERMINING THE STRENGTH
OF VOLUNTARY EFFORT

In general, the strength of contraction of a muscle may be adjusted in two ways: (1) *by increasing or decreasing the number of motor units in action* and (2) *by increasing or decreasing the frequency of activation*

54

of each individual unit. It appears that the frequency of activation responds continuously to the need for changes of tension, whereas each addition or subtraction of motor units represents a separate step.

A fast, powerful contraction is the result of a short burst of impulses from a large number of motor neurons. A slower and less powerful contraction results from a more prolonged discharge at a lower frequency and from fewer motor neurons. The terrific rate of impulse discharge required for a fast, powerful contraction cannot be maintained for more than a brief period. The heaviest weights lifted overhead by weight-lifting champions are raised by rapid movements known as the "clean and jerk," and the lifters can support these heavy weights for only a very few seconds once they are lifted. Lighter loads can be lifted slowly, and the lifts can be repeated a greater number of times. When a light load is moved by a muscle, fewer fibers need to be brought into play. The remaining fibers are at rest and are ready to act if they are needed in succeeding contractions. As the working fibers become fatigued during light work, the threshold of irritability is raised and these fatigued fibers fail to respond to the stimuli. The stimuli pass into fresh fibers whose threshold of irritability is low, and the burden of the work is thus shifted from the fatigued to the fresh fibers in the muscle.

Emotional states. Emotional states influence the strength of the stimulus by reinforcing or depressing the discharge of the ventral horn cells. Clenching the fists or contracting muscles in parts of the body not involved in the movement may increase the nervous discharge to the muscles involved in the movement by *irradiation* of nerve impulses in the central nervous system. Excitement and the cheering of spectators may intensify the nervous discharge of the muscles and may also liberate

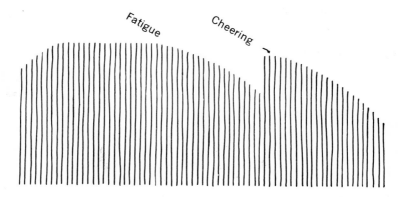

Fig. 15. Influence of cheering on performance of work as indicated by an ergogram of the movements of an arm. Vertical lines represent maximum lifts at the rate of 1 per second.

adrenaline (epinephrine), which increases the strength of the muscles and allays fatigue (Fig. 15).

Inhibition. Commencing with the thesis that the expression of human strength is generally limited by psychologically induced inhibitions, Ikai and Steinhaus (1961) examined means of increasing performance by reducing inhibitions. Using pavlovian conditioning procedures they demonstrated that maximum pull of the forearm flexors could be increased (or decreased in some instances) in a predictable fashion by a pistol shot, by a shout from the subject, by hypnosis, and by administration of alcohol, adrenaline, or amphetamine. These demonstrations are in accord with other laboratory studies which showed that maximum pulls against a tensiometer were enhanced by 12.2% when the subject shouted loudly during a random final pull.

Since the end point of a brief maximal strength effort may be set by inhibitory functions, strength training exercises should be directed toward reducing the responsiveness of inhibitory controls. This lessening of inhibitory sensitivity would permit a higher degree of tension to develop, thus increasing the strength of movement.

In a *behavioral* sense the whole organism seems to respond to maximal exertion in relation to the degree of intensity that it interprets as the severity of threat to its integrity. This homeostatic force acts to preserve the organism.

Strength is increased if the importance of the effort to the survival or well-being of the performer is believed to be great and if the effort is known by previous experiences to be nondestructive.

The deinhibition theory suggests implications for two principles of strength training. Exercises that exert repeated sharp pulls on the muscle and its tendons should be practiced to diminish the attenuating influence of the sensory organs of inhibition. The load of exercise in the training program should be progressive so as gradually to extinguish overly protective inhibitions.

MOBILIZATION AND SYNCHRONIZATION

When strength is taxed during prolonged effort, a mobilization of the higher nervous system that results in improved synchronization of motor units has been observed. The phenomenon occurs in the following manner: After 5 minutes of work consisting of supporting a 22-pound weight at the end of the forearm, the subject's motor units were activated in a disorganized manner (as shown in electromyograms); muscles trembled, the character of the breathing changed, the skin became red, sweat became visible, there was a tensing of other muscles, the position of the body was disturbed, and the subject cried out, "My arm is breaking!"

With a great effort of the will the task was continued. Then came some changes in the nervous control of the work. Gradually the activity of the motor units became rhythmic and muscle potentials became larger, indicating that mobilization of a larger number of motor units had occurred and that they were operating with a greater degree of synchronization. Now the work could be continued at a high level for a considerable time. This phenomenon is termed the "phase of overcoming fatigue."

Training is observed to expedite the mobilization and synchronization of motor units during this phase of overcoming fatigue.

Eventually, of course, despite maximum voluntary effort the work declines and becomes impossible. This is the "phase of complete exhaustion." The two phases are considered as quite separate, the first as a means of extending performance and the second as a limit of maximum work.

MECHANICAL FACTORS

Two factors influence the amount of power that a muscle can supply to its lever: (1) variation in the strength of the pull resulting from different degrees of *stretch* of the working muscles and (2) the *mechanical advantage* of the lever. The position of a muscle at contraction affects the strength of the pull of the muscle. The position of greatest pull is one in which the muscle is slightly stretched. The strength of the pull is decreased when there is no stretch on the muscle, and of course, there is no further pull in the muscle when it is completely contracted. The biceps is in the position for strongest pull when the elbow is fully extended and the biceps is stretched. The triceps is in position for the strongest contraction when the elbow is fully flexed and the triceps is stretched. However, when the elbow is fully extended, the biceps pulls the radius and ulna against the humerus, and only a small force is directed toward flexion of the joint. With the elbow at one half flexion (the lower arm at right angle to the upper arm) the force of the biceps is entirely employed in the flexion, and the lever is in the position of maximal mechanical efficiency. With the elbow three-fourths flexed the pull is again against the humerus, and the efficiency of the pull is very low; also the biceps in this position is nearly fully contracted and possesses very little additional strength for movement of the lever (Fig. 16). If a heavy book is placed on the palm of the hand when the arm is extended along the top of a table, it may be observed that it is difficult to lift the book from this position. If the upper arm is raised to one-fourth flexion at the start of the lift, the lift is easier. The lift is easiest with the elbow flexed so that the upper arm is at a right angle to the lower arm. With the elbow fully flexed it is obviously impossible to lift the load farther. The

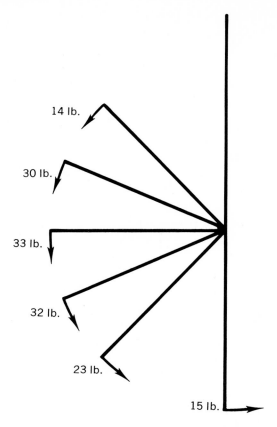

Fig. 16. Maximum steady pull of forearm against a spring scale showing the effect of the angle of pull.

combination during movement of these two factors, the advantage of muscle stretch and the mechanical advantage of the pull from a right angle, allows a great percentage of the entire force to be exerted over a wide range of movement.

As a further mechanical factor, the degree of pronation or supination in rotatory joints affects the strength of the movement. In the elbow the strength of elbow flexion is greatest when the forearm is in midposition, less when it is supinated, and least of all when it is pronated. This is probably due primarily to changes in the mechanical advantage of the pronator teres as the forearm is rotated. Flexor strength is usually stronger than extension, elbow flexion strength being more than 50% greater than elbow extension strength.

Studies of weight-lifting champions show that in general the lighter man is stronger in proportion to his *body weight* than is the heavier man. A small man cannot be expected to have as much strength as a larger one, but at the same time he needs less strength to move his smaller body.

Strength is related to *age* and *sex*. Strength scores of males increase rapidly from 12 to 19 years of age and at a rate proportional to weight increases. They then increase more slowly up to 30 years of age, after which they decline at an increasing rate up to 60 years of age. The strength scores of females increase regularly from 9 to 19 years of age, more slowly to 30 years of age, and then decrease. (See also Chapters 26 and 27.)

Adult men are about 45% stronger than women, even when allowance is made for differences in body height. The male superiority in strength is greater in the trunk, arms, and shoulders than in the legs.

MEASUREMENT OF STRENGTH OF VOLUNTARY EFFORT

The absolute strength of body musculature cannot be measured because of its interconnection with complex bony lever systems. However, the torque exerted about a joint may be conveniently measured by the use of various types of dynamometers, tensiometers, ergographs, and other instruments. *Muscular strength* is the tension developed by a single brief maximal contraction. The sum of the scores of the right and left handgrips, the back lift, and the leg lift is generally considered proportional to the total strength of the body.

The ability to sustain a muscular force or to perform continuous work is termed *muscular endurance*. This ability is significantly correlated with the strength of a brief maximum effort. See Chapter 3 in the *Laboratory Manual* for a complete discussion of the assessment of strength.

EFFECTS OF STRENGTH TRAINING

When a muscle repeatedly contracts under overload conditions several times weekly, it responds by undergoing hypertrophy. Hypertrophy of muscle is an enlargement beyond that expected in normal growth. In hypertrophy the size of each fiber is slightly enlarged, without an increase in the number of fibers. The total number of myofibrils is increased and the quantity of mitochondria is also increased.

The average diameter of fibers in most muscles is said to be 40 to 50 microns, and as a rule of thumb, fibers wider than 80 microns are considered to be hypertrophied. However, there is a rather wide variation in fiber size from one muscle to another, and the average normal diameter of muscle fibers in the thigh may exceed this figure.

It has not been proved that hypertrophy is necessarily a desirable reaction. Some students are of the opinion that it may be simply a by-product of training, perhaps a noxious one. Training of normal muscles utilizing progressive resistance exercise to produce hypertrophy does not increase strength per unit of weight. Increases in circumference after weight training correlate with increases in strength by only r = 0.422. However, patients who have regained normal muscular strength but lack normal circumference are noted to lose their strength more rapidly than those who have also regained normal muscular circumference.

Studies of the nature of hypertrophy have been made in an endeavor to understand its significance. The massive increase in the number of capillaries as the result of training may account for some of the added bulk. An increase of as much as 45% has been noted in the muscles of guinea pigs after programs of exercise. Other significant results were thickening of the sarcolemma, increase in the amount of connective tissue, increased phosphocreatine content, and increased glycogen. Working muscles are richer in water than are resting ones, but it has been determined that the amount of fluid entering the muscles would hardly increase their water content by 1%. In another study of exercised and unexercised rats it was found that the water content of the skeletal muscle was essentially the same for both groups; no significant differences were noted in nitrogen content or creatine concentration, although the myoglobin values of muscles were consistently higher in exercised animals.

Muscles hypertrophy in accordance with the specific demands imposed by exercise. Low intensity–high repetition activities such as long distance running do not cause marked hypertrophy, but high intensity–low repetition (or duration) activities such as gymnastics, wrestling, or weight lifting cause great enlargement.

In distance running the major demand is for oxygen, and this demand somehow stimulates the development of the slow oxidative skeletal muscle fibers. These are the fibers which contain a high concentration of myoglobin. Myoglobin binds with oxygen, so an increase in myoglobin should provide greater endurance. The diameter of these red fibers does not markedly increase in endurance training, but there is a significant rise in the proportion of red fibers, a significant rise in the enzymes involved in synthesizing ATP (the energy source for all work), and an increase in mitochondria. Also, there is an increase in numbers of capillaries which provides for an augmented capillary flow during exercise, thereby increasing the amounts of oxygen and nutrients that can reach the working fibers. These changes account for the restricted gains in muscle size in endurance activities.

Weight training and similar power activities utilize the white muscle fibers. These are the fast glycolytic fibers which provide energy through the breakdown of glycogen by anaerobic means, that is, without oxygen. These fast contracting white fibers are less capable of the concurrent resynthesis of ATP, so they fatigue rapidly. They do contain more myosin ATPase, which provides for rapid energy utilization. High intensity contraction of white fibers somehow stimulates an increased production of proteins in the cells. The proteins myosin, actin, and tropomyosin are synthesized on large polyribosome aggregates in the fiber sarcoplasm between the myofibrils. Apparently they then polymerize into filaments and attach in some way between the sarcomeres. It is this synthesis of filaments or myofibrils that causes the thickening of fibers.

The activation of nerves to fast and slow fibers may be part of the mechanism of adaptation to strength training. In an experimental transplantation in which the nerve to a fast fiber was attached to a slow fiber and the nerve to a slow fiber was attached to a fast one, the slow fiber speeded up and gradually attained the characteristics of a fast fiber, and the fast fiber slowed down. During the adaptation process the thickness of nerves to fast fibers increased and to slow fibers decreased. These are manifestations of the biological laws: use makes the organ, and form follows function.

When rats were injected with pituitary extracts, the quadriceps became 20 to 30% heavier and had a cross section area 6 to 12% greater than untreated animals, but this did not confer any functional benefits. In fact the muscles of the treated animals exerted less tension per gram of muscle weight than did those of the controls.

It is possible to increase the strength of muscles 3 times or more without a proportional increase in volume. This is accomplished by training with near maximal loads and using few repetitions (1 to 5). Hypertrophy without significant gain in strength results from training with moderate loads (60% of maximum) and using many repetitions (15 to 20).

Lack of use of muscles decreases the size of the fibers. The contractile strength of each fiber is diminished by disuse. Bed rest results in an almost immediate rise in the output of urinary nitrogen, and it is probable that most of the nitrogen lost in atrophy comes from muscle proteins.

RATIONALE FOR STRENGTH INCREASE DURING TRAINING

Since hypertrophy is a questionable explanation for the increased strength in trained muscles, other reasons must be examined. Using as clues the events that occur during exercise, the possible roles of such factors as oxygen deprivation, muscle temperature, and alterations in the functions of the motor nervous system were examined.

Noting that resistance exercise using heavy weights utilizes muscles in such a manner as to occlude blood flow, investigators hypothesized that periods of hypoxia may stimulate gain in strength. Accordingly, 29 college students submitted to pressure occlusions of the upper arm using a blood pressure cuff 3 times weekly. Simultaneously 28 other students performed static exercise with heavy weights. An additional 29 subjects served as controls. After 6 weeks in this regimen the group using weights demonstrated significant gain in strength, whereas the strength of the group with pressure occlusions remained the same as that of the control group. Thus oxygen deficit did not appear to be an agent in increasing strength.

Next, a similar experiment utilizing moist hot packs in place of pressure occlusion was performed in an attempt to duplicate the elevation of temperature during exercise. The purpose of this study was to see if periodic elevation of temperature would promote increase in strength. Six weeks of 3-times-weekly heating of muscles did not improve their strength. Thus elevated temperature does not appear to be an agent in increasing strength.

It is possible that agents produced locally during severe contractions may act in some way to strengthen future contractions. This is a fertile field for exploration.

The large increases in the amount of weight that can be lifted during the first 2 or 3 weeks of training appear to be the result of the acquisition of skill rather than the result of actual increases in the strength of muscle tissue. This conclusion is supported by the observation by Rasch and Morehouse (1957) that when muscles were tested in the position in which they were exercised, they showed significant gains, but when they were tested in an unaccustomed position, the gains were not present.

Improvement of strength is attained through the specific exercises that simulate the work of muscles in their exact spatial and dynamic conditions during actual performance. An explanation for the specificity of training may be that the synergic and antagonistic musculature involved in the maintenance of posture during strength efforts may be as susceptible to training as the primary muscles.

It is possible that just thinking about a movement brings about some strengthening of that movement. It is impossible to imagine bending an arm and simultaneously keep it perfectly relaxed. However, one of the advantages of using maximal or near-maximal weights in strength training may be that this form of training helps to bring some of the high threshold neurons within the orbit of voluntary activity.

In a phenomenon as yet unexplained, called "cross education," when a limb on one side of the body is exercised regularly and intensely enough to yield strength gains, the strength of the corresponding opposite limb is sometimes improved.

MUSCULAR FITNESS

The optimum amount of muscular strength for a person is slightly above that needed to meet the requirements of daily activity. A reserve of strength allows for emergency physical activity and occasional prolonged periods when adequate nutrition and hours of rest are reduced. This reserve has a dual benefit. It also enables the daily tasks to be performed with greater ease and efficiency.

On the other hand, excessive strength, especially if accompanied by massive amounts of muscular tissue, is inefficient because of the work and time required to maintain it and because the extra bulk of tissue constitutes a superfluous load to be supported and moved. Although excessive muscle does not constitute the same health hazard as excessive fat, it has the same drawbacks from metabolic and mechanical points of view.

EXERCISE FOR DEVELOPMENT OF STRENGTH RESERVE

In order to acquire and maintain the extra strength needed for his fitness reserve, a person must engage frequently and regularly in extra physical activities. This is true whether he is a professional athlete or an office worker. Fortunately for the office worker, who may find it inconvenient to fit physical exercise into his schedule of daily living, his physiological response to a small amount of exercise is of a large measure. It is the professional athlete or the heavy laborer who must work hard and frequently to keep his "edge."

Physiological considerations in the development of muscular strength and endurance are discussed in Chapter 20.

STRENGTH TRAINING IN ATHLETICS

The athlete who restricts his training to the practice of his event alone will achieve a certain degree of muscular strength by adapting in quantity and quality to the demands of the event. In endurance events the performance is within the limits of circulatory and respiratory functions, and muscular strength is not taxed to its capacity. After a period of about 6 weeks, when training loads can no longer be increased because circulorespiratory limits have been approached, no further development of muscular strength occurs. In some events, in which loading of individual muscles is low, such as swimming, strength declines during the competitive season. This results in a lack of reserve strength and can limit performance.

It is therefore necessary to include strength development as a separate component of athletic training sessions. Considerations of muscular strength in the performance of work and sport are discussed in Chapter 24.

Suggested readings

Barnard, R., Edgerton, V., and Peter, J.: Effect of exercise on skeletal muscle. I, Biochemical and histochemical properties. II, Contractile properties, J. Appl. Physiol. 28:762, 1970.

Basmajian, J.: Muscles alive, Baltimore, 1962, The Williams & Wilkins Co.

63

Broer, M.: Efficiency of human movement, ed. 2, Philadelphia, 1966, W. B. Saunders Co.

Cooper, J., and Glassow, R.: Kinesiology, ed. 3, St. Louis, 1972, The C. V. Mosby Co.

Hettinger, T.: Physiology of strength, Springfield, Ill., 1961, Charles C Thomas, Publisher.

Morehouse, L.: Neurophysiology of strength, Proceedings of the First International Congress of Psychology of Sport, Rome, 1965.

Rasch, J., and Burke, R.: The science of human movement, ed. 2, Philadelphia, 1963, Lea & Febiger.

Rasch, P., and Morehouse, L.: Effect of static and dynamic exercises on muscular strength and hypertrophy, J. Appl. Physiol. 11:29, 1957.

Snell, F.: Biophysical principles of structure and function, Reading, Mass., 1965, Addison-Wesley Publishing.

Weis, E., and von Gierke, H.: Experimental analysis of the human body as a mechanical system, New York, 1964, Plenum Press.

Wells, K.: Scientific basis of human motion, ed. 4, Philadelphia, 1966, W. B. Saunders Co.

Williams, M., and Lissner, H.: Bio-mechanics of human motion, Philadelphia, 1962, W. B. Saunders Co.

PART THREE

CIRCULORESPIRATORY
MECHANISMS IN EXERCISE

6 CIRCULATORY ADJUSTMENTS IN EXERCISE

During exercise the increased oxygen requirement of the contracting muscles is met by an increased flow of blood through the muscles. This is made possible by an increase in the amount of blood pumped by the heart each minute and by circulatory adjustments that divert a large fraction of the blood from less active tissues to the muscles. The circulatory adjustments of exercise are not, however, confined to the skeletal muscles. The oxygen requirement of the heart is increased, and the diversion of blood from the brain to the muscles must be prevented. The blood flow through the lungs must, of course, be increased in the same proportion as the flow through the systemic portion of the circulation but without an increase in the velocity of flow sufficient to prevent adequate exchange of gases. These widespread circulatory adjustments are the result of the interaction of numerous factors, both nervous and chemical, many of which are still incompletely understood.

BLOOD PRESSURE

The blood pressure is the force with which the blood distends the walls of the vessels and with which it would escape if the vessel were cut. Blood flows from one point to another along the circulatory system because of a difference in the blood pressure between the two points. The pressure thus diminishes progressively as the blood flows away from the heart and has fallen almost to zero by the time the blood reaches the right heart, completing its circulation. This is in contrast to the *velocity* of flow, which reaches a minimum in the capillaries and then increases again in the veins. The progressive fall in blood pressure along the circulatory system is caused by the loss of energy in overcoming the frictional resistance to flow offered by the walls of the vessels. The amount of friction between two moving surfaces is proportional to the area of contact and to the velocity with which one surface moves past the other. As applied to the circulation, this means that the pressure will fall most rapidly at the points of greatest friction. The blood pressure declines very little in the arteries, falls very steeply in the arterioles, and then falls more gradually in the capillaries and the veins. The great frictional resistance in the arterioles is due almost entirely to the tremendous surface of contact since a single artery gives rise to many arterioles. In the capillaries the surface of contact is still greater, but this factor, which tends to increase frictional resistance, is offset by the extreme slowing of the velocity of flow which tends to diminish friction. As a result the fall in pressure in the capillaries is much less than that in the arterioles. The rate of loss of pressure as the blood flows through the veins toward the heart is very low partly because of the additional energy imparted to the blood by the massaging action of the skeletal muscles and the siphoning effect of the respiratory movements discussed in Chapter 7.

Arterial blood pressure. A high level of blood pressure in the arteries is essential if blood is to be driven through the arterioles with their great frictional resistance and into the capillaries beyond. The ultimate source of energy for the maintenance of arterial blood pressure is, of course, the pumping action of the heart. There are, however, subsidiary factors of considerable importance for which the blood vessels themselves are responsible. Among the most significant of these are the elasticity of the large arteries, the high resistance offered by the arterioles (the so-called "peripheral resistance"), and the relation that exists between the capacity of the vascular system and the total volume of the blood that it contains. An additional factor of minor importance under most conditions is the viscosity of the blood.

When the ventricle of the heart contracts, it ejects a mass of blood into the aorta. This vessel is already full of blood that must be displaced by onward flow through the smaller arteries and arterioles into the capillaries. Because of the high resistance offered by the arterioles the flow into the capillaries cannot keep pace with the flow into the aorta. As a result the pressure in the arteries rises steadily, distending the arterial walls, until the increased velocity of flow through the arterioles is great enough to balance the inflow into the aorta. This maximal level of arterial blood pressure is called the *systolic pressure*. With the onset of ventricular relaxation and the closure of the aortic valve, the arterial pressure begins to fall since the outflow into the capillaries is no longer balanced by an inflow into the aorta. The distended arterial walls now recoil and force onward the extra mass of blood accommodated during the ejection period of the heart. The elasticity of the large arteries is thus the primary factor that ensures a flow of blood into the capillaries in the interval between beats of the heart. The fall in arterial pressure as the force of the recoil is gradually spent continues until it is checked by the next systolic ejection of blood. The lowest level reached by the arterial pressure in this decline is referred to as the *diastolic pressure*. The difference between the systolic and the diastolic pressure at any moment is the *pulse pressure*. See Chapter 9 of the *Laboratory Manual* for measurement and interpretation of arterial blood pressure.

The distention of the arterial walls at the beginning of the systolic ejection of blood is not confined to the aorta but travels down the arteries as a wave followed by a wave of recoil. In arteries that lie close to the surface of the body such as the radial artery at the wrist, the arrival of the wave of distention and subsequent recoil may be felt as a distinct throb, the *pulse*, which affords a convenient method of counting the heart rate.

If all the blood vessels in the body were to relax at the same time, the total volume of blood would be insufficient to fill them adequately. This would result in an immediate fall in blood pressure since pressure implies some distention of the vessel walls. Accordingly it is essential that a large fraction of the vessels be partly constricted at all times in order to reduce the capacity of the vascular system to a point at which the available blood volume can fill and slightly distend it. A common example of the result of a sudden widespread vasodilatation is fainting, in which the fall in blood pressure induced by dilatation of the splanchnic vessels reduces the blood flow to the brain, resulting in loss of consciousness.

An increase in the viscosity of the blood raises the general level of blood pressure since viscosity is a measure of internal resistance to flow. This factor is probably of minor importance in all but extreme cases.

An elevation of the arterial blood pressure is one of the important adjustments during exercise, providing the driving force for increasing the blood flow through the muscles. At the same time an excessively high resting blood pressure may seriously reduce the tolerance of a person for exercise. It is worthwhile then to consider briefly the influence on blood pressure of variations in the basic controlling factors just discussed. All fluctuations in blood pressure, both at rest and during exercise, are the result of alterations in one or more of these factors.

An increase in the *stroke volume* of the heart results in the ejection of a larger volume of blood into the aorta during the period of systole. If the peripheral resistance of the arterioles remains the same, the distention of the arteries must be increased to accommodate this larger mass of blood, and the systolic blood pressure rises to a higher level before outflow can be made to balance inflow. The diastolic pressure is increased to a lesser degree because the greater systolic distention of the vessel walls results in a more rapid diastolic recoil, so that the pressure may fall almost to the normal diastolic level before the next systole. An increase in the *heart rate,* on the other hand, predominantly elevates the diastolic pressure by curtailing the time available for the diastolic fall in pressure.

An increase in the *peripheral resistance* resulting from widespread constriction of arterioles elevates both the systolic and the diastolic pressures. Constriction of the arterioles diminishes the rate of outflow from the arteries. This in turn increases the systolic distention of the arterial walls and limits the speed of their recoil during diastole. If elevated arterial blood pressure due to widespread vasoconstriction is associated with localized vasodilatation in a particular organ, the conditions are ideal for an increased blood flow through that organ. It will be shown that this is, in fact, the basis of the increased blood flow through active muscles.

Measurement of arterial blood pressure in man. Measurement of the arterial blood pressure is a common clinical procedure and is part of every physical examination. An indirect method based on the measurement of the pressure that just suffices to collapse an artery is ordinarily used. The pressure is applied to the main artery of the arm by inflating an airtight rubber cuff that is wrapped around the upper arm, and a stethoscope is placed over the brachial artery below the cuff. The pressure in the cuff is rapidly raised above systolic pressure. No blood enters the artery below the cuff and no sound is heard. The cuff pressure is lowered slowly, and when it falls just below the systolic level, a spurt of blood escapes into the artery below the cuff at the peak of each systole. The impact of the small spurts of blood upon the stationary column of blood sets up vibrations that are detected as thumping sounds. The pressure indicated on the manometer is recorded as the systolic pressure. As the cuff pressure is lowered still further, more blood escapes beyond the cuff at each systole, and the sounds become louder. When the diastolic pressure is reached, blood flows through the artery under the cuff throughout the cardiac cycle, and the sounds suddenly become muffled and then disappear entirely. Direct blood pressure measurements obtained from a needle inserted in the artery indicate that indirect blood pressure measurements are accurate during rest but not during exercise. If the exercise is at all strenuous, systolic pressure may be underestimated by 8 to 15 mm. Hg and overestimated during the first few minutes of recovery by 16 to 38 mm. Hg. The errors are even greater in the measurement of diastolic pressure, and as a matter of fact, it cannot be determined at all in some subjects. As a result, much of the earlier work on changes in blood pressure during exercise and recovery must be accepted with reservation until it has been confirmed by direct blood pressure measurements.

Normal arterial blood pressure standards. The influence of *age* on the systolic, diastolic, and pulse pressures is shown in Table 1. It will be noted that there is a sharp increase in the systolic pressure about the time of puberty. After the age of 20 years there is a steady rise in both systolic and diastolic pressures as age advances, probably because of a gradual decrease in the distensibility of the arterial walls. *Sex differences* in the way in which the arterial pressure varies with age have been observed. In girls the sharp increase at puberty is less marked and is often followed by a decrease until 18 years of age, after which the increase is steady as age advances, although the absolute values are about 10 mm. Hg less than in the male.

Emotional states such as excitement, fear, and anxiety increase the arterial blood pressure and may cause falsely high results in the first of a series of blood pressure determinations. It is uncertain to what extent the effects of emotion are due to the liberation of adrenaline; a flow of nerve impulses from the cerebral cortex to the medullary centers must also be considered a possible factor.

As in the case of the heart rate, the arterial blood pressure is affected by *posture*. When a reclining subject stands up, there is a momentary fall in blood pressure caused by the diminished venous return. In most subjects the carotid sinus reflex (see Chapter 7) brings about a prompt

Table 1. Influence of age on blood pressure*

Age	Systolic pressure	Diastolic pressure	Pulse pressure
6 mo. male	89	60	29
6 mo. female	93	62	31
4 yr. male	100	67	33
4 yr. female	100	64	36
10 yr.	103	70	33
15 yr.	113	75	38
20 yr.	120	80	40
25 yr.	122	81	41
30 yr.	123	82	41
35 yr.	124	83	41
40 yr.	126	84	42
45 yr.	128	85	43
50 yr.	130	86	44
55 yr.	132	87	45
60 yr.	135	89	46

*Based on data from Allen-Williams: Arch. Dis. Childhood 20:125, 1945; and from Ponder: In Fulton, editor: Howell's textbook of physiology, ed. 15, Philadelphia, 1946, W. B. Saunders Co.

vasoconstriction in the splanchnic vessels, with a resulting rise in arterial pressure that ensures an adequate blood flow to the brain. This compensation usually overshoots the mark, and the arterial pressure is ordinarily 10 or 15 mm. Hg higher than in the reclining position. In some otherwise normal persons the compensatory vasoconstriction is inadequate or delayed, so that the blood pressure may fall when the erect posture is assumed. These persons often feel faint or dizzy upon first standing or if standing is maintained for a considerable period. This condition is called orthostatic hypotension.

The postural changes in heart rate and blood pressure are items in several tests of physical fitness. A minimal or no rise in heart rate and a moderate increase in blood pressure are interpreted as favorable circulatory adjustments, while an undue increase in heart rate and a fall in blood pressure upon assuming the standing posture are considered to indicate poor vasomotor stability. It is uncertain to what extent these postural circulatory adjustments correlate with general physical fitness.

CONTROL OF BLOOD FLOW TO ORGANS

When organs become active, they require a greater volume of blood flow. This is achieved partly by a dilatation of the arterioles supplying the active organ and a compensatory constriction of the arterioles in less active regions, so that blood is shunted from resting to active tissues. When large muscle masses contract during exercise, the vasodilatation in the muscles may be so profound that total peripheral resistance is decreased in spite of the compensatory vasoconstriction in less active regions. In this case the rise in blood pressure during exercise must be due entirely to the increased cardiac output.

All the tissues of the body do not take part in the vasoconstriction that diverts blood to active regions. The blood vessels of the skin and abdominal organs normally store large amounts of blood and can undergo the greatest amount of vasoconstriction when blood is required elsewhere. Such organs as the heart and brain, on the other hand, require a rich supply of blood at all times and hence do not participate in the compensatory vasoconstriction in exercise.

In brief, the adjustment of blood flow to the metabolic requirements of the tissues involves two distinct though interrelated processes: (1) dilatation of the arterioles in the active tissues and (2) compensatory constriction of the arterioles in certain of the less active tissues. Blood flow through the active tissues may be still further increased by an increase in cardiac output if large muscle masses are involved. The changes in caliber of the arterioles in active and inactive tissues are the result of nervous, chemical, and mechanical factors that will now be considered.

72

CONTROL OF THE BLOOD FLOW THROUGH SKELETAL MUSCLES

The vasomotor control of the blood vessels in skeletal muscles has been extensively investigated in recent years, but the situation is not yet entirely clear. The blood flow through resting muscles is relatively small because of the high degree of constriction of the blood vessels in muscles. This constriction persists after removal of the vasomotor nerve supply, so that it appears to be due to the normal intrinsic tone of the smooth muscle in blood vessels in muscles. It follows that increased blood flow in muscles during exercise must result from factors that overcome this normal constriction and bring about vasodilatation.

The blood vessels in skeletal muscle receive vasomotor fibers exclusively from the sympathetic division of the autonomic nervous system. Some of these fibers liberate noradrenaline at their endings and hence are called *adrenergic* fibers. These resemble typical vasoconstrictor nerve fibers in other parts of the body, and they are believed to exert a weak vasoconstrictor action on the blood vessels in muscle. In addition the blood vessels of skeletal muscle receive vasodilator fibers from the sympathetic nervous system. These fibers release acetylcholine at their endings (in this regard resembling parasympathetic fibers elsewhere) and hence are called *cholinergic* fibers. There is, however, no experimental evidence that these vasodilator fibers exert an increased influence on muscle blood vessels during exercise in human subjects.[4]

EFFECT OF LOCAL CHEMICAL CHANGES ON MUSCLE BLOOD FLOW DURING EXERCISE

It was mentioned previously that most of the blood vessels in resting skeletal muscles are constricted due to their intrinsic tone, largely independent of nervous control, and that the increased blood flow through exercising muscles is brought about by a decrease in this intrinsic constriction. There is much evidence to suggest that this is caused by the direct action on the blood vessels of local chemical changes. Among the agents suggested for this role are lack of oxygen,[2] increased concentrations of carbon dioxide and lactic acid, liberation of intracellular potassium,[1] and inorganic phosphate derived from the breakdown of ATP.[3] There is as yet no general consensus on this problem.

SITE OF THE COMPENSATORY VASOCONSTRICTION DURING EXERCISE

In a normal, resting man with a cardiac output of 5.4 liters per minute, the abdominal organs (gastrointestinal tract, liver, kidneys, and spleen) receive about 2.8 liters per minute, the skin about 0.5 liter, and the skeletal muscles about 0.8 liter. During exercise, along with the dilatation of the blood vessels of muscles, there is constriction of the blood vessels in the abdominal organs, so that their blood flow is decreased below resting levels despite the increase in cardiac output. The blood flow through the kidney, for example, has been shown to suffer a decrease of 50 to 80% in exercising human subjects. The blood vessels of the skin initially constrict in the same manner, but as the exercise continues, they ordinarily dilate as a part of the mechanism for eliminating the excess heat produced in the contracting muscles. The end result is a shunting of blood from the abdominal organs to the exercising muscles, heart, and skin and little change in the blood flow through other regions of the body. This shunting mechanism, together with the increased cardiac output, increases the blood flow through contracting muscles to such a degree that the oxygen uptake (milliliters of oxygen used per 100 grams of muscle per minute) may be increased from a resting value of 0.16 to an exercise value of 12, or 75 *times* the resting rate of oxygen uptake.

BLOOD FLOW THROUGH ACTIVE MUSCLES

Some of the factors that regulate the blood flow through organs, and especially through the skeletal muscles, have been outlined. Let us consider now the operation of these factors in adjusting the blood flow through muscles, first during the transition from rest to exercise, and second in work of various types and intensities.

At rest, the skeletal muscles, which constitute about 40% of the body weight, receive only about 15% of the total blood flow. Their arterioles are constricted by the intrinsic tone of their smooth muscle as well as by sympathetic vasoconstrictor nerve impulses. A large proportion of the muscle capillaries is closed; the individual capillaries probably open and close in alternation in response to the rhythmic activity (vasomotion) of the precapillary sphincters.

At the beginning of exercise, or even in anticipation, the heart rate and the cardiac output begin to increase, and the arterioles of the skeletal muscles throughout the body dilate in response to impulses from higher brain centers, transmitted by way of the sympathetic cholinergic vasodilator nerve fibers. At the same time, the blood flow to the abdominal organs and the skin is reduced through the action of sympathetic adrenergic vasoconstrictor nerve fibers. The stage is now set for the preferential shunting of blood to the muscles, but thus far without regard to the distinction between those muscles that will be active and those that will not.

The second stage of the regulation of blood flow results from the increased activity of the muscles involved in the exercise. The local increase in temperature and the release of metabolic products and other chemical agents by direct action on the arterioles cause them to dilate further, and thus the blood flow is selectively increased in the active muscles. At the same time, the arterioles in the nonactive muscles constrict, because of the disappearance of the initial sympathetic cholinergic vasodilator influence and the resumption of the normal intrinsic constriction of the smooth muscle of these arterioles. The end result of these various responses is an increase in the blood flow to the active muscles because of two factors—an increase in the total blood flow (due to an increased cardiac output) and a selective shunting of most of the increase in blood flow to the active muscles (due to vasodilatation in the active muscles and vasoconstriction in the inactive muscles, the abdominal organs, and the skin).

The amount of the increase in blood flow through active muscles varies with the type and intensity of the exercise and with the relative proportion of the total musculature involved.

Assuming maximal involvement of muscles and maximal intensity of exercise (of a rhythmic nature), some rough calculations can be made. Under resting conditions the cardiac output may be 5 liters per minute, and it may rise to 20 liters per minute during exercise. At rest, about 0.8 liter of the cardiac output goes to the skeletal muscles, and since the net flow to nonmuscular tissue probably changes little in exercise, perhaps as much as 16 liters of the cardiac output may go to the muscles during exercise. Thus the total muscle blood flow during exercise would be about 20 times greater than the muscle blood flow at rest (this relative increase might be even greater when only small muscle masses participate in the exercise). The actual increase in the delivery of oxygen to the working muscles is even greater (perhaps as much as 75 times the resting value), since a larger fraction of the oxygen is removed from each volume of blood flowing through the muscle capillaries.

The results of athletic training include an improvement in the efficiency of the shunting of blood to the active muscles (mechanism unknown) and a corresponding decrease in the cardiac output required for submaximal exercises.

BLOOD FLOW THROUGH THE HEART, LUNGS, AND BRAIN DURING EXERCISE

It has been emphasized repeatedly that muscular exercise involves widespread physiological adjustments over and above the actual contractions of the skeletal muscles. The functional activity of the heart is tremendously increased, and since the heart has a very limited capacity for anaerobic contraction, the blood flow through the coronary vessels, which nourish the heart muscle, must be correspondingly augmented.

75

The blood flow through the lungs must keep pace with the venous return or blood will accumulate in the lungs; at the same time the *velocity* of flow through the lungs must not be increased unduly if the exchange of gases in the pulmonary capillaries is to be reasonably complete. The oxygen requirement of the brain presumably varies little from rest to exercise, but it must at all times be adequate; there must be no diversion of blood from the brain to the contracting muscles. Adequate blood flow through the heart, brain, and lungs is achieved primarily by virtue of the fact that the arterioles in these organs do not participate in the compensatory vasoconstriction that diverts blood to the muscles. In the heart and the brain the principal factor determining blood flow is the level of arterial blood pressure. In addition the coronary vessels are dilated by release of vasoconstrictor tone; local dilatation by acid metabolites is probably of minor importance. The blood flow through the lung is determined by the output of the right ventricle and hence ultimately by the venous return. Dilatation of lung vessels probably results passively from the increased inflow of blood.

Blood flow through the heart. The factor of greatest importance in the control of coronary blood flow is the level of blood pressure in the aorta. The coronary arteries originate as lateral branches from the aorta just beyond the aortic valve, so that any rise in aortic blood pressure is transmitted directly to the blood in the coronary arteries. The great increase in aortic pressure during exercise thus ensures a corresponding increase in the inflow of blood into the coronary vessels. It was believed at one time that the contraction of the heart muscle in systole compresses the coronary vessels and stops the flow of blood, just as in static contraction of skeletal muscles. It now seems that this is true only for the brief isometric phase of systole when no blood is being ejected into the aorta. During the major portion of systole and throughout diastole, the blood flow in the coronary vessels is proportional to the aortic pressure.

It is technically very difficult to determine the influence of the sympathetic and vagus nerves on the coronary blood vessels because these nerves also influence the heart directly, which in turn alters the aortic blood pressure and the inflow of blood in the coronary vessels. Stimulation of the sympathetic nerves to the heart increases coronary blood flow, and stimulation of the vagus nerves decreases coronary blood flow. However, the injection of noradrenaline directly into the coronary arteries decreases coronary flow while acetylcholine increases it. It thus seems probable that the effects of stimulation of the cardiac nerves on coronary flow are indirect, by way of the influence on the rate and force of contraction of the heart.

Blood flow through the lungs. The blood flow through the lungs during exercise is increased in proportion to the increase in venous return to the heart. In spite of the considerable increase in blood flow there is no significant rise in pulmonary arterial pressure, indicating that a decrease in the resistance in the pulmonary circuit must occur. This is probably due to the passive dilatation of the pulmonary vessels and to the decrease in vasoconstrictor nervous influences on the pulmonary arterioles. Since all lobes of the lung are qualitatively identical, there is no need for a vasomotor mechanism for diversion of blood from one part to another, and the vasomotor nerves to the pulmonary vessels seem rather to regulate the total capacity of the pulmonary system.

Heavy static exercise such as weight lifting frequently involves straining, that is, forced expiration against a closed glottis. There is a considerable increase in pressure in the abdominal and thoracic cavities that may hinder the venous return to the heart, and as a direct consequence the blood flow through the lungs may be diminished rather than increased as in the case of rhythmic exercise.

Blood flow through the brain. The blood flow through the brain is steadier and more carefully safeguarded than is the flow through any other organ. The brain is enclosed within a rigid bony case, whose total volume cannot vary; hence a dilatation of the vessels in one portion of the brain must be balanced by a constriction in some other portion. There is no evidence of a significant vasomotor control of the cerebral vessels in man. Vasodilatation results from a rise in the carbon dioxide tension of the arterial blood. It is probable that the cerebral vessels have a high level of intrinsic tone which normally is reduced by the usual tension of carbon dioxide in the blood.

Cerebral blood flow is relatively unaffected by the increase in cardiac output that occurs in exercise.

BLOOD PRESSURE CHANGES DURING EXERCISE

As mentioned at the beginning of this chapter, many of the earlier studies on blood pressure changes in exercise are of little value because they were based on the indirect method of measuring blood pressure (arm cuff technique), which is now known to be unreliable during exercise. In addition, blood pressure was measured immediately after exercise in some studies, and the results do not reflect the pressures during exercise because of the sudden fall and subsequent rebound of the arterial blood pressure in the immediate postexercise period. Accurate measurements of blood pressure during standardized exercise (bicycle ergometer or treadmill) are now recorded from a needle inserted directly into an artery.

The most important determinants of arterial blood pressure are the cardiac output and the peripheral resistance to blood flow. During exercise, the arterioles in the active muscles are dilated and the peripheral resistance in these muscles is therefore reduced. It follows that the total peripheral resistance of the body may be decreased in exercise that involves large muscle masses, and that the increase in blood pressure in this case must be due entirely to the increased cardiac output. On the other hand, in vigorous exercise involving small muscle masses (for example, the arms), the total peripheral resistance may be increased because of vasoconstriction in the inactive muscles (as well as in the abdominal organs and skin) and the rise in blood pressure may be greater than in exercise involving larger muscle masses. This in turn imposes an extra burden on the heart and may explain the danger of hard work with the arms (such as shoveling snow) in cardiac patients.

During the transition from rest to work there may be a momentary fall in arterial blood pressure, lasting for a few seconds, which has been attributed to the initial generalized vasodilatation in the muscles. This is followed by a steady rise in pressure, which reaches a maximum within the first minute; this maximum is proportional to the intensity of the work. Thereafter, as the work continues at a steady rate the blood pressure usually declines slowly. The significance of this decline is not certain. During light work it is often associated with a decrease in heart rate and it may indicate a more efficient adaptation of the muscle circulation as the work proceeds. During heavy work, an additional factor contributing to the slow decline in blood pressure may be the decrease in peripheral resistance resulting from the dilatation of blood vessels in the skin; this is an essential feature of the regulation of body temperature during heavy work (see Chapter 16).

Both the systolic and the diastolic pressures follow the general pattern of changes described above. The increase in the systolic pressure usually exceeds that in the diastolic pressure, so that the pulse pressure is greater than in the resting state. The decrease in diastolic pressure reported in earlier studies was probably due to the inadequacy of the indirect method of blood pressure measurement.

With the cessation of exercise the arterial blood pressure falls abruptly, reaching a minimal value (which is often below the resting level) in 5 to 10 seconds, and then rises again. The initial fall in pressure has been attributed to the pooling of blood in the dilated muscle vessels coincident with the sudden withdrawal of the booster pump action of the contracting muscles. The secondary partial recovery of the blood pressure is probably caused by reflex vasoconstriction triggered by the initial fall in blood pressure. The rapidity and magnitude of these postexercise changes emphasize the futility of attempts to predict exercise blood pressure from postexercise measurements.

References

1. Biamino, G., and Wessel, H. J.: Potassium induced relaxation of vascular smooth muscle: a possible mechanism of exercise hyperaemia, Pflügers Arch. 343:95, 1973.
2. Guyton, A. C., and others: Evidence for tissue oxygen demand as the major factor causing autoregulation, Circulat. Res. 15 Suppl. 1:60, 1964.
3. Hilton, S. M.: Evidence for inorganic phosphate as the initiator of postcontraction hyperaemia in skeletal muscle, Scand. J. Clin. Lab. Invest. 29:135, 1972.
4. Uvnäs, B.: Cholinergic vasodilator innervation to skeletal muscles, Circulat. Res. 20 Suppl. 1:1-83, 1967.

Suggested readings

Barcroft, H.: Circulation in skeletal muscle. In Field, J., editor: Handbook of physiology, Vol. 2, Washington, D. C., 1963, American Physiological Society.

Carlsten, A., and Grimby, G.: The circulatory response to muscular exercise in man, Springfield, Ill., 1966, Charles C Thomas, Publisher.

7 THE HEART

The heart is a muscular pump that imparts sufficient kinetic energy to the blood to move it through the capillaries. The arteries conduct the blood from the heart to the capillaries, and the veins conduct the blood from the capillaries back to the heart again. As will be seen in later chapters, the arteries and veins are not simply passive conducting tubes but are also responsible, through alterations in their diameters, for the proper distribution of the blood to various organs and tissues in accordance with their metabolic requirements.

From the standpoint of the physiology of exercise the heart is primarily a respiratory organ. In the periods of rest between bouts of exercise the muscles are able to store sufficient food materials to initiate exercise and to maintain it until reserves can be mobilized. There is, however, no mechanism for the storage of oxygen in the tissues. Any increase in the oxygen requirement must be satisfied by a corresponding increase in the transport of oxygen to the tissues. This is accomplished in two ways: (1) by diverting blood to the contracting muscles from less active regions and (2) by increasing the volume of blood pumped by the heart per minute. Not only is the flow of blood to the muscles increased when they become active but also a larger volume of oxygen is removed from each volume of blood.

The increased pumping action of the heart has long been regarded as the most important of the adaptive responses that increase the delivery of oxygen to contracting muscles and as the factor that ordinarily sets the upper limit to the capacity for exercise. There is evidence that peripheral vascular changes, which increase the capacity of the muscle blood vessels to receive the increased blood flow, may also be important. Nevertheless, the increase in cardiac output remains a key factor in the physiological response to exercise.

CARDIAC OUTPUT

The degree of activity of the heart is best expressed in terms of the cardiac output; that is, the volume of blood pumped by *each* ventricle per minute. The cardiac output is the product of heart rate × stroke volume (the volume of blood ejected from each ventricle in one beat). In practice, the heart rate and the cardiac output are measured, and the stroke volume is then calculated. For example, if the cardiac output of a person is found to be 4.2 liters per minute and the heart rate is 70 per minute, the stroke volume is 4,200/70 or 60 ml.

There are several methods for measuring cardiac output. One that has been widely used is based on the Fick principle, which states that the blood flow through an organ can be calculated from measurements of the concentration of some substance in the blood entering and leaving the organ and the rate at which the organ takes up or gives off the substance. Suppose that the oxygen content of the venous blood entering the lungs is 15 volumes percent, that of the arterial blood leaving the lungs is 20 volumes percent, and the oxygen consumption of the body is 250 ml. per minute (the amount of oxygen used per minute equals the amount of oxygen absorbed by the lungs per minute). According to the

Fick principle, then, the cardiac output is $\dfrac{250}{20-15} \times 100 = 5,000$ ml.,

since the blood flow through the lungs is equal to the output of the right heart, and the output per minute of the right heart and that of the left heart are equal. The oxygen content of the arterial blood is measured in a blood sample from any convenient artery, and the oxygen consumption of the body is determined with the apparatus used to measure basal metabolism. The venous blood sample used in the calculation must represent the mixed venous blood from all parts of the body, which is pumped to the lungs by the right ventricle; it is obtained directly from the right heart through a plastic catheter that is inserted into an arm vein and then carefully threaded up the vein into the heart. This procedure is done only under medical supervision.

Another method for measuring cardiac output that is now widely used (since it does not require cardiac catheterization) is the dye dilution procedure. A known amount of a dye is injected into a vein (preferably close to the heart) and its concentration is then measured in serial samples of arterial blood. If the dye concentration in arterial blood is plotted against time, a curve is obtained whose area is inversely related to the cardiac output and the latter can be calculated from a formula.

It has been customary to regard the Fick method as the most accurate of all the techniques used in measuring cardiac output. It should be emphasized, however, that this is true only in the resting state or in a

81

steady state during exercise. The dye dilution method is more accurate when the cardiac output is changing rapidly.

Cardiac output in resting subjects. The cardiac output in resting subjects varies with posture. At rest in the supine position the cardiac output is about 4 to 6 liters per minute. If a sitting or standing posture is assumed, blood pools in the lower parts of the body under the influence of gravity. This results in a decreased venous return to the heart and a reduction in cardiac output of 1 to 2 liters per minute, despite certain compensatory mechanisms to be described later. The reduction in cardiac output in the upright position is due entirely to a decrease in the stroke volume, since the heart rate is usually increased slightly. Failure to take into account the postural changes in stroke volume has been responsible for much of the controversy concerning stroke volume changes in exercise. The resting cardiac output should be measured with the subject in the same posture as that assumed during the exercise.

Cardiac output during exercise. The obvious technical problems of injecting dyes and obtaining blood samples make the measurement of cardiac output during most types of athletic events impossible at present. Instead, cardiac output is measured in subjects exercising on bicycle ergometers and treadmills. This has the advantage that the intensity of the work can be measured at the same time, and the relation of cardiac output to work rate can be determined.

Trained athletes may attain a cardiac output of 30 liters per minute during maximal exercise, and untrained subjects about 20 liters per minute. The increase in cardiac output is due to increases in both the heart rate and the stroke volume. Furthermore, since the increase in heart rate in maximal exercise is about the same in athletes and non-athletes, the greater increase in cardiac output achieved by the athletes must be due to their greater capacity for increasing the stroke volume of the heart.

The regulation of the cardiac output involves the regulation of the two separate though interrelated components, the heart rate and the stroke volume.

REGULATION OF THE STROKE VOLUME OF THE HEART

The amount of blood that the heart pumps at each beat is limited by two factors: the volume of blood contained in the ventricle at the beginning of systole (referred to as the diastolic volume) and the completeness with which the ventricle empties during contraction. During exercise, the increased stroke volume might be the result of greater filling of the ventricle or more complete emptying or both. It was believed for many years that increased filling of the heart during diastole was responsible for the increased stroke volume in exercise. It was thought that the result of the increased filling was an increased diastolic volume, and that the associated stretching of the ventricle increased its force of contraction, resulting in the ejection of a greater volume of blood. This is in accord with a well-known principle, known as Starling's law of the heart. Starling was a famous English physiologist who observed that, in an isolated heart-lung preparation in which the filling of the heart could be artificially controlled, the stroke volume increased as the diastolic filling of the heart increased. Starling explained this result on the basis of the already well-established fact that the stretching of a skeletal muscle increases its force of contraction. It seemed reasonable, then, to suppose that the increased stroke volume of the heart during exercise was due to the operation of Starling's law. This would imply that the diastolic size of the heart is greater during exercise and it tacitly assumes that the ventricle empties completely at each beat.

However, in experiments on men working on bicycle ergometers, it was observed that the diastolic size of the heart measured on x-ray films did not increase in exercise, but that the degree of emptying was increased. This would suggest that the increase in stroke volume in exercise is due not to greater filling of the ventricles during diastole but to more complete emptying during systole, presumably because of the stimulating effect on the heart muscle of sympathetic nerve impulses and increased secretion of adrenaline.

The most recent experimental evidence (from studies of exercising dogs) indicates that whether or not Starling's law of the heart accounts for any of the increase in stroke volume during exercise depends on the severity of the exercise.[5] During mild exercise, the increase in stroke volume in their experiments was due entirely to more complete emptying of the ventricles, with no increase in diastolic filling (in keeping with the foregoing discussion). During both moderate and severe exercise, on the other hand, increases in stroke volume were accompanied by significant increases in left ventricular end-diastolic diameter (in accord with Starling's law of the heart). This has not yet to our knowledge been confirmed in man. It is best to reserve judgment on this important point.

It is difficult to obtain from the literature a complete and consistent picture of the stroke volume changes in exercise. There is fairly general agreement that exercise in the supine position produces relatively little increase in the stroke volume. When exercise is performed in the upright position, the stroke volume is increased proportionally more (with reference to the resting stroke volume in the upright position), and the maximal stroke volume is about the same in both the supine and upright positions. The following stroke volume values are approximately correct for untrained subjects: supine resting, 100 ml.; standing resting, 60 to 70 ml.; supine, maximal exercise, 125 ml.; standing, maximal exercise, 125 ml. The maximal stroke volume is increased as a result of training to average values of about 150 ml.; in exceptionally well-trained athletes, the stroke volume during maximal work may rise to 200 ml.

In summary, it is probable that when an untrained person in the upright position begins to exercise, the increase in cardiac output is achieved primarily by an increase in the heart rate, with a modest increase in the stroke volume. The more highly trained the subject, the greater is the contribution of an increased stroke volume to the elevated cardiac output of exercise.

VENOUS RETURN TO THE HEART

When a person is standing, the blood pressure in the right atrium is approximately atmospheric. In the absence of compensatory mechanisms, the blood pressure in the veins of the feet would be equal to that of a column of fluid reaching from the feet to the heart, because of the effect of gravity. This would amount to a pressure of about 90 mm. Hg in a person of average size, and it would result in marked pooling of blood in the feet and legs. In addition, the pressure in the capillaries would be increased and fluid would pass from the blood to the tissue spaces, causing edema of the feet and legs. The pooling of blood in the lower extremities, by reducing the return of blood to the heart, would cause a decrease in the cardiac output. Since these effects do not usually occur, it is clear that efficient mechanisms for compensating the effect of gravity must operate. These consist of (1) reflex vasoconstriction of the leg veins, (2) the massaging effect of the contractions of the leg muscles, (3) the presence of one-way valves in the leg veins, and (4) the effect of the breathing movements.

Reflex vasoconstriction of the leg veins. The veins are thin walled and distensible and might be capable of pooling much of the increased blood flow that results from decreased vascular resistance in exercising muscles. It has been observed, however, that the limb veins in both exercising and nonexercising limbs undergo reflex vasconstriction during exercise, so that the blood is returned promptly to the heart rather than pooling in the veins.[1]

Massaging action of skeletal muscles. The veins are thin-walled, easily collapsible vessels. When the muscle mass surrounding one of these vessels contracts, the vein is collapsed and its contained mass of blood is forced out. When the muscles relax, the vein is filled with blood. Contraction of the muscles might force blood out of the vein in both directions, that is, toward the heart and toward the capillaries, if it were not for the presence of *valves* in the veins that prevent the backward flow of blood. As a result muscular contraction squeezes the blood in the veins onward toward the heart, and relaxation of the muscles allows the veins to fill with blood from the capillaries. In this way the contracting muscles act as a "booster pump." This mechanism is constantly active to varying degrees. Even when the subject is standing at attention the muscle contractions that maintain muscle tone aid somewhat in the venous return. The fact that the mechanism may be inadequate under these conditions is indicated by the reduction in venous return, often sufficient to produce fainting by curtailment of the blood flow to the brain, which sometimes occurs in subjects standing at attention too long.

The quantitative importance of this pumping mechanism varies considerably according to the intensity and type of exercise. It is obvious that for a given type of exercise greater intensity results in a more rapid and more powerful massaging effect. During different types of exercise of the same intensity, the effect on venous return is correlated with the position of the muscles relative to the main venous channels and with the frequency of alternation between contraction and relaxation. For example, in comparing two almost equally exhausting sports, running and rowing, the movements are more rapid and rhythmical in running, and the volume flow of blood is correspondingly greater. Maintained static contractions of the muscles, as in rowing, may actually hinder the venous return of blood to the heart and make such activities exhausting out of all proportion to the amount of energy expended.

Respiratory movements. The veins of the abdominal and thoracic cavities constitute a venous reservoir largely unsupported by skeletal muscles and capable of holding 400 to 500 ml. of blood. This reservoir is closed at its lower end by the valves of the femoral veins and at its upper end by the valves of the jugular and subclavian veins. The outlet of least resistance is into the right heart. Respiratory movements exert a pumping action on the blood contained in this reservoir in the following way. During inspiration the thoracic cavity is enlarged in all dimensions by the movements of the ribs and diaphragm. This results in a fall in pressure in the thoracic cavity, which is transmitted to the thin-walled veins in that cavity. At the same time the descent of the diaphragm results in a rise in pressure in the abdominal cavity, only partly offset by the bulging of the anterior abdominal wall. This increased pressure is also exerted on the thin-walled vena cava, and since the blood is not only prevented from flowing backward by the iliac and femoral vein valves but also is aspirated into the thoracic veins by the decreased pressure in the thorax, its onward flow to the heart is promoted. Thus inspiration favors the emptying of the blood from the abdominal veins into the thoracic veins. During expiration the pressure changes are reversed. The rise in intrathoracic pressure exerted on the thoracic veins causes them to empty their blood into the right heart, while the fall in intra-abdominal pressure, because of upward movement of the diaphragm, allows the abdominal veins to fill with blood again. Alternate inspiration and expiration therefore create a pumping device similar to that caused by rhythmic contraction of the leg muscles. During exercise, this influence is increased by the greater depth and frequency of the respiratory movements.

The mechanical pumping action of respiration is not present in all forms of activity. In weight lifting and other forms of exertion in which "straining" is present, both intrathoracic and intra-abdominal pressures are elevated by the forced expiration against a closed glottis and the contraction of the abdominal muscles. As a result the blood is unable to enter the abdominal and thoracic veins and the veins of the limbs and face are engorged. The decrease in venous return no doubt accounts for the sudden fall in blood pressure that may follow the initial rise in such activities.

Electrocardiogram. Each beat of the heart is initiated by a specialized muscle mass known as the pacemaker, or sinoatrial (S-A) node. This

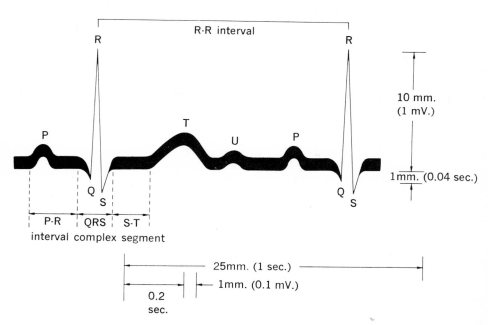

Fig. 17. The component parts of normal electrocardiogram wave forms are schematically represented, and the duration of the segments and intervals is indicated. (From Morehouse, L. E.: Laboratory manual for physiology of exercise, St. Louis, 1972, The C. V. Mosby Co.)

stimulus starts a wave of electrical negativity through a specialized conducting system, the atrioventricular (A-V) node and bundle. The progressive depolarization moving through the heart initiates atrial and ventricular myocardial contraction. These electrical changes are conducted to the body surface and can be detected there by means of an electrocardiograph, as shown in Fig. 17.

The electrical excitation of the atrium is seen as the P wave. Then there is electrical silence for 0.12-0.20 second while the impulse is spreading through the A-V node. Depolarization continues across the septum and into the walls of the ventricles and then recedes, seen as the QRS complex and lasting 0.10-0.12 second. There is normally another electrical silence between the completion of depolarization and repolarization when the T wave occurs. However, if the myocardium lacks oxygen, a condition known as ischemia, depolarization is incomplete and the ST segment is depressed. This sign of myocardial ischemia is taken as evidence of coronary insufficiency—a disproportion between coronary blood flow and the blood demands of the myocardium. This condition is exacerbated by physical exertion, making the exercise electrocardiogram useful in the early detection of coronary heart disease.

RESTING HEART RATE

The rate of beating of the heart is influenced by many factors, including posture, exercise, emotion, and body temperature. Normal heart rate under presumably controlled conditions shows a wide range in different persons. The American Heart Association suggests that the normal range should be 50 to 100 beats per minute. It is difficult to say whether the variation in heart rate from person to person is actually this great or whether it indicates lack of rigid control of the factors that modify heart rate. It emphasizes, however, the importance of careful determination of the resting heart rate in experiments and tests involving changes in heart rate during exercise.

There is said to be a tendency for the resting heart rate to be lower in subjects who are in good physical condition than in nonathletic subjects. There seems to be little relation between heart rate and body weight, stature, or body type, although the rate is ordinarily 5 to 10 beats per minute higher in women than in men.

During sleep there is a progressive slowing of the heart rate during the first 7 hours, followed by an increase before awakening. During waking hours wide variations in heart rate are associated with random activity. The average heart rate under resting (but not basal) conditions is about 78 beats per minute for men and 84 beats per minute for women. The heart rate diminishes progressively from birth (when it is about 130 beats per minute) to adolescence but increases

Table 2. Postural changes affecting heart rate*

	Heartbeats per minute		
	Lying	Standing	Difference
Average subject	74	92	18
Athletes	66	83	17

*Based on data from Schneider and Truesdell.

slightly again in old age. Methods of counting and interpreting the heart rate at rest and during exercise are described in Chapter 8 of the *Laboratory Manual.*

POSTURAL CHANGES AFFECTING HEART RATE

An extensive study by Schneider and Truesdell (Table 2) indicated postural changes affecting heart rate. These data do not support the widespread belief that greater physical fitness is associated with a smaller difference between reclining and standing heart rates, which has led to its inclusion in numerous physical fitness tests.

Actually the increase in heart rate upon changing from the recumbent to the standing position is a favorable compensatory reaction. It balances the decrease in stroke volume caused by gravity interference with filling of the heart and prevents a serious decrease in cardiac output. An excessive increase in heart rate upon standing, however, indicates inadequate compensation for the effects of gravity on the circulation and is often present in persons who stand after prolonged periods of bed rest. Excessive postural increase in heart rate may then distinguish obviously abnormal people from normal people but probably not normal sedentary people from athletes. Its value as a component of physical fitness tests is very doubtful.

HEART RATE CHANGES DURING EXERCISE

The fact that the heart rate is increased during exercise is a matter of common observation. The ease with which the pulse rate may be counted has led to a tremendous number of investigations on the changes in the heart rate resulting from different types, intensities, and durations of exercise. Many of these studies have suffered from the defect that the period of observation usually began after the cessation of exercise. However, with modern recording methods it is possible to record the heart rate continuously during exercise and recovery.

The maximal heart rate reached during exercise and the rapidity with which the maximal value is attained vary with a number of

Table 3. Mean values of maximal heart rate in 350 Swedish subjects[*]

Age	Maximal heart rate
5	205
10	220
15	205
20	200
25	190
30	185
35	180
40	180
45	175
50	165
55	165
60	160
65	160

[*]Derived from Åstrand, P.-O., and Rodahl, K.: Textbook of work physiology, New York, 1970, McGraw-Hill Book Co., p. 166.

factors, including the type of exercise (its intensity and duration), the emotional content of the exercise, environmental temperature and humidity, and the physical condition of the subject. Heart rates of more than 200 beats per minute have been reported in well men during exercise.

AGE-PREDICTED MAXIMAL HEART RATE

The average heart rate during maximal exercise is highest at age 10, 220 beats/min., as is shown in Table 3. With advancing age the maximum heart rate is seen to decrease approximately one beat per minute each year. The decline is similar in men and women. There is considerable variation in this value. For practical purposes the formula 220-age is a useful computation of one's estimated maximal heart rate, and may be used to express the individual's maximal heart rate when it is not prudent to exhaust him in order to determine it experimentally.

In using the heart rate to monitor exercise, the effort can be expressed as a percentage of the estimated maximal heart rate. Heart rate is directly related to oxygen uptake, and the percentage of maximal heart rate is a linear function of the percentage of maximal oxygen consumption.[3] This relationship is shown graphically in Fig. 18.

The acceleration of the heart rate begins immediately after the commencement of exercise; it may, in fact, begin *before* exercise starts, coincident with the tensing of the muscles, as in "getting set" for a sprint. This preliminary increase in heart rate is believed to be caused by the influence of the cerebral cortex on the cardiac centers in the medulla. The preliminary rise in heart rate usually shows a tendency

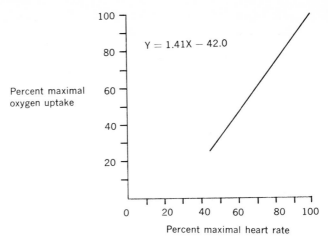

$$Y = 1.41X - 42.0$$

Percent maximal oxygen uptake

Percent maximal heart rate

Fig. 18. Relationship between percent maximal oxygen uptake, Y, and percent maximal heart rate, X. (From Hellerstein and Adler, 1971.)

Table 4. Relation between work load and heart rate[*]

Work load (foot-pounds per minute)	Heart rate per minute	Heart rate increment
Resting	75	—
2,000	105	30
4,000	132	27
6,000	154	22
8,000	177	23
10,000	198	21

[*]From Schneider: Physiology of muscular activity, ed. 2, Philadelphia, 1939, W. B. Saunders Co.

to level off after a few seconds and is followed by a more gradual rise to the final maximal level, which may be reached only after 4 or 5 minutes. This time course is subject to very considerable variation. In some persons the maximal rate may be attained within less than 1 minute; in others the rate may continue to rise slowly for more than 1 hour.

In a given subject the maximal heart rate reached during exertion, especially if the subject is in a steady state, correlates fairly closely with the *work load*. Table 4 gives the relation between heart rate and work load in the case of a man working on a bicycle ergometer. The successive increases in heart rate were 30, 27, 22, 23, and 21, respectively. It is a common observation that the successive increments in heart rate may become smaller as the limiting value of the heart rate (about 200 for most persons) is approached.

The type of exercise influences the increase in heart rate. The greatest acceleration of the heart occurs in exercises of speed (sprint running) and the smallest acceleration in exercises of strength (weight lifting and throwing). In endurance exercises (distance running) the heart rate increase is intermediate between those of speed and strength exercises, but the rate returns to normal more slowly following cessation of the exercise.

For a given work load, the increase in heart rate is less in more physically fit subjects. When subjects of varying degrees of fitness work to the point of exhaustion, the maximal heart rates are approximately the same in all, but the total work performed is greater in the more fit subjects. The greater stroke volume of the trained subject enables him to achieve the necessary cardiac output with a smaller increase in heart rate, and therefore he uses less of his cardiac reserve.

The influence of emotional and environmental factors on heart function during exercise is considered in later chapters. It is sufficient to point out here that emotion increases the heart rate at rest and in light exercise but probably has little influence on the maximal heart rate. The same is true, to a lesser degree perhaps, of an elevation in environmental temperature and humidity.

RETURN OF THE HEART RATE TO NORMAL AFTER EXERCISE

The time required for the heart rate to return to normal after exercise depends on the work load of the exercise period and on the physical condition of the subject. In men in good physical condition, recovery occurs more rapidly than in fatigued or poorly trained subjects. The return to normal occurs more slowly during very exhausting exercise, sometimes requiring as long as 1 to 2 hours.

The physiological factors that determine the time course of the recovery of the heart rate after exercise are not clearly understood. They probably include the following[4]:

1. A persistence during recovery of some of the same factors that increase the heart rate during exercise, for example, the elevated body temperature (an increase in body temperature in a resting person results in a faster heart rate) and the increased blood acidity.

2. Reflex responses to the sudden cessation of exercise with the consequent pooling of blood in the dilated muscle vessels → decreased venous return → decreased stroke volume → decreased blood pressure → increased heart rate. The increased heart rate in this case results from a decrease in the carotid sinus reflex (a reflex that slows the heart). The carotid sinus reflex is described on p. 93.

In support of suggestion 2 is the fact that the heart rate recovers more rapidly if the limbs used in the exercise are firmly bandaged at the beginning of the recovery period.

REGULATION OF THE HEART RATE

The heart rate during rest and exercise is regulated by a complex mechanism involving both nervous and chemical factors. The impulse that excites the heart to contract arises within the heart itself, in the sinoatrial (S-A) node, also called the pacemaker. The heart is thus not dependent on the nervous system for its excitation, as are the skeletal muscles; however, the nerve supply to the heart plays an important role in regulating its activity.

The pacemaker discharges rhythmic impulses that cause a rhythmic beating of the heart. The cardiac nerves, which terminate in the heart in close association with the pacemaker, belong to the autonomic division of the nervous system and are of two types: (1) the vagus nerves, which *slow* the rate of beating of the heart and (2) the sympathetic or accelerator nerves, which *increase* the heart rate. It is believed that these nerves exert their characteristic influence on the heart rate by direct action on the pacemaker. Under resting conditions the pacemaker is constantly bombarded by impulses reaching it by way of the vagus nerve, which slow the heart rate. This continuous arrival of vagal impulses is due to the constant discharge of the nerve cells in the medulla from which the vagus nerves arise. This group of nerve cells is called the cardioinhibitory center. A nervous center that is continuously discharging impulses is said to be *tonically* active or to exhibit *tone*. Thus the constant influence on the heart of the vagus nerves is referred to as *vagal tone*. If the vagus nerves in experimental animals are cut or their endings in the heart paralyzed with atropine, this vagal tone is abolished and the heart rate immediately increases. It is believed that some of the increase in heart rate in exercise is the result of a decrease in the inhibitory action of the vagus nerve on the heart (decrease in vagal tone). However, complete abolition of the vagal influence on the heart in man by the injection of atropine results in an increase in heart rate of only 30 to 40 beats per minute, whereas the increase in heart rate during exercise may amount to 100 beats per minute. Obviously decreased vagal action cannot be the only cause of the increased heart rate during exercise. There is good evidence that, especially during very strenuous exercise, increased stimulation of the heart by way of its sympathetic (accelerator) nerves is of equal or perhaps even greater importance. A certain amount of accelerator tone exists, but its influence on the resting heart is much less important than is that of the vagal mechanism. Additional factors include increased body temperature and increased secretion of adrenaline, both of which act directly on the heart.

The slow heart rate often present in well-trained athletes is believed to be caused partly by an increase in vagal tone. It is not entirely clear to what extent this is due to training; it may be partly inherent. During submaximal exercise of the same intensity, the increase in heart rate is usually less in trained athletes than in untrained subjects. This is thought to result both from greater vagal tone and lesser sympathetic stimulation of the heart in the athletes.[2]

The discharge of impulses from the vagal or cardioinhibitory center in the medulla is due to the arrival at the center of afferent impulses from several sources; in other words the control of the heart rate is predominantly through *reflexes,* the cells of the cardiac centers corresponding to the motor nerve cells in the spinal cord in the case of spinal reflexes. The most important sources of afferent impulses for the cardiac reflexes are specialized nerve endings located in the walls of the aorta and the internal carotid artery. The *carotid sinus,* a small dilatation of the internal carotid artery at its origin from the common carotid about the level of the angle of the jaw, is richly supplied with receptors that are sensitive to stretch. The ordinary level of arterial blood pressure is sufficient to stretch the walls of the sinus somewhat, so that a stream of impulses is constantly being sent over the sinus nerve to the cardioinhibitory center in the medulla. This results in tonic discharge of the cardioinhibitory center over the vagus nerves to the heart. If the nerve endings in the carotid sinus are experimentally destroyed in animals, the heart speeds up just as though the vagus nerves had been cut. A rise in blood pressure in the carotid artery, by causing greater stretching of the walls of the sinus, increases the flow of impulses to the cardioinhibitory center and thus reflexly slows the heart rate. This probably protects the heart from excessive increase in rate when the blood pressure rises, as during exercise. The reverse of this reaction also occurs; when the arterial blood pressure falls, the stretching of the sinus walls and hence the discharge of impulses to the cardioinhibitory center is diminished and the heart rate is increased by the removal of vagal tone. The *aortic sinus,* similar in structure and function to the carotid sinus, is located in the arch of the aorta.

It has been known for many years that the rate of secretion of adrenaline is increased during various emotional states (fear, anger, excitement) and during muscular exercise. The increased secretion of adrenaline during exercise may be due partly to the emotional component of the exercise. The hormone is transported in the bloodstream and upon reaching the heart increases both its force of contraction and its rate of beating.

It has been suggested that reflexes originating in the muscles and joints contribute to the increases in both heart rate and respiration during exercise. The stimulus that initiates this reflex may be the stretching of sensory receptors in the moving joints or in the contracting muscles or the stimulation of chemical receptors in the muscles (or in their blood vessels) by the acid metabolic products of muscular activity.

It should be obvious from the preceding discussion that a complete explanation of the increase in heart rate that occurs during exercise is not yet possible. A number of factors are known to be capable of increasing the heart rate under experimental conditions, but their quantitative importance in exercising human subjects is uncertain.

Even before exercise commences, the heart rate increases, probably due to psychic factors in anticipation of effort. Cardiac centers in the medulla are influenced by cerebral cortical stimuli. In a sudden maximal exercise such as sprint running, the maximal heart rate may be reached in less than 1 minute. As exercise continues, other factors come into operation, including perhaps acid metabolites liberated from the working muscles, reflexes originating in contracting muscles and moving joints, and the secretion into the bloodstream of much larger amounts of adrenaline.

Under steady state conditions in submaximal exercise such as endurance running, the heart rate correlates with the biochemical changes associated with metabolism, oxygen consumption, and carbon dioxide output. Associated functions such as respiratory minute volume are also correlated with heart rate. When unaffected by emotional and environmental (heat and altitude) factors, exercise heart rate is a reliable indicator of the effort of continuous work. The heart rate resulting from combined efforts is an index of cardiac stress. The effort or stress is mild if the rate is 100 and below, moderate at 120, heavy at 140, and strenuous at 160 and above.

References

1. Bevegård, B. S., and Shepherd, J. T.: Changes in tone of limb veins during supine exercise, J. Appl. Physiol. **20**:1, 1965.
2. Ekblom, B., Kilbom, A., and Soltysiak, J.: Physical training, bradycardia and autonomic nervous system, Scand. J. Clin. Lab. Invest. **32**:251, 1973.
3. Hellerstein, H. K., and Adler, R.: Relationships between percent maximal oxygen uptake in normals and cardiacs, Circulation 43-44, Suppl. II., October, 1971.
4. Herxheimer, H.: Heart rate in recovery from severe exercise, J. Appl. Physiol. **1**:279, 1948.
5. Horwitz, L. D., Atkins, J. M., and Leshin, S. J.: Role of the Frank-Starling mechanism in exercise, Circulat. Res. **31**:868, 1972.

Suggested readings

Aviado, D. M., Jr.: Some controversial cardiac reflexes, Circulat. Res. **10**:831, 1962.

Bolter, C. P., Hughson, R. L., and Critz, J. B.: Intrinsic rate and cholinergic sensitivity of isolated atria from trained and sedentary rats, Proc. Soc. Exp. Biol. Med. **144**:364, 1973.

Bevegård, B. S., and Shepherd, J. T.: Regulation of the circulation during exercise in man, Physiol. Rev. **47**:178, 1967.

Braunwald, E., and others: An analysis of the cardiac response to exercise, Circulat. Res. **20** Suppl. 1: 1-44, 1967.

Rowell, B.: Circulation, Med. Sci. Sports **1**:15, 1969.

8 PULMONARY VENTILATION

The term respiration includes all the processes involved in transporting oxygen from the atmosphere to the tissue cells and carbon dioxide from the cells to the atmosphere. These processes together are sometimes referred to as *external* respiration, and the utilization of oxygen in the cells as *internal* respiration. In this and the following chapter, we shall be concerned with external respiration, including the adjustments that occur in exercise. For convenience of discussion we shall consider respiration as involving three separate processes: (1) pulmonary ventilation or breathing, (2) the exchange of oxygen and carbon dioxide in the lungs and tissues, and (3) the transport of oxygen and carbon dioxide in the blood. We shall also be concerned with the effects of exercise on all three processes. A convenient starting point is to consider the mechanism of breathing, what it accomplishes, and how it is regulated to meet changing metabolic requirements for oxygen uptake and carbon dioxide elimination.

MECHANICS OF BREATHING

Structure of the lung. Functionally, the lung consists of two portions—the alveoli, in which gas exchange occurs between air and pulmonary capillary blood, and the conducting system of trachea, bronchi, bronchioles, and so on, by means of which air reaches the alveoli during inspiration and leaves the alveoli during expiration. Since the conducting system is not involved in gas exchange, it is called the respiratory dead space. The analogy with the arteries and the capillaries in the circulatory system is obvious. The alveoli constitute about 95 percent of the volume of the lungs, and their appearance is shown in Fig. 19 as resembling clusters of grapes at the end of the conducting bronchioles. Each alveolus is invested with a network of pulmonary capillaries, so that the total surface

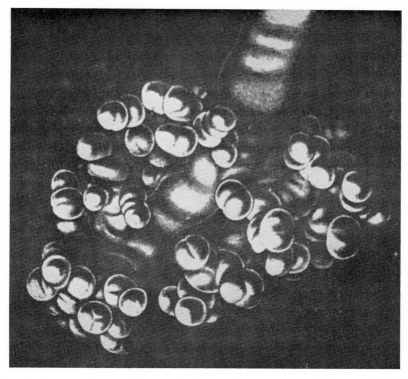

Fig. 19. Portion of a metal cast of a human lung showing the arrangement of alveoli and alveolar sacs (air sacs) and the branching alveolar duct. (After Bender; from Maximow and Bloom: A textbook of histology, ed. 4, Philadelphia, 1944, W. B. Saunders Co.)

of contact between air in the alveoli and blood in the capillaries is very large, making possible a rapid exchange of gases.

Inspiration and expiration. The two lungs lie one on either side of the mediastinum (the central compartment of the thorax, which contains the heart and great vessels, trachea, and esophagus). Each lung is covered with a thin membrane, the *visceral pleura,* which is reflected at the root of the lung onto the walls of the mediastinum, the inner surface of the chest wall, and the upper surface of the diaphragm to form the *parietal pleura.* A thin film of fluid separates the two layers of pleura from one another.

Inspiration is initiated by a discharge of nerve impulses from the respiratory center in the medulla to the inspiratory muscles (primarily the diaphragm and external intercostals). The contraction of these muscles enlarges the thorax, and since the lungs are essentially "glued" to the inner surface of the chest wall and upper surface of the diaphragm by the intervening fluid film, the volume of the lungs is also increased. (The volume of the lungs may be said to increase during inspiration by the

97

force of hydraulic traction.) With the enlargement of the lungs, the pressure within the lungs (the intrapulmonic pressure) falls below atmospheric pressure and air enters the lungs, constituting the act of inspiration. The lungs are elastic structures and tend constantly to pull away from the chest wall (exerting what is known as "elastic recoil"). As a result, the pressure in the film of fluid between the two layers of pleura (the intrapleural space) is slightly subatmospheric at all times. Inspiration enlarges the lungs and thus increases their force of elastic recoil, which makes the intrapleural pressure still more subatmospheric. When the respiratory center ceases to discharge impulses, the inspiratory muscles relax, and the increased elastic recoil of the lungs and chest wall returns them to their smaller resting volume, raising the intrapulmonic pressure above atmospheric pressure, so that air leaves the lungs (expiration). Thus, under normal resting conditions, inspiration is *active*, depending on the contraction of the inspiratory muscles, while expiration is *passive*, depending on the increased elastic recoil of the lungs and chest wall that is produced by the preceding inspiration. It should be emphasized that the changes in intrapleural pressure associated with breathing have nothing to do with *causing* changes in lung volume (as taught in some texts), but are the *result* of changes in lung volume and hence in the elastic recoil of the lungs.

THE RESPIRED AIR

In quiet breathing, about 500 ml. of air moves in and out of the lungs at each breath. This is the tidal volume, so called because it goes in and out like the tides of the ocean. The tidal volume may be greatly increased in exercise. The air conducting portions of the respiratory tract constitute a dead space, having an average capacity of 150 ml. in the resting subject. This means that of the 500 ml. of air in a normal inspiration only 350 ml. actually mixes with the 2,000 to 3,000 ml. of air in the alveoli; the rest remains in the dead space. With the onset of expiration, the first portion of air to be expelled is that filling the dead space. Since it has not participated in respiratory exchange, its composition is essentially the same as that of atmospheric air. The rest of the air exhaled comes from the depths of the lungs where gas exchange has occurred. By convention this air, which has participated in respiratory exchange, is called *alveolar air*. It is believed to approximate the composition of the air in the alveoli very closely. The expired air is thus a mixture of atmospheric (dead space) air and alveolar air, and its composition is intermediate between the two.

Alveolar air. As just mentioned, the term "alveolar air" is used to identify the air in those portions of the respiratory tree in which gas exchange occurs. It is with this air and not with that of the outside atmosphere that the blood flowing through the capillaries of the lungs come into diffusion equilibrium. The average composition of the alveolar air is oxygen, 14.5%; carbon dioxide, 5.5%; and nitrogen, 80%.* This composition remains reasonably constant in a given subject at rest, indicating that ventilation of the alveoli is so adjusted as to balance the gas exchange between the alveolar air and blood in the pulmonary capillaries.

It is of considerable significance that the alveoli are not completely flushed out at each inspiration. If this did occur, the composition of the alveolar air would fluctuate widely from inspiration to expiration, with a corresponding fluctuation in the gaseous composition of the blood leaving the lungs.

Expired air. The expired air is a mixture of atmospheric air from the dead space and alveolar air. Its composition varies with fluctuations in that of the alveolar air and in the depth of breathing. It is obvious that the smaller the tidal volume (that is, the shallower the breath), the more closely will the expired air approach the composition of atmospheric air. For example, with a tidal volume of 450 ml. and a dead space of 150 ml., the expired air will consist of one-third atmospheric air and two-thirds alveolar air, whereas a reduction of the tidal volume to 300 ml. would result in an equal mixture of atmospheric and alveolar airs in the expired air. Since the composition of the expired air and the alveolar air and the volume of the dead space are mutually dependent variables, if the values of any two are known, that of the third may be calculated. This is a valuable procedure in many types of research dealing with the physiological adjustments to exercise. This and other procedures for measuring pulmonary ventilation and respiratory gases are discussed in Chapters 10 and 11 in the *Laboratory Manual*.

PULMONARY VENTILATION DURING EXERCISE

Minute volume of breathing. Ventilation of the lungs during exercise is probably always adequate for normal saturation of the blood flowing through the lungs and in moderate exertion there is a linear relation between the minute volume of breathing and the amount of oxygen absorbed. This is illustrated in Fig. 20.

The approximately linear relation between work load and minute volume of breathing is maintained as the work load is increased until the intensity of work is so great that a steady state cannot be achieved. With the accumulation of lactic acid, pulmonary ventilation becomes excessive

---

*The composition of atmospheric air is oxygen, 20.93%; carbon dioxide, 0.03%; and nitrogen, 79.04%. The rare gases are included in the nitrogen fraction.

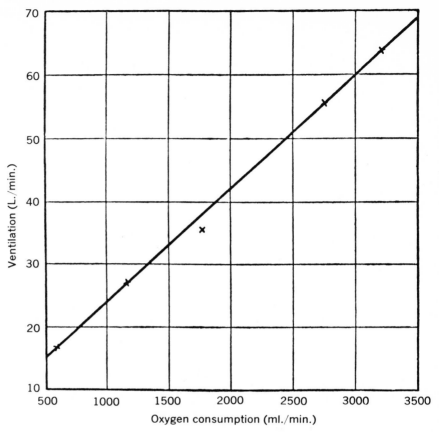

Fig. 20. Relation between oxygen consumption and pulmonary ventilation during exercise. (From Bainbridge: The physiology of muscular exercise, rewritten by Bock and Dill, London, 1931, Longmans, Green & Co.)

and no longer bears a constant relation to oxygen consumption. This excessive ventilation serves no useful purpose since the delivery of oxygen to the tissues is now limited by the maximal output of blood by the heart and by the capacity of the blood vessels in the contracting muscles for receiving the increased flow of blood. It does indicate that pulmonary ventilation is capable of further increase at a time when the limit of circulatory adjustment has been reached, emphasizing the fact that the minute volume of breathing is unlikely to be a limiting factor in exercise. However, when breathing becomes excessive, the energy cost of breathing (that is, the oxygen requirement of the respiratory muscles) may become excessive, and this may be a limiting factor in exercise. Also, the feeling that breathing is difficult (dyspnea) in severe exercise may in itself make prolongation of the exercise impossible.

The minute volume of breathing in exercise is influenced by the physical condition of the subject and by training. The trained subject demonstrates (1) a decrease in the minute volume of breathing required for the performance of a given load, indicating an improvement in the efficiency of ventilation, and (2) an increase in the maximal respiratory minute volume that can be achieved during very strenuous exertion.

It is probable that the respiratory superiority of the trained athlete lies not so much in a larger vital capacity as in a greater ability to utilize his maximal lung capacity. As the depth of breathing approaches the limit imposed by the vital capacity, subjective feelings of discomfort develop. This stage is reached sooner by an untrained man than by a trained man, and the subject is said to be "out of breath" or "winded." The physiological basis of this phenomenon is not clearly understood. It may be correlated with certain differences in the breathing patterns of trained and untrained men. In an untrained man there is a tendency toward a greater frequency of breathing to attain a given minute volume of ventilation. This may be caused by his inability to achieve both rapid and maximal enlargement of the thoracic cage because of the lesser strength of his respiratory muscles. Another characteristic of the respiratory pattern of untrained men is the relatively greater role of costal as opposed to diaphragmatic enlargement of the chest. Since costal enlargement is executed against a greater resistance as the elastic limits of the chest wall are approached, fatigue of the respiratory muscles and the accompanying subjective feelings of distress appear more quickly than in predominantly diaphragmatic breathing.

The cause of the stabbing pain in the side, called a "stitch," is not definitely known. It has been thought by some to be caused by an inadequate supply of oxygen to the diaphragm. It has also been attributed to engorgement of the liver,[4] which might explain the relief said to be experienced when the victim of a stitch bends forward and presses upon the liver area in order to "squeeze out the excess blood." Since the blood flow to the liver, like that to other visceral organs, is thought to be decreased in exercise, this explanation is difficult to accept.

Time relations of the respiratory changes during exercise. With the beginning of exercise an immediate augmentation of breathing occurs. When the excitement of competition is involved, there may occur an anticipatory increase in breathing just before the work is started. For a given work load there are two phases to the respiratory response, the rapid initial increase just mentioned, followed by a slow rise to the final value which is maintained throughout the exercise. Since the onset of the initial phase is very rapid, occurring before any metabolic products from the contracting muscles could possibly reach the respiratory center, it is thought to be the result of impulses from the cerebral cortex influencing the respiratory center.

There may be a considerable lag in the attainment of the final maximal level of breathing, indicating a steadily mounting chemical and reflex drive to the respiratory center. With moderate exertion a steady state is usually reached in 3 to 5 minutes, which is approximately the same as the time required for completion of the circulatory adjustments. This suggests that certain factors of control are common to both types of adjustment.

When exertion is severe, both the minute volume and the frequency of breathing may continue to increase throughout the period of work, although there may be a slight decrease in the tidal volume. It will be recalled that the adjustment of heart function during severe exercise follows a similar pattern, that is, a continuing rise in heart rate associated with a slight decrease in the stroke volume.

Aftereffects of exercise on breathing. The time required for breathing to return to the preexercise level is determined by the severity and duration of the exertion and by the physical condition of the subject. After work of moderate intensity the minute volume of breathing falls off rapidly, more or less duplicating in reverse the time required for the attainment of maximal ventilation at the beginning of exercise. Following very severe exertion the return of breathing to the preexercise level may be greatly delayed. The respiratory rate usually returns to normal more slowly than does the depth of breathing.

REGULATION OF BREATHING

Regulation of breathing at rest. An important factor in the control of breathing is the chemical composition of the arterial blood. Breathing is increased by a rise in the carbon dioxide tension or the acidity of the arterial blood and is decreased by a fall in arterial carbon dioxide or acidity. The neurons of the respiratory center are not stimulated directly by these changes in the blood; instead the blood changes act on chemoreceptors located in the lateral walls of the medulla. These receptors can also be stimulated by changes in the acidity of the cerebrospinal fluid. When these chemoreceptors are stimulated, they send increased numbers of nerve impulses to the respiratory center and breathing increases. If the acidity of the blood or cerebrospinal fluid is decreased, fewer impulses are transmitted to the respiratory center, and breathing decreases. Under normal conditions the carbon dioxide tension in the arterial blood is nicely adjusted to give exactly the right amount of stimulation to the respiratory center; any change in the arterial carbon dioxide tension results in appropriate changes in breathing, which restore the blood carbon dioxide tension to normal. The chemoreceptors in the carotid and aortic bodies are also stimulated by increased arterial carbon dioxide tension or acidity; however, their most important function is to stimulate breathing in response to a fall in the arterial oxygen tension, something of which the central (medullary) chemoreceptors are incapable.

The rhythmic alternation of inspiration and expiration probably results from an inherent rhythmicity of discharge of the neurons of the respiratory center. This rhythm is adjusted to give the appropriate rate and depth of breathing by the chemical factors already mentioned and by nerve impulses from many parts of the body. Among the important sources of the nerve impulses which act on the respiratory center are other portions of the brain, including the cerebral cortex and the chemoreceptors in the carotid and aortic bodies and medulla.

Increased breathing during exercise. Exercise increases the metabolism of the body and the requirement for oxygen. In response to this demand for more oxygen, the rate and depth of breathing are promptly increased. The nature of the stimulus that causes increased breathing during exercise has been the subject of much speculation. The answer might seem obvious—the increased carbon dioxide produced by the working muscles stimulates the respiratory center. That this is not so is indicated by two lines of evidence:

1. Strenuous exercise produces a greater increase in respiration than can be induced by breathing the highest concentration of carbon dioxide that can be tolerated.
2. Although the arterial blood carbon dioxide tension often rises slightly during mild exercise, it actually falls below normal during more strenuous exercise because it is eliminated in the lungs at a faster rate than it is produced in the muscles.

There seems to be little doubt that stimuli arising in the joints involved in exercise constitute an important source of impulses which excite the respiratory center. The exact location of the receptors and the nature of the agents that stimulate these receptors are uncertain. There is experimental evidence that proprioceptors (receptors sensitive to tension or stretching) in the moving joints contribute to the increased stimulation of the respiratory center during exercise. In addition, chemical agents liberated by the muscles as a result of their increased metabolism may stimulate local chemoreceptors, which in turn send impulses to the respiratory center.[1-3,7] The nature of these chemical stimuli is in doubt, but one that is currently receiving much attention is potassium. There have been many suggestions of chemoreceptors in the venous side of the circulation that are supposed to be stimulated by the increase in carbon dioxide tension and acidity, and perhaps other changes in the venous blood leaving working muscles; however, such receptors have never been demonstrated. The existence of reflex stimulation of breathing in exercise resulting from chemical changes in the contracting muscles remains highly controversial. It has also been claimed that the sensitivity of the peripheral (carotid) chemoreceptors to changes in arterial carbon dioxide and oxygen tensions is increased in exercise, so that at normal blood gas tensions there is greater stimulation of the respiratory center.[6]

A rise in body temperature from any cause (fever, hot baths, exercise) results in increased breathing, probably because impulses are sent to the respiratory center from the temperature regulating center in the hypothalamus. Impulses from temperature receptors in the skin may also affect the respiratory center as they pass through the medulla on their way to higher brain centers. It is difficult to say how important is the rise in body temperature during exercise in the increase in breathing; it may be especially important during exercise in the heat.[5]

Impulses from the cerebral cortex are thought to be responsible for the anticipatory increase in breathing, which is sometimes seen just prior to the onset of exercise having a high emotional content (for example, track events). This influence is probably not important in sustaining the increased breathing during the exercise.

Let us now attempt to integrate the various factors which may contribute to the increased breathing of exercise. Before the exercise begins there may be an anticipatory increase in breathing due to impulses from the cerebral cortex. Stimulation from this source probably ceases shortly after the exercise begins, but breathing continues to increase. This early phase of the respiratory response to exercise occurs before sufficient time has elapsed to permit chemical substances formed or liberated in the working muscles to be carried in the blood to the respiratory center, so that the stimulus must be neurogenic, possibly involving proprioceptors or chemoreceptors in the joints and muscles. Since the arterial oxygen tension is usually well maintained during exercise, and since the arterial carbon dioxide tension is normal or, more often, a little below normal in exercise, we can probably dismiss the carotid and aortic chemoreceptors and the central chemoreceptors as important sources of increased excitation of the respiratory center, at least until the blood lactic acid concentration begins to rise. As exercise continues, the body temperature begins to rise, and this contributes to the stimulation of breathing.

While, as we have seen, a rise in arterial carbon dioxide tension cannot be involved as a direct factor in the increased breathing rate during exercise (since such a rise does not ordinarily occur); nevertheless, the arterial carbon dioxide tension serves in a regulatory capacity through a negative feedback mechanism. If the increase in breathing due to other factors becomes excessive during exercise, the lowering of the arterial carbon dioxide tension which results has a damping effect on the increase in breathing, permitting enough retention of carbon dioxide to restore the arterial level to normal. Similarly, if the increase in breathing is not adequate to eliminate the excess carbon dioxide formed in exercise, the rise in arterial carbon dioxide tension causes a further stimulation of breathing, which lowers the arterial level to normal. Thus the breathing during exercise is accurately adjusted to maintain a near normal arterial carbon dioxide tension, even though it is not directly controlled by the blood carbon dioxide level. It may be suggested that the coarse adjustment of the breathing during exercise is due to neurogenic factors, including proprioceptor and chemoreceptor reflexes from the working muscles and moving joints, and that these adjust the breathing to the intensity of the muscular contractions. The fine adjustment, on the other hand, is due to chemical changes in the blood, which adjust the breathing to the metabolic needs of the body. The exact role of the rise of body temperature in exercise on the regulation of breathing is unclear.

There is a natural tendency while straining against a heavy load to close the glottis and hold the breath at end-inspiration. Although this act tends to stabilize the thorax and abdomen, it is potentially harmful. When executed forcefully, this act, called the "Valsalva maneuver," changes intrathoracic pressure from the normal subatmospheric level to a high positive one and interferes with venous return. If held long enough, fainting may occur.

While moving heavy loads the functions of circulorespiratory systems are enhanced if the rhythm of breathing is coordinated with the rhythm of movement. Using the normal movements of the thorax as a cue, inhalation is performed while the weight is being lifted, exhalation while it is being lowered.

During continuous high workloads, adjustment of breathing to the demands of exercise is most efficient if it is involuntary. Hyperventilation (overbreathing) can cause giddiness, sensations of numbness, tingling, weakness, and pain in the arms and chest. This is due to excessive "blowing off" of carbon dioxide, resulting in a fall in hydrogen ion concentration, which in turn affects brain function by reducing the cerebral blood flow.

Hyperventilation is followed by a period of reduced breathing. It is possible to hold the breath longer after a few rapid deep breaths. This practice can be dangerous in underwater swimmers because the respiratory receptors are not highly sensitive to oxygen deficit. A rapidly decreasing oxygen tension during underwater swimming may cause fainting and drowning before ventilation is stimulated.

EFFECT OF ATMOSPHERIC POLLUTION

Irritation of mucous membranes by airborne pollutants such as hydrocarbons and sulphur oxides causes increased secretion. These mucous secretions narrow the air passages in the respiratory tract and increase airway resistance. The effects are a reduction in respiratory function, an increase in the energy cost of breathing, a reduction in oxygen uptake, and chest pain. There seems to be no acclimatization to these pollutants.

During times of high pollution heavy aerobic exercise accompanied by high ventilation rates could cause damage to the respiratory tract. Therefore, aerobic training should occur in clear air if possible.

NATURE OF "SECOND WIND"

During the first few minutes of violent exercise, such as rowing or running, there is often a feeling of distress, characterized by breathlessness, a throbbing of the head, and an impression that the work is very difficult. The distress eventually subsides and the individual is said to have his "second wind." Neither the factors responsible for the initial distress nor those that bring the relief are known for certain. No significant physiological differences have been found in individuals before and during second wind, or between individuals who claim to experience it and those who do not. There is no evidence that performance is improved or that fatigue is lessened by an episode of second wind. It is generally believed, however, that the early distress is a reflection of an intense stimulus to breathing due to an accumulation of metabolites in the working muscles (including the respiratory muscles) and the blood, because of inadequate transport of oxygen to the muscles. The relief of the distress may then be attributed to improved oxygen transport as the breathing and cardiac output increase and the blood vessels in the working muscles dilate.

References

1. Coote, J. H., Hilton, S. M., and Perez-Gonzalez, J. F.: The reflex nature of the pressor response to muscular exercise, J. Physiol. **215**:789, 1971.
2. Dejours, P., Mithoefer, J. C., and Raynaud, J.: Evidence against the existence of specific chemoreceptors in the legs, J. Appl. Physiol. **10**:367, 1957.
3. Dejours, P., Mithoefer, J. C., and Labrousse, Y.: Influence of local chemical change on ventilatory stimulus from the legs during exercise, J. Appl. Physiol. **10**:372, 1957.
4. Evdokimova, M. M.: Painful liver syndrome in athletes. Quoted by Karpovich, P. V., and Sinning, W. E.: Physiology of muscular activity, ed. 7, Philadelphia, 1971, W. B. Saunders Co., p. 152.
5. Peterson, E. S., and Vejby-Christensen, H.: Effect of body temperature on steady state ventilation and metabolism in exercise, Acta Physiol. Scand. **89**:342, 1973.
6. Weil, J. V., and others: Augmentation of chemosensitivity during mild exercise in man, J. Appl. Physiol. **33**:813, 1972.
7. Wildenthal, K., and others: Potassium-induced cardiovascular and ventilatory reflexes from the dog hindlimb, Am. J. Physiol. **215**:542, 1968.

Suggested readings

Dejours, P.: Control of respiration in muscular exercise. In Field, J., editor: Handbook of physiology, Vol. 1, Washington, D. C., 1964, American Physiological Society.

Grimby, G.: Respiration in exercise, Med. Sci. Sports 1:9, 1969.

9 GAS EXCHANGE AND TRANSPORT

A gas is a state of matter in which the kinetic energy of the molecules is greater than their intermolecular forces of attraction; the result is that gas molecules tend to spread apart and fill the space available to them. They exert a force against the walls of their container, and the force per unit area is the *pressure* of the gas; it is proportional to the concentration of gas molecules and to their energy (which in turn is proportional to the temperature of the gas). The concept of gas pressures dominates respiratory physiology, since the exchange of oxygen and carbon dioxide in the lungs and tissue capillaries results from pressure differences.

It will be recalled from other science courses that each gas (including water vapor) in a mixture of gases exerts a pressure proportional to its concentration in the mixture (Dalton's law of partial pressures), and that the solution of gases in liquids depends on the pressure of the gas, its solubility in the particular liquid, and the temperature. These relations are important in understanding the transport of respiratory gases in the blood. The following example illustrates these principles, as applied to alveolar air:

$$
\begin{aligned}
\text{Assume} \quad \text{barometric pressure} &= 760 \text{ mm. Hg} \\
\text{water vapor pressure} &= 47 \text{ mm. Hg} \\
\text{pressure of } O_2 + CO_2 + N_2 &= 713 \text{ mm. Hg} \\
\% \, O_2 = 15 = 0.15 \times 713 &= 107 \text{ mm. Hg} \\
\% \, CO_2 = 5 = 0.05 \times 713 &= 37 \text{ mm. Hg}
\end{aligned}
$$

Note that the analysis of a gas mixture always refers to *dry* gas, and that water vapor, when present, simply dilutes the other gases.

108

GAS EXCHANGE IN THE LUNGS

At rest, the mixed venous blood that the right ventricle pumps to the lungs has an oxygen tension of about 40 mm. Hg and a carbon dioxide tension of about 45 mm. Hg. Assuming for convenience that the composition of the air in all the alveoli is the same (this is not strictly true), we may say that alveolar oxygen pressure is about 100 mm. Hg and alveolar carbon dioxide pressure is about 40 mm. Hg. Therefore, the oxygen pressure difference between alveolar air and the mixed venous blood as it enters the lung capillaries is 100 − 40 = 60 mm. Hg, and oxygen immediately diffuses from alveolar air to capillary blood. This diffusion continues as the blood flows through the length of the capillaries (about 1 mm.), and the blood leaving the capillaries has nearly the same oxygen tension as that of the alveolar air. The diffusion of carbon dioxide from blood to alveolar air results from the higher tension of this gas in the blood entering the lungs than in the alveolar air, and the blood leaving the lungs has a carbon dioxide tension of about 40 mm. Hg, the same as that of the alveolar air.

GAS EXCHANGE IN THE TISSUES

The arterial blood, with an oxygen tension of about 100 mm. Hg and a carbon dioxide tension of about 40 mm. Hg, is pumped by the left ventricle into the systemic arteries. In the tissue capillaries oxygen diffuses from blood to tissues, and carbon dioxide diffuses from tissues to blood under the driving force of the respective pressure differences, just as in the lungs.

A quantitative analysis of gas exchange in the tissues is difficult because of the influence of local factors. If an organ becomes active, for example, its oxygen consumption increases and the average tissue oxygen tension is diminished. This increases the oxygen pressure differences between blood and tissues and hastens the diffusion of oxygen. The increased production of carbon dioxide associated with activity likewise accelerates the passage of this gas into the blood. The tissue pressure differences are also influenced by the volume flow of blood and the number of open capillaries. Under resting conditions many capillaries in skeletal muscles are closed. This means that each muscle fiber receives blood from a small number of capillaries. If additional capillaries open during exercise, each muscle fiber receives oxygen from a greater number of capillaries. This partially offsets the fall in the oxygen tension of tissue that results from the greater rate of oxygen consumption in the active tissues.

The oxygen tension in the tissue cells is influenced by the rate at which the cells are using oxygen, by their location relative to the

109

arterial or the venous end of their nearest capillary, and by the number of open capillaries. Assume for the sake of simplicity that a particular cell is supplied by one capillary only, that the length of the capillary is great in comparison to the diameter of the cell, and that the blood oxygen tension falls linearly as the blood flows through the capillary. It is clear that the most favorable conditions are enjoyed by cells near the capillary and near the arterial rather than the venous end of the capillary, while cells far from the capillary and nearer the venous than the arterial end of the capillary are in the least favorable situation. The term "lethal corner" has been applied to the cells in the latter category; in many cases these cells obtain barely sufficient oxygen under normal conditions, and they are the first to suffer when oxygen becomes less available to the organ.

It should be clear from this discussion that the concept of a "tissue oxygen tension" is a meaningless abstraction. Oxygen tension in a tissue varies from cell to cell and in the same cell from time to time.

The diffusion of carbon dioxide from the tissues into the blood is subject to the same influences. Because of the high diffusion rate of carbon dioxide, it is probable that its tension in the tissues never exceeds that in the venous blood more than 5 to 10 mm. Hg.

TRANSPORT OF OXYGEN BY THE BLOOD

Reaction between oxygen and hemoglobin. Each 100 ml. of arterial blood contains on the average about 20 ml. of oxygen. At the oxygen tension of arterial blood and at body temperature, only about 0.2 ml. of oxygen can dissolve in this volume of blood, so that 99% of the oxygen must exist in some form other than physical solution. This nondissolved oxygen exists in loose chemical combination with the pigment hemoglobin. Dissolved oxygen reacts reversibly with hemoglobin according to the equation $Hb + O_2 \rightleftharpoons HbO_2$, in which Hb is the symbol for a molecule of reduced hemoglobin. The reaction is of the mass action type; that is, its velocity is proportional to the product of the active masses of the reacting constituents. Since the amount of hemoglobin remains fairly constant, the direction of the reaction is actually determined by the concentration (the tension) of oxygen. If the concentration of dissolved oxygen decreases (as in the tissue capillaries because of diffusion of oxygen from the blood into the tissues), the oxygen tension falls, and the reaction $Hb + O_2 \rightleftharpoons HbO_2$ proceeds to the left, so that more oxygen goes into solution and is available for diffusion out into the tissues. In the lung capillaries the diffusion of oxygen from the alveolar air raises the oxygen tension in the blood, and the reaction proceeds to the right, with the result that almost all Hb is converted to HbO_2.

Oxygen dissociation curve. The proportion of the hemoglobin in the form of HbO_2 is expressed as percent saturation. This is a more convenient characterization of the degree of oxygenation than is the oxygen *content* of the blood, since the content varies not only with the oxygen tension but also with the hemoglobin concentration. The oxygen saturation of different samples of blood having widely different hemoglobin concentrations is the same if all samples have the same oxygen tension.

Although the oxygen saturation of blood is determined primarily by the oxygen tension, it is influenced by two other factors—temperature and acidity. An increase in temperature or acidity favors the reaction $HbO_2 \rightarrow Hb + O_2$, so that the oxygen saturation at a given oxygen tension is decreased. A fall in temperature or acidity has the opposite effect.

The effect of acidity (and carbon dioxide tension) on the affinity of hemoglobin for oxygen is known as the Bohr effect. A third factor that affects the affinity of hemoglobin for oxygen is the concentration in the erythrocytes of the organic phosphorus compound 2, 3 DPG (2, 3-diphosphoglycerate), which is a byproduct of glycolysis in the erythrocyte. This compound has the same effect as increased temperature and acidity on the affinity of hemoglobin for oxygen. It is uncertain whether the result is a direct one on the hemoglobin molecule, or an indirect effect through the increase in intra-erythrocyte acidity due to a Donnan effect on the distribution of H^+ ions.[1,2] The evidence that erythrocyte 2, 3 DPG concentration has a significant effect on the delivery of oxygen to the muscles in exercise is scanty and conflicting.

If temperature and acidity are held constant, the relation between oxygen tension and oxygen saturation may be determined. Samples of blood having the same hemoglobin content are exposed to gas mixtures having different pressures of oxygen. When equilibrium has been reached, the oxygen content of each sample is determined. The oxygen content of a sample of blood completely saturated with oxygen is used as a reference; the saturation of this sample is 100%. A sample having one half the oxygen content of the reference sample is 50% saturated, and so on. If the percent saturation is plotted against the oxygen tension, a curve called the *oxygen dissociation curve* is obtained (Fig. 21). The use of this curve makes possible a quantitative analysis of the gas exchange in the lungs and in the capillaries of tissues during both rest and exercise.

Reference to the dissociation curve indicates that blood returning to the lungs with an average oxygen tension of 40 mm. Hg is approximately 75% saturated. As oxygen diffuses from the alveoli into the blood, the oxygen tension rises steadily, with the result that more and more of the reduced hemoglobin combines with oxygen to form oxyhemo-

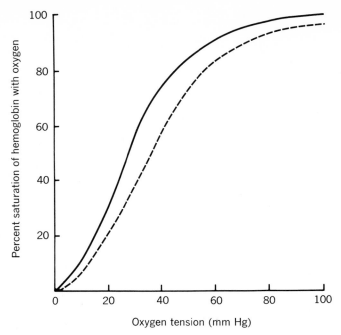

Fig. 21. The oxygen dissociation curve of hemoglobin. Solid line, "normal" curve (37° C.; pH, 7.4; Pco₂, 40 mm. Hg). Dotted line, shaft of the curve to the right as occurs with increase in temperature or acidity of the blood.

globin. The blood leaves the lungs with an oxygen tension of about 100 mm. Hg and an oxygen saturation of about 98%. No oxygen is lost from the blood until it reaches the capillaries (or perhaps the small arteries, according to evidence reported by Duling and Berne[3]). There it comes in contact with extravascular fluid having a lower oxygen tension, and dissolved oxygen in the blood immediately begins to diffuse across the vessel membrane. Since the amount of dissolved oxygen in the blood is very small (about 1% of the total), the oxygen tension drops as oxygen diffuses into the tissues. The fall in blood oxygen tension initiates the reaction $HbO_2 \rightarrow Hb + O_2$, and the oxygen thus liberated goes into solution, raising the oxygen tension and increasing the rate of diffusion. This process of diffusion of the oxygen made available by the breakdown of oxyhemoglobin continues as the blood flows along the capillary, and the blood finally leaves the capillary with an oxygen tension of about 40 mm. Hg and an oxygen saturation of about 75%. It is apparent that, in passing through the capillary, the blood has lost 98% − 75% = 23% of its total oxygen; this fraction of the total oxygen that is delivered to the tissues is known as the *coefficient of oxygen utilization*. An increase in this coefficient would increase the volume of oxygen delivered to the tissues in unit time, and this occurs during exercise. Under conditions of strenuous exertion, more than 90% of the oxygen may be removed from blood flowing through the contracting muscles. The large amount of oxygen remaining in the venous blood under resting conditions thus constitutes a factor of safety that can be called on in times of increased need.

The carbon dioxide tension influences the position of the dissociation curve. An increase in the carbon dioxide tension shifts the curve to the right, so that the oxygen saturation at any given oxygen tension is diminished—in other words, carbon dioxide "drives" oxygen out of the blood. The same is also true for any acid. In the tissue capillaries carbon dioxide enters the blood from the tissues and increases the breakdown of oxyhemoglobin. During exercise this effect is increased because of the larger amounts of acid metabolites formed in the active muscles. The quantitative importance of this factor (the Bohr effect) in increasing the delivery of oxygen to muscles in exercise has been questioned by recent investigators. It seems likely that the fall in muscle oxygen tension and the opening of previously closed capillaries may be of considerably greater importance. In the lungs the diffusion of carbon dioxide into the alveoli lowers the acidity of the blood, which hastens the combination of oxygen with hemoglobin.

Oxygen exchange during exercise. Most of the physiological adjustments during exercise are directed toward the delivery of a greater volume of oxygen to the working muscles. The increase in blood flow through the muscles has been discussed in previous chapters. For this adjustment to be fully effective, there must be provision for maintaining a normal saturation of the blood with oxygen in spite of the greater blood flow through the lungs. Ideally this would mean that blood would leave the lungs about 98% saturated with oxygen, as under resting conditions.

The blood flowing through the lungs must remain in the pulmonary capillaries long enough to permit the diffusion of an amount of oxygen sufficient to saturate the hemoglobin. Analyses of arterial blood samples taken during exercise usually indicate that the hemoglobin saturation is normal, despite the greater flow of blood through the lungs, so effective compensations must occur. The most important of these compensations are (1) a dilatation of the blood vessels in the lungs, which prevents the flow from becoming too rapid, and (2) a better ventilation of the alveoli due to the deeper breathing.

In the capillaries of the working muscles local metabolic conditions greatly facilitate the delivery of large amounts of oxygen. In the first place, the lowered oxygen tension of tissues, which results from their increased rate of oxygen consumption, increases the oxygen pressure difference between blood and tissues. At the same time the large quantities of carbon dioxide and lactic acid produced in the

113

contracting muscles diffuse into the capillaries where they facilitate the breakdown of oxyhemoglobin with the liberation of freely diffusible oxygen. The local rise in temperature resulting from the increased production of heat by active muscles has the same effect on the breakdown of oxyhemoglobin as does the increased acidity. The net result of these local factors is to increase the coefficient of oxygen utilization from the resting value of about 0.3 up to 0.7 to 0.9.

The interplay of the various factors that influence the delivery of oxygen to the muscles during exercise may be illustrated by the following quantitative example: (1) The cardiac output may be increased 4 times. (2) Dilatation of muscle vessels with compensatory vasoconstriction elsewhere may increase the relative blood flow through the muscle as much as fivefold. Factors 1 and 2 together may increase the total blood flow through the active muscles to 20 times the resting value. (3) The coefficient of oxygen utilization may be increased to 3 times the resting value (which is usually low in skeletal muscles). Thus the combination of all three factors permits an oxygen delivery to the muscles that may be $4 \times 5 \times 3 = 60$ times as great as during rest. These are conservative figures. There is good evidence that the consumption of oxygen during maximal activity of muscles may be as much as 75 to 100 times that of the resting muscles.

FACTORS LIMITING THE SUPPLY OF OXYGEN TO EXERCISING MUSCLES

Theoretically, the limiting factor in the delivery of oxygen might be the capacity for ventilating the lungs or for pumping blood.

Pulmonary ventilation is still capable of further increase when the maximal cardiac output has been reached, so that the supply of oxygen to exercising muscles is not ordinarily limited by the breathing capacity. In extreme cases, as pointed out in Chapter 12, the energy cost of breathing might limit exercise to some extent. The importance of this factor has not been determined precisely. By implication, circulation rather than respiration is the limiting factor, but this does not necessarily mean that the cardiac activity is inadequate. The ability of the heart to increase its output may be greater than the capacity of the muscles for receiving the blood, at least in exercise that involves only a portion of the musculature, as in rowing. What is important, of course, is not the absolute amount of oxygen delivered to the working muscles, but the relation of oxygen supply to oxygen requirement. When exercise does not involve large muscle groups, the oxygen supply to the active muscles may be inadequate to meet their requirement simply because there are not enough capillaries in the muscles[4]; in this connection it is of interest that one of the results of training is an increase in the number of capillaries in the muscles involved in the training. When, however, a large proportion of the total musculature is involved in exercise, the oxygen supply to the working muscles may be limited by both the cardiac output and the capacity of the circulation in the muscles.

If exercise involving large muscle masses (as in treadmill running) is progressively increased in intensity, the oxygen uptake also increases up to a certain point; beyond this point, further increase in exercise intensity is not accompanied by an increase in oxygen uptake, and this rate of oxygen uptake is referred to as the "maximal oxygen uptake," for which the symbol $\dot{V}O_2$ max is often used. The $\dot{V}O_2$ max is widely regarded as the best indication of the cardiovascular fitness of an individual for exercise lasting more than 1 to 2 minutes (in brief exercise much of the energy may be obtained from non–oxygen-requiring metabolism). The measurement of $\dot{V}O_2$ max by the procedure described above is not a very convenient one in practice. It has been established, however, that increase in the heart rate parallels the increase in oxygen uptake in exercise of increasing intensity, and furthermore that the maximal oxygen uptake can be predicted fairly accurately from the heart rate measured during submaximal exercise. One of the beneficial effects of training is an increase in $\dot{V}O_2$ max.[5]

ADMINISTRATION OF OXYGEN BEFORE, DURING, AND AFTER EXERCISE

Athletic coaches and trainers frequently administer oxygen to athletes during time-out periods, with the objectives of increasing the rate of recovery from previous exercise and improving the subsequent performance. The rationale of this procedure is based more on testimonials than on experimental evidence.

In laboratory tests nearly all workers agree that the administration of oxygen following exercise has little influence on the rate of recovery. This would be expected since the decrease in cardiac output after the cessation of exercise makes it possible for the blood to remain in the pulmonary capillaries long enough to achieve equilibrium with the alveolar air. There is less agreement concerning the beneficial effects of breathing oxygen just before exercise. It is difficult to explain the occasional report claiming such benefit in view of the fact that the arterial blood is virtually saturated with oxygen when room air is breathed during rest.

By contrast, it is fairly generally agreed that the administration of oxygen *during* exercise is beneficial, although there is disagreement concerning the degree of benefit. Since the administration of oxygen during exercise is not feasible in most types of athletic events, the question is of academic rather than practical importance. The psychological aspects of reported benefits from oxygen inhalation during sporting events should not be underestimated.

TRANSPORT OF CARBON DIOXIDE IN THE BLOOD

We have seen that nearly all the oxygen present in blood is in a bound form, and the same is true of carbon dioxide. Most of the carbon dioxide in blood is in the form of bicarbonate. Of the remainder, a portion exists in direct combination with hemoglobin, and another portion is in solution. The mechanisms involved in the transport of carbon dioxide are best visualized by a description of the events occurring with the uptake of carbon dioxide in the tissue capillaries and its elimination in the lung capillaries.

Blood enters the tissue capillaries with a carbon dioxide tension of about 40 mm. Hg. Under resting conditions the average tissue carbon dioxide tension may be assumed to be perhaps 45 to 50 mm. Hg, and accordingly carbon dioxide diffuses from the tissues into the blood. This increases the carbon dioxide tension in the blood plasma, and some of it therefore diffuses from the plasma into the erythrocytes, where about 20% of the carbon dioxide combines directly with hemoglobin. Another 10% remains in solution, and about 70% combines with water to form carbonic acid. This reaction occurs to only a slight extent in the plasma because it is a very slow reaction unless catalyzed by an enzyme. This enzyme, known as carbonic anhydrase, is present in the erythrocytes (and in certain other cells such as the kidney tubule cells and the gastric gland cells that secrete hydrochloric acid); none is present in the plasma. The carbonic acid formed under the influence of carbonic anhydrase must be neutralized in order to prevent a dangerous rise in acidity. Some of the neutralization is effected by the buffer action of hemoglobin in the following manner. Hemoglobin is a weak acid, and it exists partly in the form of free acid and partly as the potassium salt of the acid. Since a weak acid and its salt constitute a buffer system, hemoglobin can act in the same manner as any other buffer system. Since hemoglobin is a weaker acid than carbonic acid, the following buffer reaction will take place: $KHb + H_2CO_3 \rightleftharpoons HHb + KHCO_3$. This reaction proceeds from left to right in the tissue capillaries because of the increasing concentration of H_2CO_3. The result is the substitution of a weaker acid (HHb) for a stronger acid (H_2CO_3) that is the essence of any buffer reaction.

Hemoglobin contributes in a second way to the uptake of carbon dioxide, by what is known as the isohydric reaction. Oxyhemoglobin is a stronger acid than is reduced hemoglobin. Thus, when oxyhemoglobin gives up some of its oxygen in the tissue capillaries, its capacity to bind

116

hydrogen ions is increased, and a large proportion of the hydrogen ions from the newly formed carbonic acid is bound by the hemoglobin, according to the following reaction: $K_2HbO_2 + H_2CO_3 \rightleftharpoons KHHb + KHCO_3 + O_2$. In this reaction, 1 molecule of carbon dioxide (as carbonic acid) can be neutralized for each molecule of oxygen liberated from hemoglobin.

The end result of the reactions within the erythrocytes is the direct combination of about 20% of the extra carbon dioxide with hemoglobin and the conversion of about 70% to bicarbonate. Many of the newly formed bicarbonate ions diffuse out of the erythrocytes into the plasma (in exchange for an equal number of plasma anions—mostly chloride), so that although most of the bicarbonate is formed in the erythrocytes, much of it is transported in the plasma. A small amount of carbonic acid is formed from carbon dioxide in the plasma and is buffered there, mostly by the plasma proteins, to form a little additional bicarbonate. All the reactions just discussed are, of course, exactly reversed in the lung capillaries.

It is apparent that hemoglobin accounts in one way or another for the binding or neutralization of about 90% of the extra carbon dioxide that is taken up by the blood flowing through the tissue capillaries. It is thus almost as important in the transport of carbon dioxide as it is in the transport of oxygen.

A final statement should be made about the blood buffer systems because of a common misunderstanding. The most important blood buffer for carbon dioxide (as carbonic acid) is hemoglobin. The most important blood buffer for all other acids is the bicarbonate system (carbonic acid and its salt, sodium or potassium bicarbonate in the plasma and erythrocytes, respectively).

The transport of larger amounts of carbon dioxide from the muscles in exercise presents no particular problem since all of the reactions discussed previously can be increased within rather wide limits. The extra lactic acid formed when the oxygen supply is not entirely adequate is buffered by all the blood buffers but chiefly by the bicarbonate system since it is present in the largest amount. This reaction is as follows:

$$HL \text{ (lactic acid)} + NaHCO_3 \rightleftharpoons NaL + H_2CO_3$$
$$H_2CO_3 \rightleftharpoons H_2O + CO_2$$

Since the CO_2 formed in the second reaction is "blown off" in the lungs, this is an extremely efficient buffer reaction. Nevertheless, the blood does become more acidic during strenuous exercise, since the rise in blood lactic acid concentration gradually depletes the bicarbonate buffer level in the blood.

117

References

1. Brewer, G. J., and Eaton, J. W.: Erythrocyte metabolism: interaction with oxygen transport, Science **171**: 1205, 1971.
2. Duhm, J.: Effects of 2, 3-diphospho-glycerate and other organic phosphate compounds on oxygen affinity and intracellular pH of human erythrocytes, Pflügers Arch. **326**:341, 1971.
3. Duling, B. R., and Berne, R. M.: Longitudinal gradients in periartereolar oxygen tension. A possible mechanism for the participation of oxygen in local regulation of blood flow, Circulat. Res. **27**:669, 1970.
4. Gleser, M. A.: Effects of hypoxia and physical training on hemodynamic adjustments to one-legged exercise, J. Appl. Physiol. **34**:655, 1973.
5. Morehouse, L. E.: Laboratory manual for physiology of exercise, St. Louis, 1972, The C. V. Mosby Co.

Suggested readings

Craig, F. N.: Oxygen uptake at the beginning of work, J. Appl. Physiol. **33**: 611, 1972.

Ekblom, B.: Effect of physical training on oxygen transport system in man, Acta Physiol. Scand. 1969, Suppl. 328.

Lawson, W. H., Jr.: Rebreathing measurements of pulmonary diffusing capacity for CO during exercise, J. Appl. Physiol. **29**:896, 1970.

Ouellet, Y., Poh, S. C., and Becklake, M. R.: Circulatory factors limiting maximal aerobic exercise capacity, J. Appl. Physiol. **27**:874, 1969.

PART FOUR

ENERGY METABOLISM

10 METABOLISM IN EXERCISE

During rest the energy requirement of the body is met by the breakdown of ATP, and the supply of ATP is continuously restored by energy derived from the oxidation of the foodstuffs (aerobic metabolism). During exercise the energy requirement may be increased many times, but it is still met by the breakdown of ATP just as it is during rest. If the exercise is not too severe, the restoration of ATP may continue to depend on energy derived from aerobic metabolism, as reflected in an increased rate of oxygen consumption, and the organism is said to be in a steady state. If the maximal rate of oxygen consumption does not provide sufficient energy to restore the ATP as rapidly as it is broken down, the balance of the energy needed is derived from anaerobic metabolism, in which the pyruvic acid formed in glycolysis is reduced to lactic acid instead of being oxidized to carbon dioxide and water. In exercise of this type, the rate of oxygen consumption remains elevated after the exercise is ended and returns gradually to normal during the recovery period. This chapter will be devoted to a discussion of the energy metabolism during exercise and recovery, with emphasis on the mechanisms and the limiting factors.

MEASUREMENT OF METABOLIC RATE

Aerobic metabolism is associated with the consumption of oxygen and the production of carbon dioxide and heat, and the rate of metabolism can be expressed in terms of any of these reactions. The measurement of heat production (direct calorimetry) was used almost exclusively in early studies on metabolism, and metabolic rate was accordingly expressed in terms of Calories per minute or hour. The measurement of heat production requires elaborate and expensive equipment and is seldom used today. Instead, oxygen consumption is measured (indirect calorimetry), and metabolic rate is expressed in terms of liters of oxygen per minute. Since the

121

consumption of 1 liter of oxygen is associated with the liberation of about 5 Calories of heat, the two units of metabolic rate are easily interconverted. Metabolism is seldom measured in terms of carbon dioxide production because this is influenced by numerous nonmetabolic factors.

Oxygen consumption can be measured by either closed or open circuit methods. In the closed circuit method the subject breathes in and out from a spirometer containing oxygen. The carbon dioxide in the expired air is absorbed by soda lime and the rate of oxygen consumption is calculated from the rate of fall of the spirometer bell as the oxygen in the bell is used up. In the open circuit technique the subject inhales air or oxygen and exhales into a collecting bag or spirometer. At the end of a suitable period of time the volume and oxygen concentration of the expired air are measured, and the oxygen consumption is calculated as total volume of oxygen inhaled (volume inspired $\times$ O_2 concentration of inspired gas) minus the total volume of oxygen exhaled (volume expired $\times$ O_2 concentration of expired gas). Further details concerning these methods are given in Chapter 12 in the *Laboratory Manual.*

ENERGY COST OF EXERCISE

The energy requirement of an activity may be expressed either as the rate of oxygen consumption during the activity or as a multiple of the resting rate of metabolism. The term MET (the rate of metabolism during rest) is the unit used for expressing metabolic rate in the latter method.

For exercise performed in a steady state, the energy requirement may be expressed as liters of oxygen used per minute (gross energy requirement) or as the increase over the resting level in the liters of oxygen used per minute (net energy requirement). When the exercise is too strenuous to be performed in a steady state, the oxygen consumption remains elevated during recovery, and the energy cost of the activity is the extra oxygen used during both exercise and recovery. An approximate classification of work intensity for a male college physical education student is given in Table 5. Values for older, unconditioned subjects would be lower.

FACTORS INFLUENCING THE ENERGY COST OF EXERCISE

The oxygen requirement of exercise is determined by a combination of factors, including the intensity, duration and speed of the work, the size of the muscle mass involved, the economy of muscular activity (a reflection of motor skill), fatigue, and environmental conditions.

Intensity of work. It was pointed out in Chapter 3 that the tension

Table 5. Metabolic classification of effort

Classification	MET	$\dot{V}O_2$ (liter/min.)	Kcal./min.
Very light	Under 2.5	Under 0.5	Under 3.5
Light	2.5-5.0	0.5-1.0	3.5-5.5
Moderate	5.0-7.5	1.0-1.5	5.5-8.0
Heavy	7.5-10.0	1.5-2.0	8.0-10.5
Very heavy	Over 10.0	Over 2.0	Over 10.5

exerted by a contracting muscle is dependent on two factors—the number of fibers contracting and the frequency of their contraction. Muscle tone, which is based on the low-frequency activation of a small proportion of the total number of muscle fibers, requires a very small oxygen intake. The same is true of a weak voluntary contraction. If a stronger contraction is needed, additional muscle fibers must be brought into activity, and the frequency with which each fiber contracts must be increased; both of these adjustments increase the oxygen requirement of the muscle.

Duration of work. Within certain limits the oxygen requirement of work is directly proportional to its duration. If, however, the intensity is great enough or the duration long enough to induce a state of fatigue, the oxygen requirement per unit of time usually begins to increase rapidly. As a muscle begins to tire, the tension developed by each fiber is reduced, and hence more fibers must be brought into activity if the same level of work is to be maintained. The oxygen requirement is increased in proportion to the increased number of active muscle fibers.

Rate or speed of work. The relation between the oxygen requirement of work and the speed of performance is complex. For many types of work there is an optimal speed at which the oxygen requirement is minimal. If the work is performed at a slower or a faster rate, the mechanical efficiency is diminished and the oxygen requirement increased. Fig. 22 illustrates this relation for the act of climbing stairs in which the body weight is lifted at each step. The net result of two opposing factors determines the optimal speed of performance:

1. A rapidly contracting muscle has been shown to develop less tension than does a muscle contracting more slowly, because of the limited rate at which the chemical and mechanical changes underlying muscle contraction can occur.
2. A definite amount of energy is required to *maintain* tension in a muscle once it is developed, and the slower the contraction, the greater is the proportion of the total energy used for this purpose (that is, tension must be maintained over a longer pe-

123

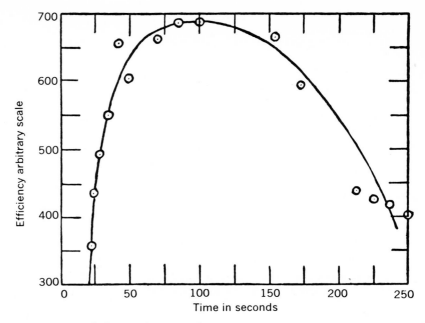

Fig. 22. Curve of the mechanical efficiency of the body during stair climbing at different speeds.

riod of time to accomplish a given amount of work at a slower rate of contraction).

The first factor tends to make work more economical (lower oxygen requirement) at low speeds, but the second factor results in a smaller oxygen requirement at high speeds.

In some types of work, the slowest speed is the most economical. An example (running 100 yards) is shown in Table 6. The reason is that even at the lowest speed listed, the subject is already exceeding the optimal speed for horizontal locomotion. In walking, on the other hand, there is a definite optimal speed of about 100 yards (120 steps) per minute for a person of average size.

Economy of muscular activity. In activities involving an element of motor skill, the same amount of work is usually performed with a smaller oxygen requirement by the trained athlete. This is due primarily to the fact that the acquisition of motor skill results in the suppression or elimination of extraneous muscular movements which, while contributing nothing to the performance of the task, require oxygen.

Environmental factors. The mechanical efficiency of the body is apparently little altered by rather wide changes in external temperature and humidity. For example, in one study there was found to be little

Table 6. Oxygen requirements for running 120 yards at different speeds

Speed (yards per second)	Oxygen requirement	
	Liters per 120 yards	Liters per minute
5.56	1.83	5.08
6.45	2.71	8.75
7.15	2.94	10.50
7.24	3.08	11.13
7.70	3.85	14.81
8.40	4.33	18.17
9.10	6.27	28.46
9.23	7.36	33.96

difference in the oxygen requirement of men working on a bicycle ergometer in a cold room (54° F.) and in a warm room (93° F.).[2] It is quite possible, however, that in activities requiring skill high temperatures might result in a lowered mechanical efficiency by diminishing the accuracy of neuromuscular coordination. There is no doubt that working capacity (output of work is a given time) is diminished by unfavorable environmental factors, especially by a combination of high temperature and high humidity.

AEROBIC AND ANAEROBIC METABOLISM

In order to understand the metabolic adjustments that occur during exercise we should briefly review the basic reactions from which cells derive their energy.

During rest and moderate exercise, all the energy required is provided by aerobic metabolism in which ATP is formed with great efficiency, and carbon dioxide and water are the metabolic end products. When the supply of oxygen is not adequate for producing all the ATP required, the deficit is made good by anaerobic metabolism, in which the efficiency of ATP production is low, and the metabolic end product, lactic acid, accumulates in the cells and blood.

A *steady state* is a condition in which the utilization of some constituent is balanced by a corresponding input of that constituent. With reference to metabolism, in a steady state the utilization of oxygen is balanced by a corresponding intake of oxygen. Under these conditions, exercise can continue until it is terminated by some other factor, such as exhaustion of the glycogen stores, muscle soreness, or blisters.

When a resting subject begins to exercise, a new steady state is not achieved immediately. The circulatory and respiratory adjustments that make possible a greater oxygen intake come into play gradually, and in heavy work several minutes may be required for the

125

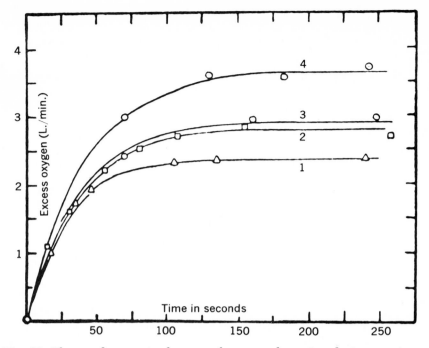

Fig. 23. The steady state in the rate of oxygen absorption during running at speeds of *1*, 193.5 yards per minute; *2* and *3*, 135 yards per minute; and *4*, 169 yards per minute. Note the lag of approximately 100 seconds in reaching the steady state; during this lag period an oxygen debt is being incurred.

oxygen intake to reach the level of the steady state. During this preliminary period a small oxygen deficit is incurred that is repaid during the recovery period that follows the exercise. Fig. 23 illustrates this lag in reaching the steady state, as well as the constant rate of oxygen consumption during the maintenance of the steady state.

The rate of oxygen intake may rise from 250 ml. per minute at rest, to a value of 2.5 to 4.5 liters per minute during a steady state of exercise, depending on the size, strength, and other characteristics of the subject. The American middle distance runner, Lash, was able to achieve an oxygen intake of 5.35 liters per minute during an exhausting run on a treadmill; this was 21.4 times his resting level. In 1955 the Swedish cross-country skier, Jernberg, reached an oxygen intake of 5.9 liters per minute. Since then the record has remained in Sweden. In 1967 Saltin and Åstrand reported an oxygen uptake value of 6.17 liters/min.[10] The next year a new record of 6.24 liters/min. was registered by Ekblom and Hermansen in a top athlete trained in orienteering.[3] When maximal oxygen uptake was calculated on the basis of body size, the values were 85.1 and 81.1 ml./kg./min.

There is evidence that in the steady state the upper limit for performing work under truly aerobic conditions corresponds to about 70% of the maximal oxygen consumption.[6] It should be pointed out in this connection that a constant level of oxygen intake during exercise is not sufficient evidence in itself to establish the existence of a steady state. The oxygen consumption may be constant simply because the subject has reached his maximal level of oxygen intake and lactic acid may be accumulating. This can be checked by successive determinations of the concentration of lactic acid in the blood or more simply by noting whether or not the oxygen intake increases further with a slight increase in the intensity of the work.

OXYGEN DEBT

The oxygen debt concept has long dominated considerations of metabolism in exercise. The term was coined many years ago by the English physiologist A. V. Hill as a convenient expression of the idea that the deficit in oxygen intake in strenuous activity represents a debt that is repaid during recovery. In the early days it was thought that the lactic acid that accumulates during exercise forces the consumption of extra oxygen during recovery, the extra oxygen being used for the oxidation of some of the lactic acid. The energy so produced was then believed to be used to convert the remainder of the lactic acid to glycogen. As the years passed, additional experimental evidence required successive modifications of this simple theory, and the present concept is quite different from Hill's original proposal. The reader is referred to the paper by Harris for an elegant description of these successive modifications.[5]

Let us begin by considering the experimental evidence without any preconceptions about its interpretation. If a person engages in mild exercise, there is no oxygen deficit during the exercise, that is, a steady state exists, and there is no excess oxygen consumption during recovery. If the exercise is somewhat more strenuous, the oxygen consumption during recovery is above the resting level, indicating an oxygen deficit during the exercise. The blood lactic acid concentration is not increased, however, indicating that no extra lactic acid was formed during the exercise. It is obvious, in this case, that lactic acid has nothing to do with the extra oxygen consumption during recovery. If the exercise is made even more strenuous, the excess oxygen consumption during recovery is greater and the blood lactic acid concentration is elevated. During the recovery period, the rate of oxygen consumption and the blood lactic acid concentration gradually return to normal. However, the rate at which the oxygen consumption decreases usually bears no relation to the rate of disappearance of lactic acid

127

from the blood. In exercise lasting only a few minutes, the blood lactic acid concentration remains elevated long after the oxygen consumption has returned to the resting state, while the reverse may be true during recovery from long-lasting exercise, in which the oxygen consumption may remain elevated for many hours. The conclusion to be drawn is that the magnitude of the excess oxygen consumption of recovery is in no way related to the lactic acid formed during exercise. What, then, is the cause of the extra consumption of oxygen during the recovery from exercise? In the discussion that follows it should be borne in mind that this extra oxygen consumption may amount to as much as 20 liters during a 60-minute recovery period.

1. The oxygen stores of the body may be partially depleted during exercise and they must be refilled during recovery. Since alveolar and arterial oxygen levels are not appreciably altered during exercise, these may be disregarded. In a man weighing 70 kg., there are about 600 ml. of oxygen in the venous blood, 50 ml. of oxygen dissolved in the tissues, and 300 ml. of oxygen combined with myoglobin. If these stores were entirely depleted during exercise, their refilling during recovery would account for only about 1 liter of the excess oxygen consumption.

2. ATP and creatine phosphate are broken down in muscle during exercise, and the products of ATP breakdown (ADP and P) are known to stimulate both glycolysis and oxidative metabolism, resulting in the restoration of ATP and creatine phosphate to their normal levels. If all the ATP and creatine phosphate in the entire skeletal muscle mass were broken down in exercise (experimental evidence indicates that this does not occur), their restoration, in a man weighing 70 kg., would require the consumption of about 2.5 liters of oxygen. Thus far, we have accounted at the most for only about 3.5 liters of excess oxygen consumption.

3. Exercise is associated with increased secretion of adrenaline and related compounds and with an elevation of body temperature. These changes persist for a time after the cessation of exercise, and both are known to stimulate oxidative metabolism. Their quantitative contribution to the excess oxygen consumption of recovery is difficult to estimate.

4. Does disposal of the lactic acid formed during exercise account for any of the excess oxygen consumption of recovery? The answer to this question is not clear. The portion of the lactic acid that is oxidized may simply take the place of some other fuel, and this would not increase the overall rate of oxygen consumption. The glycogen stores of the body may be considerably reduced during exercise, especially if it is of long duration, and the resynthesis of glycogen during recovery

requires oxygen. It has been observed, however, that lactic acid is a poor precursor for glycogen formation. When labeled lactate is infused into the bloodstream in laboratory animals, very little of it is incorporated in muscle glycogen, and after heavy exercise in man, restoration of muscle glycogen may require several days if the subject is kept on a carbohydrate-free diet.[7] It would be interesting to know what effect this delay in restoration of muscle glycogen would have on the excess oxygen consumption following exercise.

The general conclusion to be drawn from the experimental evidence is that the increased oxygen consumption during recovery from exercise reflects the replenishment of the stores of oxygen and high energy compounds (ATP and creatine phosphate) and the persisting stimulation of metabolism by the increased level of circulating adrenaline and related compounds, the elevated body temperature, and perhaps other factors as yet unidentified. It probably does not reflect the energy required to replenish muscle glycogen, since in the experiments of Hultman the muscle glycogen measured several hours after exercise was just about as low as it was immediately following the exercise. Finally, the excess oxygen consumption during recovery seems to be unrelated to the metabolic removal of the lactic acid formed during exercise.

POWER AND CAPACITY OF THE AEROBIC AND ANAEROBIC METABOLISM OF MUSCLE

Margaria has introduced a useful characterization of the energy metabolism of muscle in terms of its power and its capacity.[8] The *power* defines the rate of delivery of energy, while the *capacity* defines the total amount of energy that can be delivered. Aerobic and anaerobic metabolism differ in each of these two energy characteristics. *Aerobic metabolism* is characterized by a relatively low power (measured by the maximal oxygen uptake, about 5 to 6 liters [25 to 30 Cal.] per minute in highly trained athletes), but a high capacity (virtually unlimited since oxygen and food can be replenished continuously as they are used up). *Anaerobic metabolism,* on the other hand, has a high power (determined by the maximal rate of splitting of ATP) but a low capacity (about 0.2 Cal./kg.), presumably because of the limited tolerance of the muscles to the accumulation of lactic acid and the rapid exhaustion of glycogen stores.

These characteristics of muscle metabolism help to explain the sequence of metabolic changes during the shift from rest to exercise. The immediate increase in energy utilization requires a rapid delivery of energy, but the total amount of energy required is only that which is sufficient to cover the transition from the initial breakdown of ATP and creatine phosphate to the achievement of a steady state of oxygen uptake. These features (high power and low capacity) are precisely those of anaerobic metabolism. For long-lasting exercise, which must be performed in a steady state, the requirement is for high capacity but not necessarily high power, and these are the features of aerobic metabolism.

The reader is referred to the paper by Margaria for further details, including the practical applications of the concepts of energy power and capacity to athletics. Methods of measuring aerobic and anaerobic capacity are found in Chapters 17 and 18 in the *Laboratory Manual*.

FUEL OF MUSCULAR EXERCISE

The fuel of muscular exercise can be estimated in several ways, including (1) measurement of the respiratory quotient (R.Q.), (2) measurement of the difference in the concentration of a substrate in the blood entering and leaving a contracting muscle (A-V difference), and (3) analysis of biopsy samples of muscle before and after exercise. Each of these methods has yielded useful information. The R.Q. method, for example, has demonstrated that only about 2% of the energy requirement of activity is derived from protein; there is thus no scientific basis for the belief that heavy work, including athletics, requires an increased intake of protein. The nonprotein R.Q. of a resting subject on an average diet is about 0.8, indicating that about two-thirds of his energy requirement is derived from fat and about one-third from carbohydrate. In light to moderate exercise, the proportions of carbohydrate and fat utilized are about the same as during rest. In more strenuous exercise the R.Q. rises toward 1.0, indicating a greater use of carbohydrate, but as hard work is continued for hours, the R.Q. begins to fall and eventually approaches 0.7. This suggests that carbohydrate is used preferentially by working muscles as long as it is available, but that continued hard work may exhaust carbohydrate stores (principally liver and muscle glycogen) and force the muscles to derive their energy from fat. In extreme cases, as in marathon races, depletion of the carbohydrate reserve may result in a serious lowering of the blood sugar level, and exhaustion and collapse may follow because of impairment of the function of the central nervous system, which requires an adequate supply of glucose at all times. This prediction of the type of foodstuffs being utilized by the body, and more particularly by the contracting muscles during exercise, is open to criticism since it can be influenced by many other factors.

It is now generally agreed that fatty acids are important fuel for the aerobic metabolism of muscles. Skeletal muscles can oxidize fatty acids in vitro, and the rate of oxidization is increased if the muscle is

130

made to contract. It has been both claimed and denied that the lipid stores of the muscles themselves can be used during exercise.[12]

Perhaps the most striking demonstration of the utilization of carbohydrate by skeletal muscles during exercise is the virtual disappearance of glycogen in needle biopsy samples of human muscle following exhausting exercise.[9,11]

While there is some difference of opinion in the papers quoted in the preceding section, the general conclusion seems justified that both glycogen and fatty acids are utilized during heavy, prolonged work, that glycogen stores are probably depleted before lipid stores, and that after depletion of glycogen stores, prolonged work of reduced intensity can still be performed, provided the supply of fatty acids is adequate.

A field that currently is under active investigation is the histochemical study of the rate of depletion, during exercise, of glycogen and other compounds in different fiber types. Gollnick and associates studied the effect of exercise on the glycogen content of slow twitch and fast twitch fibers in human muscles after prolonged, severe exercise.[4] Total muscle glycogen was very low at the end of exercise, but depletion occurred earlier in slow twitch fibers. "These data may suggest a preferential utilization of slow twitch fibers during prolonged intense exercise, with a secondary recruitment of fast twitch as the slow twitch fibers become depleted of their glycogen stores."[4] This topic is further analyzed by Baldwin and co-workers, who also claim that liver glycogen is more important than muscle glycogen as a source of fuel for exercise.[1]

References

1. Baldwin, K. M., and others: Substrate depletion in different types of muscle and in liver during prolonged running, Am. J. Physiol. **275**:1045, 1973.
2. Dill, D. B., and others: Physical performance in relation to external temperature, Arbeitsphysiol. **4**:508, 1931.
3. Ekblom, B., and Hermansen, L.: Maximal oxygen uptake in athletics, J. Appl. Physiol. **25**:16, 1968.
4. Gollnick, P. D., and others: Glycogen depletion patterns in human skeletal muscle fibers during prolonged work, Pflügers Archiv. **344**:1, 1973.
5. Harris, P.: Lactic acid and the phlogiston debt, Cardiovasc. Res. **3**:381, 1969.
6. Hesser, C. M.: Energy cost of alternating positive and negative work, Acta Physiol. Scand. **63**:84, 1965.
7. Hultman, E.: Physiological role of muscle glycogen in man, with special reference to exercise, Circulat. Res. **20-21**:99, 1967.
8. Margaria, R.: Capacity and power of the energy processes in muscle activity: their practical relevance in athletics, Int. Z. angew. Physiol. **25**:352, 1968.
9. Pernow, B., and Saltin, B.: Availability of substrates and capacity for prolonged exercise in man, J. Appl. Physiol. **31**:416, 1971.
10. Saltin, B., and Åstrand, P. O.: Maximal oxygen utpake in athletics, J. Appl. Physiol. **23**:353, 1967.
11. Taylor, A. W., Lappage, R., and Rao, S.: Skeletal muscle glycogen stores after submaximal and maximal work, Med. Sci. Sports **3**:75, 1971.
12. Therriault, D. G., and others: Intramuscular energy sources in dogs during physical work, J. Lipid Res. **14**:54, 1973.

Suggested readings

Drummond, G. I.: Microenvironment and enzyme function: control of energy metabolism during muscle work, Am. Zoologist 11:83, 1971.

Hermansen, L.: Anaerobic energy release, Med. Sci. Sports 1:32, 1969.

Karlsson, J.: Lactate and phosphagen concentrations in working muscle of man, Acta Physiol. Scand. Suppl. 358, 1971.

Pernow, B., and Saltin, B., editors: Muscle metabolism during exercise, New York, 1971, Plenum Publishing Co.

Saltin, B.: Metabolic fundamentals in exercise, Med. Sci. Sports 5:137, 1973.

11 ENERGY COST AND EFFICIENCY OF WORK

Estimates of the energy expenditure during various activities such as those listed in Table 7 are useful for computing dietary requirements, for assessing the severity of activities, and for determining optimum means and rates of work. Considerations of human performance in work and sport usually involve some combination of the three applications.

COMPUTATION OF DIETARY REQUIREMENT

The quantity of foodstuff required to sustain physical activity depends upon the intensity and the duration of the activity. A normal 150-pound man requires approximately 1,200 Calories daily to sustain his body processes in a resting condition. Vigorous physical labor continued throughout the day may raise the daily dietary requirement to 7,000 Calories. If the caloric intake does not balance the caloric expenditure, substances that compose body tissues will be consumed as energy fuels, and a loss in body weight will ensue. Conversely, an excessive dietary intake will cause substances to be stored in the body tissues, and the body weight will be increased. Lacking the apparatus to measure energy metabolism accurately, one can use a careful record of the body weight to provide an index of the caloric balance between the food intake and the energy requirement for a program of physical activities.

ASSESSING SEVERITY OF EXERCISE

The severity of a calisthenic exercise, a sport, or an occupation must be determined before it can be used during convalescence or as a therapeutic measure. The amount of stress caused by the activity may be estimated by measuring the energy requirement.

The following scale of the severity of exercise in terms of oxygen consumption is commonly used:

Classification	Oxygen uptake (liters/min.)
Light	Less than 1.0
Moderate to heavy	1.0 to 2.0
Very heavy	Greater than 2.0

Such a cost list must be used with caution because of wide fluctuations in values from patient to patient and in a given patient from one exercise period to another. In addition the condition of the specific system that has been affected by the disease should be assessed by observing its adjustment to exercise. Some types of slow, heavy work such as weight lifting or wrestling cause a strain on the heart and circulation, especially if they are performed with the glottis closed. In these exercises the intrathoracic pressure may be increased to a level that reduces the flow of venous blood to the heart. This imposes a strain upon the heart by interfering with its oxygen supply. This type of stress is not assessed by energy determinations and should be considered separately.

WORK EFFICIENCY

The efficiency of performance of a piece of work may be evaluated by computing its energy requirement. A more efficient worker accomplishes a certain piece of work with less expenditure of energy. Evaluation of a task such as flying an airplane can be accomplished by measurement of energy utilization. As a worker's duties increase in complexity, his muscular tension is increased, resulting in an increased metabolic rate. The level of skill of a performer may be assessed by observing his energy utilization during work. Generalized increases in skeletal muscular tension that elevate metabolism are characteristic of an inexperienced worker.

The energy requirement for a particular task may be reduced by (1) improving the skill elements of the task, (2) reducing extra movements, (3) improving the physical condition of the worker, and (4) adjusting the rate of work to an optimum rate. Observations on the energy requirements of various rates of work demonstrate that two factors are involved. There is an optimum rate at which a given piece of work is accomplished with the least expenditure of energy. There is also a maximum rate of work that can be sustained for a given period of time. In many instances when quantity of work is not a factor, the most rapid rate is the most economical, even though exhaustion may occur early, since the work period is so short that only a very small amount of the total energy is used for supporting the body processes. Work done at a rapid rate may be within the range at which skill is not limited, yet beyond the range of intensity at which a steady state can be established. At this rapid rate of work there is a progressive development of fatigue, and exhaustion becomes inevitable. Even though this rapid rate may require the least energy for the unit output of work, the work must soon be slowed considerably or stopped to allow a period of recovery during which time little or no work is accomplished. Thus it is evident that a definition of the optimum rate of work must involve a consideration of the steady state level as well as of the economy of energy.

MAXIMUM STEADY STATE WORK

The maximum rate of sustained work is a function of a person's ability to attain a steady state at high levels of exertion. In distance running, swimming, bicycling, skiing, or rowing the competitor must adjust his speed to a rate that is within his ability to maintain a steady state of physiological activity. An athlete raises his steady state level by three procedures.

1. He improves his *general physical condition* so that the organs may function to sustain a physiological equilibrium at higher levels of activity.
2. He improves his *skill* in the activity he is to perform so that there is an economy of expenditure of energy and so that the movements will be skillful even at very rapid rates.
3. He learns to recognize the maximum rate that can be maintained in a physiological steady state. This is accomplished through *pacing*. Pacing is usually the last to be perfected. A characteristic of an inexperienced athlete is his inability to maintain a steady pace. He tends to exhaust himself early in the race by surpassing his maximum physiological steady state.

The energy required for maintaining the body functions at rest and during work is derived ultimately from the oxidation of foodstuffs. In a steady state of rest or moderate work the rate of oxygen consumption is an expression of the rate of energy production. In hard work in which the oxidation of the foodstuffs cannot keep pace with the energy requirement, energy is also liberated by anaerobic processes and an oxygen debt is accumulated (see Chapter 10). This oxygen debt is paid off during recovery. In steady state work the oxygen consumption during work is a measure of the energy requirement of the work. During exhausting work, however, the energy requirement is the sum of the oxygen consumed during work and the amount of the oxygen debt.

The manner in which Table 7 can be used is illustrated in **Table 8.**

Table 7. Energy required by a 70-kg. (154-pound) person for various physical activities*

Activity	Total Calories per hour
Sleeping	70
Lying quietly	80
Sitting	100
Mental work seated	105
Standing	110
Seamstress, handwork	115
Singing	120
Croquet	135
Driving a car	140
Office work	145
Light housework	150
Calisthenics	160
Walking, 2 m.p.h.	170
Piloting an airplane	175
Walking up stairs, 1 m.p.h.	180
Riding a bicycle, 5.5 m.p.h.	190
Walking down stairs, 2 m.p.h.	200
Bricklaying	205
House painting	210
Bowling	215
Carpenter work	230
Billiards	235
Pitching horseshoes	240
Dancing, moderate	250
Volleyball, 6-man (noncompetitive)	255
Swedish gymnastics	260
Laundress work	270
Baseball (except pitcher)	280
Horizontal walking, 3.5 m.p.h.	290
Gardening	295
Rowing for pleasure	300
Wand drill	310
Dancing, vigorous	340
Table tennis	345
Horizontal walking, 3 m.p.h., carrying 43-lb. load	350
Walking up 3% grade, 3.5 m.p.h.	370
Baseball pitcher	390
Basketball	395
Pick and shovel work	400
Shoveling sand	405
Swimming breaststroke, 1 m.p.h.	410
Bicycle riding, rapid	415
Swimming crawl stroke, 1 m.p.h.	420
Walking up 8.6% grade, 2.4 m.p.h.	430
Chopping wood	450

*The oxygen consumptions from which the caloric values in this table have been calculated are only approximations. These values include resting metabolic needs. Variables that must be considered in any interpretation of this table are size, body type, and age of the subjects, differences between individuals of the same build, physical fitness, and skill in the particular activity, nutritional condition, and environmental conditions (whether they help or hinder the individual).

Table 7. Energy required by a 70-kg. (154-pound) person for various physical activities—cont'd

Activity	Total Calories per hour
Skating, 9 m.p.h.	470
Sawing wood	480
Swimming breaststroke, 1.6 m.p.h.	490
Swimming backstroke, 1 m.p.h.	500
Snowshoeing (bearpaw), 2.5 m.p.h.	520
Skiing, 3 m.p.h.	540
Swimming sidestroke, 1 m.p.h.	550
Walking up 8.6% grade, 3.5 m.p.h.	560
Figure skating	570
Walking up 10% grade, 3.5 m.p.h.	580
Walking up stairs, 2 m.p.h.	590
Mountain climbing	600
Snowshoeing (trail snowshoes), 2.5 m.p.h.	620
Fencing	630
Skating, 11 m.p.h.	640
Rowing, 3.5 m.p.h.	660
Walking up 36% grade, 1 m.p.h., carrying 43-lb. load	680
Swimming crawl stroke, 1.6 m.p.h.	700
Parallel bar work	710
Horizontal running, 5.7 m.p.h.	720
Walking up 14.4% grade, 3.5 m.p.h.	740
Walking in 12-18 in. snow	760
Skating, 13 m.p.h.	780
Wrestling	790
Swimming backstroke, 1.6 m.p.h.	800
Horizontal running, 5 m.p.h., carrying 43-lb. load	820
Horizontal running, 7 m.p.h.	870
Walking up 36% grade, 1.5 m.p.h., carrying 43-lb. load	890
Running up 8.6% grade, 7 m.p.h.	950
Rowing, 11 m.p.h.	970
Marathon running	990
Football	1,000
Rowing, 11.3 m.p.h.	1,130
Swimming sidestroke, 1.6 m.p.h.	1,200
Horizontal running, 11.4 m.p.h.	1,300
Rowing, 12 m.p.h.	1,500
Swimming crawl stroke, 2.2 m.p.h.	1,600
Swimming breaststroke, 2.2 m.p.h.	1,850
Swimming backstroke, 2.2 m.p.h.	2,000
Horizontal running, 13.2 m.p.h.	2,330
Swimming breaststroke, 2.4 m.p.h.	2,530
Horizontal running, 14.8 m.p.h.	2,880
Swimming sidestroke, 2.2 m.p.h.	3,000
Swimming breaststroke, 2.7 m.p.h.	3,690
Horizontal running, 15.8 m.p.h.	3,910
Horizontal running, 17.2 m.p.h.	4,740
Horizontal running, 18.6 m.p.h.	7,790
Horizontal running, 18.9 m.p.h.	9,480

Table 8. Estimate of daily energy expenditure of a 70-kg. (154-pound) college student

Time	Hours	Activity	Calories per hour	Total
12:00- 7:00	7.0	Sleeping	70	490
7:00- 7:30	0.5	Morning toilet	110	55
7:30- 8:00	0.5	Breakfast	110	55
8:00- 8:15	0.25	Walking	290	73
8:15- 9:00	0.75	Study and writing	140	105
9:00-12:00	3.0	Class work (150 min.), standing and walking between classes (30 min.)	200	600
12:00- 1:00	1.0	Lunch	110	110
1:00- 3:00	2.0	Laboratory	130	260
3:00- 6:00	3.0	Team practice	600	1,800
6:00- 6:15	0.25	Walking	290	73
6:15- 7:00	0.75	Rest	80	60
7:00- 8:00	1.0	Dinner	110	110
8:00- 8:30	0.5	Conversation	110	55
8:30-10:30	2.5	Study and writing	140	350
10:30-12:00	1.5	Sleeping	70	105
Total expenditure in 24 hours				4,301

INEFFICIENCY OF ANAEROBIC WORK

When work is first started, it is carried on in a partly anaerobic condition. During light and moderate work this lag in the increasing rate of oxygen consumption in the initial stages of work is slightly less than the lag in the decreasing rate of oxygen consumption after the work has stopped. A consequence of this postexercise deficit plus "interest" is that the efficiency of short periods of work is lower than the efficiency of work of longer duration. During very brief and heavy exertion the anaerobic part of the work is greater than during moderate exertion, and the excess oxygen consumed after the exercise may be 20 times that consumed during the work. Hence very severe work, which is performed mainly anaerobically with a subsequent aerobic recovery, may be as little as 40% as efficient as aerobic work.[5]

METHOD OF MEASURING WORK METABOLISM

Energy expenditure is commonly determined by calculations from respiratory data. The subject is connected to a Douglas bag or Tissot gasometer through a face mask or mouthpiece and a suitable length of tubing. A system of valves allows the subject to inspire atmospheric air and to expire into the container for about 5 minutes. At the end of the period the volume of the air collected is noted and corrected to the volume of dry gas at standard temperature and pressure.

Samples of the expired air are collected from the bag or gasometer before it is emptied and analyzed for oxygen and carbon dioxide. From these various data the oxygen consumption per minute is calculated. The caloric value of 1 liter of oxygen when the fuel is carbohydrate is 5 Calories. Each Calorie has the energetic equivalent value of 3,086 foot-pounds. Thus when the fuel is predominately carbohydrate, the energy requirement during muscular work may be calculated from the oxygen consumption. Similar calculations can be made when fat or protein is utilized.

ENERGY REQUIREMENT OF ACTIVITIES

Table 7 gives a tabulation of the energy requirements of various activities. The figures in the table show the total metabolism during each activity. Work at a rate of over 900 Calories per hour is followed by a large oxygen debt. This debt is included in the figure representing the total energy requirement in such cases. Treadmill experiments in the Harvard Fatigue Laboratory showed that work which results in an expenditure greater than 700 Calories per hour cannot be continued for much longer than 1 hour by the average man. Champion marathon runners are able to run over 2 hours at a rate slightly faster than 11 m.p.h. They possess such superior physical equipment and are in such a fine state of training that they can attain a steady state of physiological activity at about 90% of their maximal oxygen intake capacity, using energy at the rate of approximately 1,300 Calories per hour.

Trained and untrained woodcutters, working hard all day for several days, were observed to expend an average of about 300 Calories per hour. Although the daily work (cutting and stacking cords of wood) accomplished by the trained woodcutters was over 4 times greater than that of the untrained workers, the caloric requirement was nearly the same.

SEXUAL ACTIVITY

Regardless of the technique of stimulation during coitus, physiological responses increase progressively during erotic excitement and intromission, rapidly attain a maximum at orgasm, and decline markedly during resolution. During the ejaculation and orgasm phase, which usually lasts less than 15 seconds, heart rates of middle-aged, long-married couples average fewer than 120 beats per minute and seldom exceed 140. The systolic blood pressure typically rises from 130 to a maximum of 160 mm. Hg. Higher values are recorded during extramarital intercourse. Oxygen uptake during sexual activity has not yet been reported and thus the energy cost of the exertion has not been assessed. It is probable that oxygen uptake does not parallel

139

cardiopulmonary changes because the emotional nature of sexual activity makes it essentially a sympathetic nervous system stimulant. Yet, the cardiac cost in terms of myocardial oxygen consumption may be somewhat high as indicated by the increased heart rate and blood pressure. The effort of sexual intercourse is usually the equivalent of climbing a flight of stairs or walking briskly. It ordinarily does not exceed the performance of everyday tasks.

Sexual activity is not a bodily exercise in terms of its effectiveness in enhancing physical condition. Improved physical condition due to exercise training, however, does seem to enhance sexual drive; both frequency and quality of sexual activity are increased.[3]

EFFICIENCY

Work is accomplished by the expenditure of energy. When more work is done with the same energy expenditure or when a given amount of work is accomplished at a smaller energy cost, the *efficiency of the performance is higher.* Other factors that must be considered in an appraisal of the overall efficiency of performance include (1) the *rate* of work, (2) the *load*, (3) the *duration* of the work, (4) the *quality* of the work, and (5) the *speed of recovery* following the work period. It is apparent that efficiency is a complex measurement involving many variables. If the influence on efficiency of a single variable is to be estimated, the other variables must be kept constant.

ESTIMATION OF WORK EFFICIENCY

Efficiency is expressed by the formula:

$$\text{Efficiency (in percent)} = \frac{\text{Energy output}}{\text{Energy intake}} \times 100$$

"Energy output" is usually expressed in terms of foot-pounds or Calories (1 Calorie = 3,086 foot-pounds). For example, if a man weighing 150 pounds climbs stairs to a height of 20 feet, he performs 20 × 150 = 3,000 foot-pounds of work. The "energy intake" in performing muscular work is ordinarily expressed in terms of the liters of oxygen consumed or in terms of the equivalent value in Calories of heat energy (1 liter of oxygen is equivalent to 5 Calories). If the efficiency of work is to be calculated from the formula just given, the work done and the energy used must be expressed in terms of the same unit. For example, if the 150-pound man uses 8 Calories of energy for his 20-foot climb, his energy expenditure is 8 × 3,086 = 24,688 foot-pounds, and the efficiency of his performance is as follows:

$$\frac{3,000}{24,688} \times 100 = 12.1\%$$

EFFICIENCY OF WORK ALONG A HORIZONTAL PLANE

In many of the physical activities of man movement occurs along a horizontal plane. In this type of work the arms and legs are raised and lowered with each step while the trunk is propelled along a steady plane with only a slight rise and fall at each step. In horizontal movement the external work accomplished is rather small. Other factors that require the expenditure of energy, such as the overcoming of muscle viscosity, the inertia of the bony levers, and external wind resistance, are practically impossible to measure. As a result of these complications, the efficiency of work along a horizontal plane is usually expressed not by the ratio of work done to energy used but rather by a consideration of the energy requirement for the particular distance and at the particular speed. The lower the energy requirement, the higher the efficiency.

LEG LENGTH AND STRIDE LENGTH

Each person makes characteristic adjustments in length of stride for various speeds of walking. This adjustment is close to the optimal stride length as measured by the energy cost of locomotion. Leg length has no significant effect on the energy cost of walking; a person with short legs walks about as economically as one with long legs.[4]

Apparently, any loss in efficiency due to increased stride length in long-legged persons tends to be offset by a gain in economy due to decreased work in lifting the body in these subjects.[2] Subjects with long legs take fewer steps in walking a standard distance and lift themselves less frequently.

EFFICIENCY OF GRADE CLIMBING

In walking or running up a slight grade most of the energy expended is used in movements of the arms and legs and is dissipated as heat; very little is used in actually raising the body. As the grade becomes steeper, more of the total energy expenditure is applied to raising the body, and the work efficiency is accordingly increased.

Estimates of the work efficiency of movement up a slight grade are practically useless for assessing the mechanical efficiency of the entire body. They are of some value when the efficiencies of two or more persons are to be compared. For this purpose, the energy expenditure of each subject performing the same run is measured; the lower the energy expenditure, the higher the efficiency. Steeper grades or higher rates of climbing differentiate more clearly among different persons because of the greater stresses involved.

Balke and Ware measured the cost of grade walking of U. S. Air Force personnel and found an average of 1.8 ml. oxygen per kg.-meter

141

of work done and the corresponding *absolute efficiency* was 27%.[1] The energy expenditure per unit weight was nearly constant in different subjects.

ENERGY COST OF PROGRESSION

The comparative efficiencies of walking, running, climbing, and other forms of progression at various speeds along a horizontal plane or up varying grades may be evaluated by comparing the energy expanded in traveling a fixed distance such as a mile. Very slow rates of progression that are performed with low expenditures of energy are not efficient. Moving slowly to "save energy" is false economy when a certain distance has to be traversed.

Table 9 demonstrates that fewer Calories are used in walking a mile at 3.5 m.p.h. than when the speed is slowed to 2.3 m.p.h. or in-

Table 9. Energy expenditures at various speeds and grades of different types of progression*

Type of progression	Speed (m.p.h.)	Grade (%)	Energy expenditure 70-kg. (154-lb.) man	
			Calories per hour	Calories per mile
Horizontal walking	2.3	0	210	90
	3.5	0	290	85
	4.6	0	470	100
Grade walking	2.0	5.0	250	125
	2.5	5.0	290	115
	2.3	5.5	350	150
	3.5	5.5	450	130
	2.4	8.6	430	180
	3.5	8.6	560	160
Horizontal walking carrying 43-lb. load	1.0	0	210	210
	2.0	0	270	135
	3.0	0	350	115
	4.0	0	540	135
(Running)	5.0	0	820	165
Grade walking carrying 43-lb. load	0.5	35.8	370	740
	1.0	35.8	680	680
	1.5	35.8	890	595
Skiing along level	3.0	0	540	180
	5.0	0	720	145
	7.5	0	950	125
Swimming (breaststroke)	1.0		410	410
	1.6		490	305
	1.9		820	430

*Based on data from Harvard Fatigue Laboratory in Morehouse and Cherry: Energy cost of progression, National Academy of Science, Washington, D. C., July, 1946, Government Printing Office. The same precautions should be used in interpreting these data as are noted in Table 7.

creased to 4.6 m.p.h. Speeds of grade climbing below 2.5 m.p.h. require the expenditure of more Calories each mile than do speeds of
2.5 to 3.5 m.p.h. Less energy is expended when a 43-pound load is
carried at 3 m.p.h. than at either slower or faster speeds. In carrying
the load up a steep grade, the faster speed is more economical, but at
the greater speed the rate of energy expenditure becomes so high that
a steady state of physiological activity cannot be established, and exhaustion occurs within a short distance. In the case of walking up a
grade carrying a 43-pound load, it would appear that 1 m.p.h. is the
optimal speed if the load is to be carried more than a mile, but 1.5
m.p.h. is optimal if the load is to be carried less than a mile. The same
principles apply to skiing along a level. The faster speed is more economical, but the high-energy requirement at speeds above 5 m.p.h.
prevent these rates from being continued for more than 1 hour. The
rapidly increasing energy requirement as swimming speed is increased
necessitates a moderately slow rate of swimming if the distance to be
covered requires more than 1 hour. Extremely slow rates of swimming
are uneconomical.

LOW ECONOMY OF SLOW WORK

The reason for the low economy of progression at a slow rate is
that a large part of the energy used during the work is required for
the maintenance of body functions (digestive, glandular, and so on)
that do not contribute directly to the performance of the work. When
the distance is traversed in a shorter time, the energy cost of maintenance of these supportive functions is correspondingly reduced.

The increase in energy cost when work is performed at slow rates
is shown in Table 10. The 1-mile climb at 0.5 m.p.h. requires 2 hours.
At 1.5 m.p.h. the climb can be completed in 40 minutes. At the slow
rate of work the energy cost of maintaining the human machine must
be met for 80 minutes longer than at the faster rate of work. This increased energy cost, amounting to 145 Calories, reduces the work
efficiency from 24 to 6%.

A dominant factor in human efficiency is the time spent in perform-

Table 10. Relation of efficiency to rate of work—70-kg. (154-pound)
man carrying 43-pound load up 35.8% grade*

Speed (m.p.h.)	Climbing 1 hour		Climbing 1 mile	
	Calories per hour	Efficiency	Calories per mile	Efficiency
0.5	370	13%	740	6%
1.0	680	14%	680	14%
1.5	890	16%	595	24%

*Data from Table 9.

ing the work. The longer the work period, the lower the efficiency. In order to achieve the highest efficiency work should be performed at the most rapid rate within the limits of skill and endurance.

INFLUENCE OF WORK LOAD ON EFFICIENCY

An additional factor in work efficiency, as shown in Table 10, is the total work accomplished when climbing one hour and climbing one mile. When the speed was increased from 0.5 to 1 m.p.h., the work load was increased by 145,548 foot-pounds per hour and the efficiency improved from 13 to 14%. At 1.5 m.p.h. the work load was 436,444 foot-pounds per hour and the efficiency was 16%.

The increase in efficiency as the load is increased demonstrates that the percentage of energy utilized for the work is greater when fairly heavy work is done than when light work is done.

Net efficiency, in which the energy cost of recovery is added to the energy cost during work, is lowered as the load of brief bouts of heavy work is increased.

MAXIMUM RATE OF WORK

Work that requires an energy expenditure greater than 700 Calories per hour cannot be continued for much longer than 1 hour by an untrained man. Unless the man carrying the 43-pound load up the 35.8% grade (Table 10) was well trained, he could not be expected to climb at 1.5 m.p.h. for more than 1 hour since the energy expenditure at this rate is 890 Calories per hour. If the speed is reduced to 1 m.p.h., the energy requirement is reduced to 680 Calories per hour, and the work can be sustained for a longer period. If the distance is great, the speed should be reduced so that the climber is not exhausted by the work. Efficiency must be sacrificed for endurance in order to accomplish work of long duration. If the distance is short, greater speed or heavier loads are necessary if the work is to be performed with the greatest efficiency. A well-trained person is able to carry on work at a higher level of energy expenditure; thus he is able to perform work at higher speeds for longer periods.

RACING PLAN

Steadiness in the rate of work is also a factor in efficiency. Work is done more efficiently if it is carried on at a steady rate. As shown before, it costs energy to accelerate. In distance races, whether running, swimming, rowing, or bicycling, energy must be conserved and a steady state established at a dangerously high level of energy expenditure. Under these conditions the race will be finished in the shortest time if the athlete has maintained a speed at which a maximum steady state level has been established for the number of minutes required for the event. Then, at the proper distance before the end of the race, he increases the speed so that the maximum oxygen debt is reached at the finish. In this race plan the maximum energy is expended in the most economical manner.

Physiological factors are not the only ones that enter into the efficiency complex. Other important factors are heredity, environment, and economics.

With these limitations in mind the following summary of calculations may be used to compare the efficiency of various physical activities:

Event	Efficiency (%)	Reference
Sprint running	22.7	Fenn
60-yard run	mean 37.7	Furasawa et al.
	range 27.8 to 44.5	
Swimming, crawl stroke	0.5 to 2.2	Karpovich et al.
Swimming, backstroke	0.88 to 1.35	
Bicycle ergometry	11.4 to 21.5	Dickenson
Grade walking on treadmill	24.8 to 40.3	Erickson et al.
	15.3 to 16.9	Knehr et al.
Running up incline greater than 20%	25	Margaria et al.

References

1. Balke, B., and Ware, R.: An experimental study of physical fitness of Air Force personnel, U.S. Armed Forces Med. J. **10**:675, 1961.
2. Cotes, J. E., and Meade, F.: The energy expenditure and mechanical energy demand in walking, Ergonomics **3**:97-119, 1960.
3. Hellerstein, H., and Friedman, E.: Sexual activity and the postcoronary patient, Med. Aspects Hum. Sexuality, March, 1969.
4. van der Walt, W. H., and Wyndham, C. H.: An equation for prediction of energy expenditure of walking and running, J. Appl. Physiol. **34**:559, 1973.
5. Whipp, B., and Wasserman, K.: Efficiency of muscular work, J. Appl. Physiol. **26**:644, 1969.

Suggested readings

Brody, S.: Bioenergetics and growth—with special reference to the efficiency complex in domestic animals, New York, 1964, Reinhold Publishing Corp.

Brouha, L.: Physiology in industry, ed. 2, New York, 1967, Pergamon Press.

Consolazio, C. F., and Johnson, H. L.: Measurement of energy cost in humans, Fed. Proc. **30**:1444, 1971.

Costill, D.: Metabolic responses during distance running, J. Appl. Physiol. **28**: 251, 1970.

Dickenson, S.: The efficiency of bicycle-pedalling as affected by speed and load, Am. J. Physiol. **67**:242, 1929.

Fenn, W.: Frictional and kinetic factors in the work of sprint running, Am. J. Physiol. **92**:583, 1930.

Kamon, E.: Negative and positive work in climbing a laddermill, J. Appl. Physiol. **29**:1, 1970.

Soule, R., and Goldman, R.: Energy cost of loads carried on the head, hands or feet, J. Appl. Physiol. **27**:687, 1969.

12 MAXIMAL EFFORT AND FATIGUE

In Chapter 11 we studied man as a work animal. Now we shall look at man's physiological capacity for maximal effort, and see the effects of fatigue on his ability to perform.

ENDURANCE

Endurance may be considered as the ability of the body to withstand the stresses set up by prolonged activity. Factorial techniques of analysis have resulted in the isolation of four factors in endurance: circulorespiratory, velocity, muscular structure, and body build. Endurance for *exhausting* work depends mainly on the ability of the body to supply and use oxygen and to dispose of the rapidly mounting concentrations of lactic acid and carbon dioxide. Training for endurance results in an increased capillarization of the muscle, thus providing more channels for the delivery of oxygen and food and the removal of wastes. Distance runners and other athletes participating in endurance-type athletics do not possess the hypertrophied muscles typical of athletes who are engaged in activities requiring great strength. Hypertrophy involves reduction of the diffusion surface area per unit volume of muscle fiber and thus a reduction in the oxygen supply to the fibers. In addition, compared with a muscle containing an optimum amount of contractile tissue, there is a loss in efficiency because of the necessary passive deformation of inactive parts of the muscle mass; this in turn causes a relative increase in the metabolism in proportion to the work performed and therefore a reduction in efficiency.

Endurance for *moderate* (steady state) activity depends upon the supply and utilization of fuels such as sugar. The fuel factor is recognized to be so critical in prolonged moderate work that it has been suggested that moderate work should be preceded by 2 days of rest from strenuous work in order to permit filling of the glycogen stores in the body. During prolonged work without food, as in running or swimming distances requiring more than 2½ hours to complete, the depletion of these stores is indicated by a marked fall in the blood sugar (hypoglycemia) and the appearance of fatigue. In such events an athlete benefits by light feeding at frequent intervals during the race. In order for sugar feeding to have a beneficial effect, it must be taken well before hypoglycemic changes occur, due to the time required for its absorption.

Cardiovascular responses to static muscular effort are different from those found during rhythmic exercise. During rhythmic exercise there is a large increase in heart rate, a rise of systolic pressure but usually a reduction of diastolic pressure, and a large fall in systemic vascular resistance.

Sustained contractions lead to dramatic rises of both systolic and diastolic pressures, and only moderate rise in heart rate. There is little or no change in systemic vascular resistance. It is the degree of muscle tonus, not the amount of muscular involvement, that is the important factor in inducing these responses, As in rhythmic exercise, a rising blood pressure indicates that static effort is fatiguing. Using this response as a criterion, it was found among stretcher bearers that only 10 kg. loads could be carried by the hands without fatigue, whereas 80 kg. could be carried in a shoulder harness.[2]

Anaerobic capacity. Anaerobic capacity is important for brief activities of high intensity, or for activities that require more energy than is available from the oxygen transporting system. As discussed in Chapters 1, 2, 3, and 10, this anaerobic energy is derived from high-energy phosphate compounds produced during the breakdown of glycogen to lactic acid. These nutrients are exhausted in less than 60 seconds during all-out effort. Repetitive work of the fast-acting white fibers, as employed in sprinting, is limited by the dearth of capillaries which supply them with oxygen. White fibers also contain too few mitochondria to support intensive effort for long periods.

A method for measuring anaerobic capacity is described in Chapter 18 in the *Laboratory Manual.*

Aerobic capacity. Given an adequate oxygen supply and a source of nutrient such as glucose to be broken down to provide contractile energy, the muscle will contract indefinitely.

When large groups of muscles are brought into continuous action as in running uphill, the demand for oxygen exceeds the supply. The point at which the supply can no longer keep pace with the demand for oxygen represents the performer's aerobic capacity. This is termed *maximal oxygen uptake* and is expressed as $\dot{V}O_2$ max. Methods of measuring maximal oxygen uptake and determining aerobic capacity are described in Chapter 17 of the *Laboratory Manual.*

STRENGTH

The strength of the working muscles is a limiting factor in endurance. A load easily carried by strong muscles may quickly exhaust weak ones. When a strong muscle lifts a comparatively light load, relatively few fibers need to be brought into play. As these become fatigued, their threshold of irritability is raised, and they fail to respond to the stimuli. The stimuli then arouse fresh fibers, and they take over the work while the fatigued fibers recuperate and resume the burden later on if necessary.

FAT

Since fat increases the load the worker must move with each motion, it becomes a limiting factor in endurance. Athletes trained for endurance contests usually reduce the fat content of the body to a minimum. An exception to this is distance swimmers, in whom the increased buoyancy and decreased heat loss due to a layer of subcutaneous fat more than offset the disadvantage of the greater weight to be moved. A certain amount of fat is also desirable under conditions of prolonged restricted food intake.

MAXIMAL OXYGEN CONSUMPTION

Maximal oxygen consumption is reached when the oxygen intake per unit time is at the maximum and the rate remains constant. In normal subjects the maximal oxygen consumption achievable is usually taken as an index to maximal cardiovascular function. (Description of the methodology of measuring maximal oxygen consumption is found in Chapter 17 of the *Laboratory* Manual.)

Maximal oxygen consumption increases with age up to 20 years and then declines. It can be increased about 10% by rigorous physical training. It is 12% greater at sea level than at 6,000 feet above sea level.

Since maximal oxygen consumption is related to body size, it is usually expressed in terms of milliliters (ml.) of oxygen per kilogram (kg.) of body weight per unit time. A maximal oxygen consumption above 50 ml./kg./min. for young men, and above 40 ml./kg./min. for young women is considered to indicate a good level of endurance fitness.

Short bouts of maximal activity, in which the event is completed within 30 seconds, are performed using only the immediate fuels of contraction and are concluded before the oxidative recovery processes are fully in action. Endurance for activities requiring violent exertion for 1 to 3 minutes is limited by the concentration of lactic acid and other metabolites that can be tolerated. A lactate concentration exceeding 100 mg. per 100 ml. of blood is a common finding after maximal exercise involving large muscles.

In more prolonged events of maximal exertion requiring more than 4 minutes to complete, the limiting factor appears to be the ability of the circulorespiratory system to supply the oxygen needed by the muscles. Trained individuals have a greater "aerobic capacity" than do others. In prolonged events requiring 2½ or more hours to complete, the work rate is reduced so that a steady state is reached in which oxygen needs are easily met. Men who completed the Boston marathon had only average vital capacities for their size, and there was no significant relationship between the size of the vital capacity and the order in which the runners finished the race.

RESPIRATION

Although lung capacity and other features of ventilation are not likely to become limiting factors in endurance, there may be other respiratory factors that impinge upon the nicety of physiological adjustments necessary to support continued physical activity. The excessive hyperventilation in untrained persons, which undoubtedly restricts their ability to continue work, is little understood. The complexity of the stimuli controlling respiration, discussed in Chapter 8, may be further complicated by substances yet unidentified that are produced during exercise and that stimulate chemoreceptors.

Adequate respiration requires not only that oxygen be available in the lungs but also that it be taken up by the blood and transported to the muscles. Present evidence suggests that when the blood flow is maximal, as during heavy exercise, oxygen uptake in the lungs may be inadequate, and the blood may have a suboptimal oxygen tension when it passes from the lung.

CIRCULATION

The rate at which the oxygen is supplied to the muscles depends also on the rate of circulation of the blood. The increased stroke volume during muscular work is produced by a more complete emptying of the ventricles during systole. Nervous and hormonal effects are suggested as reasons for the increase in the power of the systolic contraction. The increase in heart rate is equally important in increasing the cardiac output in exercise. These topics are discussed at length in Chapter 6.

MOTIVATION

Possibly the most important factor in endurance is the willingness to endure the discomfort that accompanies fatigue. Studies of participants in sports with severe endurance demands, such as rowing, have served to emphasize that many participants are motivated by a need to resolve personal problems. It is possible that measures of endurance are quite largely measures of the compulsive drives that motivate a person. Step tests, treadmill running, and similar measurements very seldom give a true estimate of the endurance of the subject being tested since he is seldom motivated to put forth his best efforts. Laboratory findings indicate that significant cardiorespiratory changes occur when motivational stress factors are evident and that a greater work output is elicited.[7]

SKILL

A trained person benefits from a reduction in unnecessary movements. He achieves a greater net mechanical efficiency by using fewer muscles and by employing those used to better advantage. The least skillful runner uses half again as much oxygen as the most skillful person in performing the same task.

DISTRIBUTION OF ENERGY

Adjustment of speed. Records of running events given in Table 11 illustrate the adjustment of speed necessitated by an increase in the length of a race. The 100-yard and 220-yard dashes are run at full speed. The 220 is run at a faster average rate than the 100-yard dash because maximal speed is not attained until the runner is at least 50 yards from the start. During the first 50 yards the runner must accelerate from zero speed at the start to the maximal speed. Thus at

Table 11. Adjustment of speed in running to length of race

Event	Speed (m.p.h.)
220 yd.	22.5
100 yd.	22.0
440 yd.	19.5
880 yd.	16.6
1 mi.	15.2
2 mi.	14.0
3 mi.	13.3
6 mi.	12.9
10 mi.	12.45
Marathon (26 mi. 385 yd.)	11.0

least half of the 100-yard dash is completed before maximal speed is attained. When the race is continued to 220 yards, the sprinter can maintain maximal speed for the last 150 yards. Sprinters probably run faster than 24 m.p.h. during the later portion of the dashes.

The maximal distance that trained sprinters are able to sprint at full speed is about 300 yards. In races beyond this distance the runner must conserve his energy by reducing speed in order to run the distance in the fastest possible time. If he attempts to run beyond 300 yards at full speed, he will soon collapse. Thus running events beyond the 300-yard distance must be considered endurance contests.

Since the 440-yard dash cannot be run at full speed all of the way, the speed must be adjusted slightly. The speed must be lowered about 3 m.p.h. (14%) below maximum, or the runner will exhaust himself before the 440 yards have been run. If the runner should sprint the first 300 yards, he would have to reduce his speed the remainder of the distance to such an extent that his time for the race would be slow. He would also run the risk of collapsing during the latter portion of the race. Running the first 150 yards at an easy speed and then running the remainder of the race at full speed would be equally ineffective and hazardous. Acceleration during a race is exceedingly costly in energy; a steady pace is the most efficient. During the latter portion of a 440-yard or 880-yard run, the stride is somewhat shortened because of the poorer rate of muscular relaxation and the occurrence of contractures in the working fibers. For this reason, in this range runners are able to achieve their best times by running the early part of the race somewhat faster than the latter.

In order to run 880 yards a runner must reduce his speed about 5.5 m.p.h. (25%) below the maximum. In order to complete the mile distance a runner must reduce his speed nearly one third (33%) below the maximal rate. In races of this distance a steady state of physiological activity must be established. High concentrations of lactic acid must be endured, and large quantities of oxygen must be utilized.

In races 2 miles and longer the rate of physiological activity attained is well below the maximal level at which the trained athlete can maintain physiological equilibrium. The lactic acid concentration and the oxygen debt are small, and the runner finishes the race in a condition that would permit him to run farther. Races of 15 miles and longer are run at approximately the same rate, which is about one half the maximal speed. This rate is well tolerated by a trained athlete. He finishes with the heart rate and blood pressure only mildly elevated, and his breathing is fairly easy. The limiting factors in long-distance races appear to be the nutritional status and the condition of the feet and legs.

The relationship between the homeostatic mechanism and the rate of energy liberation is sufficiently constant to permit a mathematical prediction of speed as a function of time.

Pace. The most economical distribution of effort in running a distance of 0.5 mile or more or in swimming, cycling, or rowing equivalent distances is obtained by performing at a constant rate over the entire distance. The racing distance is covered in the shortest time when the total available energy is distributed evenly over the distance. Acceleration is so costly that changes in speed are too expensive to employ as deceptive tactics.

The achievement of proper pace requires extensive training. Pace training may be facilitated by the use of a pacing machine which enables the athlete to follow a marker that is traveling at a fixed rate.

Cheering. Environmental stimuli, such as a competitive situation, the encouragement of the coach and teammates, and the cheering of the spectators, strengthen the movements of trained athletes and extend their endurance by raising the threshold of sensitivity to fatigue and by reinforcing nerve impulses to working muscles. These phenomena account for the fact that trained athletes usually perform better during competition than during practice. In laboratory studies using an arm ergograph subjects performed 1½ times as much work when they were observed as when they worked alone. When they were cheered by the observers at the first sign of fatigue, work output increased to 2½ times that of solitary work.

The same factors that improve the performance of a trained athlete may diminish the performance of a novice. Instead of distributing his energy evenly over the distance of the race, a novice responds to cheering by increasing his speed to such an extent that he approaches exhaustion early in the race. A novice often runs better in practice than he does in competition.

Hypnosis. Hypnosis has been observed to improve physical performance of strength and endurance events. An explanation for the increased performance during the hypnotic state is offered on the basis of the removal of inhibitory influences.

Training for endurance events. In addition to pace training endurance may be improved by bettering general physical condition, increasing muscular strength, achieving greater neuromuscular coordination, and making physiochemical adjustments. In order to improve endurance the activities may be either speeded up or prolonged and preferably should include the same movements that will be used in competition. Through exposure the athlete increases his resistance to feelings of fatigue until physiological limits are reached. The ability to endure fatigue is probably the greatest factor in endurance for prolonged muscular work.

Through practice of endurance events the circulatory and respiratory systems become more efficient in supplying oxygen and in removing the waste products of metabolism. The temperature-regulating system enables the body to adjust effectively to the heat of muscular work. The skeletal and cardiac muscles become stronger and more efficient. Through training of the nervous system the movements become better coordinated, wasted motions are eliminated, and the action between synergic and antagonistic muscles is refined. Through exercise training the oxygen-carrying capacity of the blood is improved, and the body is better able to mobilize and transport foodstuffs necessary for the support of physical activity.

MEASURES OF ENDURANCE

At rest the physiological differences between an athlete with a high level of endurance and a person with poor endurance are negligible. When they both start working, however, the differences quickly appear. They are most striking during the most vigorous work. An athlete with great endurance is characterized by the ability to produce higher levels of lactic acid and to use larger volumes of oxygen and by a lower heart rate during prolonged work. The return of the heart rate and lactic acid concentration to normal is faster in a trained athlete.

To summarize, an athlete with great endurance can carry on exhausting work for a longer period and can establish a physiological steady state at higher levels of work. He can recover from work more quickly and is thereby enabled to start a second piece of hard work sooner than can a person with poor endurance.

FATIGUE

Severe muscular exercise diminishes the capacity of muscles for further activity. This depressant action of strenuous activity is called *muscular fatigue*. It must be distinguished from the subjective sensations of tiredness, sleepiness, and muscular soreness which frequently accompany it. Continued stimulation of sensory organs, such as those of vision and hearing, may result in a diminished response, a process known as *adaptation*. It is not the same as fatigue, however, since changing the strength of the sensory stimulus slightly usually restores the full vigor of the sensory response. The synapses between neurons in the central nervous system and the junction between nerve fibers and muscle fibers (motor end-plate) are readily fatigued by continued activity, and it is probable that so-called muscular fatigue in an exer-

153

cising subject is the result of loss of the capacity for transmission of nerve impulses to the muscle as well as exhaustion of the muscle itself.

GENERAL FATIGUE

The development of fatigue in a single organ that is subjected to repeated stimulation can be followed, and the extent of the reduction in its functional capacity can be predicted with a high degree of accuracy. This is not so easy in the case of so-called *general fatigue*. The fatigue resulting from the tedious repetition of dull, easy work is akin to boredom and it eludes measurement. General fatigue results from the stress of performing activities lacking in personal satisfactions. It may carry over into other types of activity, so that life itself seems to lack satisfaction. If the attitude persists, the outcome may be a flight into mental illness.

Symptoms. The onset of fatigue in a person doing light work is seldom noticed by the subject. He is unaware that his standards of performance are deteriorating, and he may even believe that his efficiency is steadily increasing. His sense of timing is the first to fail, and errors and accidents begin to appear. As fatigue advances, the worker's grasp of the overall plan of the operation begins to fade so that eventually only the most prominent features of the task are performed and the rest are ignored. Attention is finally shifted from the performance of the task to the discomfort of the body. Deterioration in skill now proceeds rapidly.

Physiological fatigue is not the only factor that influences work performance. The importance of psychological, social, and socioeconomic factors is gradually being realized by industrial physicians and management officials. Under certain favorable conditions industrial output may actually increase toward the end of the working day in spite of fatigue. Music, for example, facilitates the social contacts among workers and relieves their boredom. It is most appreciated by those doing repetitive manual tasks but may hinder those whose work demands a high degree of mental effort. To be most effective music should be presented on two or three occasions during the working day but for comparatively short periods of time. Music time should be adjusted to industrial output curves in order to offset decrements ascribable to ennui or fatigue.

Chronic fatigue (staleness). Fatigue is chronic when it is not relieved by a good night's sleep. Some of the prominent symptoms of this very common condition are subjective feeling of tiredness, loss of interest in work and other daily activities, increase in the effort that is necessary to perform the usual work, increased irritability and general emotional instability, loss of weight, poor appetite, increase in resting pulse rate and lowered blood pressure, a tendency to sigh frequently, tremor of the outstretched hands, pallor, and increased consumption of coffee, tobacco, and alcohol.

In chronic fatigue a vicious cycle may be set up. A person who is unable to sleep because he is worried may become worried because he is unable to sleep. Eventually he may resort to barbiturates or other drugs in order to sleep or to Benzedrine or other stimulants in order to stay awake and do his work. Anxiety in such states produces tension in the muscles, and these residual contractions have been suggested as a cause of fatigue.

The energy costs of physical work seldom lead to chronic fatigue. The problems involved in chronic fatigue are emotional and situational, not physiological. Under normal conditions overwork is itself a symptom of maladjustment.

The most frequent causes of chronic fatigue are long hours of work, lack of sleep, maladjustment, and worry. The symptoms usually disappear after a period of rest away from work.

Anxiety state. The effect of severe fright, such as might occur in battle or in a tragic accident, is occasionally a disorganization of a person's motor nervous system that renders him incapable of skillful movement. This motor disorganization frequently persists, and the victim behaves continually as if the original traumatic situation were still in existence. Tremor of the hand may be so intense that he is incapable of buttoning a coat. There is a reduction of muscular strength, and in severe anxiety states there is often a loss of kinesthetic sense resulting in an incapacity to stand and walk. Recovery does not occur until improvement in the mental state is made.

Effort syndrome. A person with subnormal tolerance for exercise experiences breathlessness, rapid beating of the heart, sweating, and dizziness on even such mild exertion as climbing a short flight of stairs. Such effort intolerance may be caused by a constitutional inferiority present since infancy or it may have developed from emotional disturbance.

The effort syndrome may not be recognized if a person avoids heavy physical work. Possessing a frail physique and a conviction that he has always had a "weak heart" or "lung trouble," he has always dreaded the supposed ill effects of vigorous physical exercise. The response of the heart and respiration to exercise is usually as poor as if he possessed the supposed heart and lung disorders.

The effort syndrome is seen under pressure of a job requiring occasional physical exertion. Under such a condition of pressure the feelings of insufficiency may be exaggerated until the person is out of harmony with his surroundings. Recovery commences when he is

155

restored to an environment that is within his effort capacity and when no further intense pressures are anticipated. The effect upon this person of a program of physical education that did not consider individual differences in response to exercise would probably be to increase emotional conflict and would result in further motor disorganization.

MUSCULAR FATIGUE

The term *muscular fatigue* refers to an impairment of the muscles' ability to respond to stimuli. This sort of fatigue may be measured by means of a strength decrement index, which has been used for such practical purposes as studying the effects of various types of Army packs. Muscular fatigue is a normal phenomenon and should be viewed as a normal response to a normal stress. Rest and sleep allow an opportunity for the reestablishment of homeostasis.

The physiological causes of muscular fatigue, however, are not well understood. The laborer does not accumulate lactic acid or any other product of metabolic breakdown, and anaerobic reserves are not drawn on except during strenuous work or sport.

Site of fatigue. Changes in the functional properties of nerve cells, the myoneural junction, and the muscle itself have been suggested as the basis of muscular fatigue. One theory is that the general fatigue that reduces the range and power of voluntary muscular activity is largely an affair of the central nervous system. However, if the circulation to a fatigued muscle is occluded, there is no recovery of strength. Recovery occurs only after blood flow is restored. If fatigue were a phenomenon of the central nervous system, it is unlikely that recovery would be delayed by occluding the blood flow to muscle. The nerves themselves are believed to be indefatigable, but there is evidence that after repeated stimulation a spinal reflex may diminish and its pattern may alter. Skilled activity is the first thing to suffer as an individual becomes fatigued.[3]

The impairment of muscle function in fatigue may be due in part to the decreased rate of formation and release of the transmitter substance acetylcholine at the neuromuscular junction. This would result in failure of some of the impulses arriving over the motor nerves to stimulate the muscle fibers, and would increase the impairment due to fatigue of the muscle itself.

Cortical motor and sensory centers. The fatigue that influences performance in muscular work and sport is more directly related to the motor centers of the brain. Fatigue of the sensory centers is more significant in certain types of work involving small, accurate movements or requiring continual visual or auditory attention. There is little or no correlation between fatigue of motor centers and fatigue of sensory centers in different types of work.

Fatigue of the motor and sensory centers may be measured by several techniques. In the *tapping test* the maximal frequency with which a telegraphic key can be tapped gives an index of the functional condition of the motor centers. The results of this test are not influenced by peripheral factors such as circulation or metabolism. Fatigue of the retinocortical (visual) center is indicated by a decrease in the *fusion frequency of flicker* (the rate at which alternating periods of light and dark produced by an electronic tube can be discriminated before "flicker" disappears, being replaced by a visual impression of uniform grayness). In truck driving, which has a considerable manual component, the results of the tapping test and other tests of motor function such as simple reaction time, reaction coordination ability, and manual steadiness bear a closer relation to the number of hours of driving time than do tests of sensory function. The same is true of laundry workers.

Procedures for conducting the tapping test and for measuring the fusion frequency of flicker are presented in Chapter 6 in the *Laboratory Manual.*

Fatigue occurs within the reflex arcs during both mental and physical work. The stimulus threshold of the Achilles tendon reflex and of the knee jerk gradually rises during the working period. The rise in threshold accelerates slightly during mental work and markedly during physical work. Determination of the stimulus threshold for the Achilles tendon reflex before work is resumed indicates whether or not the fatigue of the previous work period has been relieved by rest.

EFFECT OF EXERCISE ON MENTAL WORK

While fatigue of motor centers is important in the performance of muscular work and sports, fatigue of the sensory centers appears to be more important in the general sensation of fatigue. Although fatigue of motor and sensory centers are not related to one another, there is some spreading of fatigue from one type of center to the other. Flicker-fusion frequency is depressed after exhausting muscular work (700-yard run) and increased after 30 knee-bends or static work. This indicates that hard muscular work produces a certain degree of central nervous system fatigue, whereas light or moderate exercise, performed during pauses in sedentary occupations, improves the functional state of the central nervous system. Physical training in the schools should be administered in such a way as to avoid interference with the educational program. The activities during the school period should be

157

short and moderate in order to have a stimulating effect on the capacity for mental work. Severe muscular work should be performed after school in order to avoid the depressing effect on the capacity for classroom work.

EFFECT OF SENSORY FATIGUE ON MUSCULAR WORK

Systematic studies of sensory fatigue induced by a lack or curtailment of sleep show that there are no significant physiological changes with up to 200 hours of sleeplessness. Reaction time and body steadiness are impaired by lack of sleep, but hand steadiness and handgrip strength are not affected. Subjective estimation of well-being also bears little relation to work performance. The lack of correlation between fatigue of sensory centers and fatigue of motor centers may explain the confusing experiences of athletes who have performed exceedingly well on days when they have complained of feeling too ill to enter competition, whereas their performance was unsatisfactory on other days when they had such a feeling of well-being that they felt capable of breaking records.

VISUAL FATIGUE

Visual fatigue may be observed by the use of several different procedures. The fusion frequency of flicker, as stated previously, indicates the excitability of the retinocortical system. In office, laboratory, and dispensary work the fusion frequency of flicker was lower in the late afternoon than it was in the morning, but the decrement was much more pronounced in laboratory work including 3 hours' work with the microscope than in laboratory work without the use of the microscope. After 2 hours of hard inspection work at a very inadequate illumination, the fixation time and the corrective movements increased, whereas the rate of movements decreased. One manifestation of oculomotor fatigue is a blocking of eye movements for a fraction of a second, which enforces involuntary rests. Performance between these blocks is little affected. In very severe stress, such as requiring the eyes to move at the maximal attainable rate for 2 or more minutes, watering of the eyes may make reading impossible. The secretion of tears is interpreted as a spread of innervation to other effectors.

AUDITORY FATIGUE

Exposure to noise results in a hearing loss that is proportional to the duration of exposure. The cumulative effect of noise may finally result in permanent hearing loss. The recovery of acoustical threshold in riveters after a full day's work may take 15 hours. The recovery is considerably accelerated when the lunch pause of 1 hour is spent in noiseless surroundings; also the increase of the acoustical threshold at the end of the working day is much less under these conditions. Cotton plugs saturated with mineral oil introduced into the ear canal are recommended for protection.

Typists working under office conditions of high noise level from a busy street had a greater expenditure of energy than when the noise level of the same office had been reduced by acoustical methods. Reduction of the noise level increases the work output and diminishes errors, absenteeism, and employee turnover.

A varying noise causes a greater drop in work output than a steady noise. Pure tones of uniform loudness reduce output less seriously than does complex noise of equivalent loudness. Tones of frequencies above 512 CPS (cycles per second) reduce production more than lower frequencies of the same loudness, and above 512 CPS each increase in frequency is followed by further loss in production.

FOOT FATIGUE

Standing not only increases fatigue by cerebral anemia and reduction in cardiac output but also produces local fatigue of the feet, which frequently interferes with production in jobs that require prolonged standing. Change in posture from the upright to varying degrees of the recumbent position and periodic elevation of the feet serve as practical measures to reduce cardiovascular strain and fatigue, especially in hot environments.

FATIGUE AND INFECTIONS

Extreme fatigue lowers the general resistance of the body to pathogenic microorganisms and appears especially to predispose the subject to respiratory infections such as the common cold. The basis of this relation is not clear.

EXHAUSTION

At the outset of physical exhaustion there is a significant lymphocytosis suggestive of an "irritation phenomenon" such as is frequently seen in infections or other debilitating conditions. After a short but exhausting performance athletes frequently exhibit a syndrome consisting of pronounced weakness, profuse sweating, blurred vision, a throbbing headache, nausea, and vomiting. This has been termed *athletic sickness* and is due to the fact that sugar is withdrawn from the blood into the muscle tissue so rapidly that it cannot be replenished at once from the glycogen stores of the liver, and hypoglycemia results. This condition soon disappears with rest and has no unfavor-

159

able prognostic significance. Occasionally there is slight bleeding from the oral, nasal, and pharyngeal mucous membranes.

In more prolonged events such as a marathon run an exhausted athlete may display symptoms similar to those of insulin shock. Some of these runners show muscular twitching, extreme pallor, cold moist skin, nervous irritability, cyanosis, incoordination of muscular movements, extreme exhaustion, collapse, and unconsciousness. It is impossible to say which part of the athlete fails first since the whole organism breaks down together. Final physical exhaustion is reached when the cerebral distress from peripheral stimuli becomes so great that the athlete is unable to initiate any voluntary effort. Frequently the onset of exhaustion may be indicated by a clouding of the consciousness. The runner may continue to run but to do so reflexly, with complete amnesia concerning the events that transpire. A case has been recorded in which a tennis player was informed by his friends after the game that he had continually done foolish things, such as trying to give or throw his racket away. He had no recollection of this. This episode was also attributable to hypoglycemia, which may lead to confusion, epileptiform attacks, abdominal distress, migrainous headaches, vertigo, or precordial distress.

After vigorous exercise the muscles may go into contractures more readily than do rested muscles or it may not even be possible to relax them completely, and the presence of tremor may reveal a residue of activity. In some cases muscular spasm within a muscle may render an area ischemic or press on intramuscular pain fibers, resulting in myalgia. Hypersensitive muscles often develop myalgia, and once it appears the sensitivity of the muscle and its disposition to contract without apparent cause are increased.

Examination of the urine of athletes after severe exercise reveals the presence of formed elements (protein, epithelial, and red and white blood cell casts) that might under other circumstances be indicative of kidney disease. Albumin may be present in quantities varying from traces to a heavy cloud. The urine may be coffee colored or bloody after severe exercise because of the presence of hemoglobin.

During exercise accompanied by high velocity blood flow and concomitant intravascular friction there is some destruction of the blood cells. The more serious the disturbance of the general circulatory system, the more marked are the evidences of blood destruction found in the urine. In body-contact sports the factor of actual trauma to the kidneys is superimposed upon the effects resulting from exercise alone.

It is interesting that fatigue and exhaustion of the kind just described virtually never seem to result in lasting injury to a trained athlete. This is not true in the case of untrained men or convalescents.

A "generalized neuromuscular exhaustion syndrome" has been noted when victims of poliomyelitis and certain other patients have been exercised at or near their maximal capacity, resulting in a long-lasting decrement of performance.

APPRAISAL OF FATIGUE

Under ordinary conditions of exercise individuals can rate their own degree of fatigue, impending exhaustion, and subsequent recovery with fair accuracy. Those experienced in exercise, such as athletes, are more accurate in their estimates than nontrained persons. It is unclear whether this appraisal is based on kinesthetic perception of force, a sense of the activity of physiological systems at the time, or the approach of a point at which expiration cannot be completed. In the exotic environments of space and ocean depths astronauts and aquanauts lose their ability to judge their own load of work or state of fatigue and require external monitoring of their energy levels and physiological responses.

Indices of approaching exhaustion that can be employed for monitoring are:

1. Progressive fall of the systolic blood pressure
2. Rapid rise in respiratory rate
3. Rise in respiratory quotient (R.Q.)
4. Rise in body temperature (heat storage)
5. Reduction in work output
6. Rise in heart rate
7. Reduction in coordination, steadiness, and accuracy

Further and more detailed outlines of the endpoints of tolerance to exercise are presented in Chapter 2 in the *Laboratory Manual*.

PERCEIVED EXERTION

The sensation of physiological effort during the performance of a task is related to the workload and the heart rate. This perception of exertion is so acute that it can be used reliably as an indicator of somatic stress. Borg (1970) has constructed a scale of perceived exertion, using a number system based on the typical heart rate at efforts which appear to be light and hard.[1] On his scale 9 represents a 90 heart rate, 17 a 170 heart rate, and so on. His scale is as follows:

6		14	
7	very, very light	15	hard
8		16	
9	very light	17	very hard
10		18	
11	fairly light	19	very, very hard
12		20	
13	somewhat hard		

In performance terms a 12, or a 120 heart rate, represents a moderate effort, one which is about 50% of maximal capacity. Further guides to the classification of work and effort are found in Chapter 15 in the *Laboratory Manual.*

STRESS

Mechanism. Stress consists of the bodily changes produced by physiological or psychological conditions that tend to upset the homeostatic balance. Our understanding of how this comes about and whether exercise may elicit some features of the alarm reaction is by no means complete. In Selye's theory a stressor produces a generalized stress reaction in the body through either neural or hormonal pathways.[4] Acting through the nerves, it stimulates the secretion of adrenaline. Acting through the pituitary gland, the stressor produces an increased secretion of ACTH (adrenocorticotropic hormone). This in turn stimulates the adrenal cortex to produce glucocorticoids that increase gluconeogenesis, raising the concentration of liver glycogen and blood sugar. The pituitary gland secretes STH (somatotropic hormone), which Selye believes may act upon the adrenal cortex to stimulate production of mineralocorticoids that cause the retention of sodium and the loss of potassium. Under stress the pituitary secretions also intensify the production of TSH (thyroid-stimulating hormone), stimulating metabolism as a whole.

Measurement. Certain bodily changes are characteristic of increased corticoid activity—the disappearance of the white blood cells termed eosinophils, involution of the lymphatic tissue, and a generalized loss of body weight. The inverse relationship between the adrenal cortical activity and the number of circulating eosinophils in the blood has been utilized by a number of investigators as a convenient method of measuring the effects of stressors on the homeostatic balance. Eosinophil counts are lower in exercising than in resting men, signifying that exercise causes an activation of the adrenal cortex. In a study of university oarsmen it was found that on race days the coxswains and the coach also showed an eosinophil response comparable to that of the oarsmen, leading to the conclusion that emotional factors, not physical considerations alone, seem to be an important stimulus for the stress mechanism.

ROLE OF EXERCISE

Since exposure of the body to a given stress may result in the development of an adaptation that enables it to withstand that stress, it has been suggested that exercise may act to stabilize the homeostatic balance by providing a means of offsetting the physiological consequences of emotional stress.[6] A possible mechanism for this is that exercise may increase the size and lower the threshold of stimulation of the adrenal glands, thereby resulting in a greater reserve of antistress steroids and a shorter time of response to stress.

According to Selye one can discriminate between what he terms "superficial" and "deep" adaptation to stress.[5] The energy required for a superficial stress, such as moderate recreational exercise, is rapidly regenerated and the organism is strengthened by the experience. A deep stress, such as in incessant exhausting effort under continuous emotional strain, makes irreparable inroads on the organism and the adaptation energy is never regenerated. Such deep stress can be pleasurable, as when "burning the candle at both ends," or painful, as in suffering under concentration camp conditions. This "wear and tear" of an excessively stressful life is presumed by Selye to be responsible for a shortened life span.

PRESTART PHENOMENON

An explanation of physiological processes that underlie the stress response of athletes in competition has been offered. This explanation does not rely on hormonal mechanisms but turns toward Pavlov's doctrine of higher nervous activity. It is from the standpoint of conditioned reflex regulation of body functions in exercise that the attempt to elucidate the stressful effect of competitive conditions in athletic activities is made.

The competitive setting is regarded as a conditioned stimulus that causes body activities to increase even before the event starts. These elevations in body functions prior to activity are known as *prestart* increases. They can be made to disappear simply by discontinuing preliminary exercises—in other words, stopping the "warming up" activities before the contests. By doing this, functional depression is sometimes seen instead of the former prestart elevations in function when preliminary exercises had been the athlete's habit before competition.

These studies suggest that the competitive setting influences the state of the organism before the start and also affects its activity during the period of the effort and in the restorative period after its termination.

This theory has been used to explain various peculiarities of function regulation in athletes, such as individual differences in cardiovascular response. Greater increase in pulse rate and blood pressure are found among individuals of the "weak" or "quiet" type because of their higher nervous activity according to Pavlov's classification. The "active" or "unrestrained" athletes do not overreact this way and perform better than the former group in important competitions such as the Olympic games. Training does not reduce the prestart responses; in fact the "weak" type tends to get worse.

163

Age is a factor, adolescents showing higher prestart reactions than adults. The explanation is given that overreaction may be caused by the increased excitability of the growing individual, particularly in the period of sexual maturation. During adolescence functional efficiency is less than in adulthood.

Reduction of blood eosinophils during the prestart state and during competitive effort is explained on the basis of a linkage between conditioned reflex reactions and the increased activity of endocrine glands.

STRESS SYNDROME IN TRAINING AND OVERTRAINING

Well-spaced periods of regular light exercise are thought to benefit the individual by increasing his nonspecific resistance to such unfavorable stresses as overheating, cooling, hypoxia, irradiation, and infections. On the other hand, athletes in competition in the presence of great emotional tensions often work too hard to obtain this benefit. As a result their nonspecific resistance to stress is lowered, certain vegetative functions, that is, sleep and appetite, are disrupted, and motor skills that are not fixed or automatized are coordinated with difficulty.

In forced training under high emotional tensions the nonspecific resistance to stress is lost first, the vegetative functions deteriorate second, and finally the motor coordinations are affected—eventually resulting in a decrement in performance. This is seen as the mechanism of *overtraining,* and it may be the cause of increased morbidity observed in a number of top athletes.

Since in severe athletic competition physical work or emotional tensions cannot be removed, means of meeting these stresses are sought such as diet, pharmacological and physiotherapeutic media, and improved routines of training, work, and relaxation.

References

1. Borg, G.: Perceived exertion as an indicator of somatic stress, Scand. J. Rehab. Med. **2**:92, 1970.
2. Lind, A., and McNicol, G.: Cardiovascular responses to holding and carrying weights by hand and by shoulder harness, J. Appl. Physiol. **25**:261, 1968.
3. Molbech, S., and Johansen, S.: Endurance time in static work during partial curarization, J. Appl. Physiol. **27**:44, 1969.
4. Selye, H.: The stress of life, New York, 1956, McGraw-Hill Book Co.
5. Selye, H.: Personal communication, 1974.
6. Steadman, R., and Sharkey, B.: Exercise as a stressor, J. Sports Med. Phys. Fitness **9**:230-235, 1969.
7. Wilmore, J.: Influence of motivation on physical work capacity and performance, J. Appl. Physiol. **24**:459, 1968.

Suggested readings

Åstrand, P., and Rodahl, K.: Textbook of work physiology, New York, 1970, McGraw-Hill Book Co.
Bartley, S.: Fatigue: mechanism and management, ed. 2, New York, 1962, McGraw-Hill Book Co.
Costill, D., and Fox, E.: Energetics of marathon running, Med. Sci. Sports **1**:81, 1969.

Falls, H., and Richardson, R.: Comparison of recovery procedures for the reduction of exercise stress, Res. Quart. 38:550, 1967.

Jacobson, E., editor: Tension in medicine, Springfield, Ill., 1967, Charles C Thomas, Publisher.

Johnson, W. H., and Buskirk, E. R., editors: Science and medicine of exercise and sports, ed. 2, New York, 1973, Harper & Row, Publishers.

Pierson, W., and Rich, G.: Energy expenditure and fatigue during simple repetitive tasks, Human Factors 9:563, 1967.

Shephard, R.: Endurance fitness, Toronto, 1969, University of Toronto Press.

Simonson, E., editor: Physiology of work capacity and fatigue, Springfield, Ill., 1971, Charles C Thomas, Publisher.

Williams, C. G., and others: The capacity for endurance work in highly trained men, Inter. Z. angew. Physiol. 26:141, 1968.

Wyndham, C. H., and others: Physiological requirements for world-class performances in endurance running, South Afr. Med. J. 9:996, 1969.

13 NUTRITION AND ERGOGENIC AIDS

NUTRITION

Any diet that contains a wide variety of foods in sufficient quantity to maintain normal body weight and to support growth is adequate for individuals in all categories of exercise habits—from sedentary to athletic. This concept is generally true, but there are certain dietary modifications that affect body functions in vigorous exercise.

Also, exercise affects the nutritional state of an individual. It is with these phenomena that this chapter is principally concerned.

QUANTITY OF FOOD

The increased energy metabolism during muscular exercise must be supported by an equivalent increase in energy supply. If the demand exceeds the supply, body energy stores and eventually the body tissues themselves are consumed in the course of the activity. The depletion of body tissues impairs the functions of the organs of which these tissues are a part.

The quantity of food required by active men varies to such an extent among the individuals in a group and also in a single person from day to day that the establishment of a standard dietary requirement for a group or a person would be meaningless. The total daily energy requirement for an active man may range from 3,000 to 8,000 Calories, depending upon his size and physical condition and the severity of the work performed each day. An experiment on rats demonstrates some of the variables that affect the daily energy requirement. Twelve female albino rats from 4 to 12 months old were observed while quantitative variations in activity, food intake, and environmental temperature were induced. When activity was increased, the weight decreased if food intake was constant. When the food intake was increased, there was an increase in body weight when activity was constant. When environmental temperature was increased, there was a decrease in body weight when activity was constant. The quantity of food required to support increased physical activity and environmental stress is soon indicated by alterations in body weight.

A similar demonstration has been obtained in man. Light workers, clerks, and mechanics, were observed to have the least caloric intake. The intake was greater among workers who performed heavier work. Of interest also was an elevated food intake among the extremely sedentary individuals, the stallholders and supervisors.

BODY FAT

Various types of competitive athletics require different proportions of fat to muscle for maximum performance. A minimum amount of fat is desirable in a distance runner, a high jumper, and a gymnast. These athletes must move their own weight in a highly economical fashion, and any added weight taxes the strength and endurance. Distance swimmers need a certain amount of fat distributed near the skin surface to diminish the heat loss to the water. Football players, especially linemen, employ the fat portion of their mass in achieving momentum and also as a cushion to absorb the shocks of repeated contact.

During severe athletic training the normal amount of fat is reduced to a minimum because this tissue is considered an encumbrance. It is an extra load to be carried and it impedes the violent contraction of muscles. Reduction of fat in obese persons increases work efficiency. This results from the reduced metabolic cost of maintaining a decreased tissue mass, rather than from a modification of intrinsic energetic mechanisms of muscle.

During a season of athletic training a slight loss in body weight may be expected at first due to a loss of fat. The initial loss is followed by a slow gain attributable to increased muscular development. One evidence of *staleness* or *overtraining* is a gradual loss of weight; that is, the weight loss during exercise is not regained as it should be. Rest and feeding are indicated when weight continues to decline.

WEIGHT AND BODY FAT REDUCTION BY EXERCISE

Exercise alone, without cutting down on food intake, can reduce body weight and fatness in overweight persons if the energy expenditure is high enough. While eating as much as usual, performance of a daily exercise program consisting of covering about 5 miles at any speed will reduce body weight and skinfold thickness. Apparently caloric intake regulated by appetite and satiety fails to compensate for the increased Calories expended by exercise, with the result that fat stores are reduced.

"MAKING WEIGHT"

"Making weight" by wrestlers, boxers, weight lifters, and jockeys is accomplished by profuse sweating and by abstaining from food and liquids for a few hours before weighing in. Weight loss up to 10 pounds (representing 5% of the body weight) was accomplished without any measurable deleterious effects in six wrestlers. Weight loss was induced by a procedure considered orthodox by wrestling coaches. Food and water were withheld. The wrestlers, wearing heavy sweat suits, worked on the mats and alternated this with sitting in a heated cabinet. This abnormal loss of weight is regained in part after weighing in by eating and drinking. More than 5 pounds may be regained in a few hours.

WEIGHT LOSS IN ATHLETICS

Losses of weight exceeding 10 pounds in 1½ hours have been reported during football games at the beginning of training. During especially exciting games a substitute who has been "sweating out" the entire game on the bench has been observed to lose 5 pounds. This weight is entirely and rapidly regained after eating and drinking.

SEMISTARVATION

A diet that is inadequate to support the needs of the body will soon result in a deterioration in fitness for exercise. When the daily caloric intake is reduced, the day-to-day output of voluntary work is reduced proportionally. A substandard diet causes a reduction in the performance of the physiological systems.

DIETARY NOTIONS AMONG ATHLETES

The problem of what constitutes the optimal diet for athletes in training for competitive contests is probably older than organized sports. Many of the dietary superstitions of primitive tribes are based on the idea that certain foods—in particular the meat of certain animals—endow the consumer with the qualities of strength, endurance, and courage with which his prey was identified. Trainers and coaches have inherited something of this theory and have applied it to the athletes under their tutelage.

One of the most widespread of such practices has been the advocacy of eating large quantities of meat to replenish "muscle substance" following the "losses" supposedly incurred during severe muscular work.

This particular practice was first recorded in Greece during the fifth century B.C. and ascribed to two athletes who had deviated from the hitherto traditional (chiefly vegetarian) diet of the time to a regimen entailing the intake of large quantities of meat and leading to increased body bulk. The fifth century B.C. also saw a change in cultural outlooks on physical fitness. Instead of being considered essentially a broad prerequisite in the defense of the country, physical fitness became subordinate to training for specific sports, excellence in which was considered superior to almost all other values.

There are many dietary notions among athletes, and athletes have turned in championship performances after training on diets that in the light of accepted dietary standards would be considered inadequate in many respects. Many champions are vegetarians, others eat large quantities of meat, some of it raw. Most athletes reduce the intake of fat in their training diets, but others make no changes whatsoever and eat what they please or what is served to them with no regard to the possible effect of nutrition upon performance. These experiences are in line with recent experimental evidence that the ratio of fat, carbohydrate, and protein in the diet may be altered considerably before changes in work performance appear.

Within wide limits there appear to be certain dietary principles that are associated with improved performance in work and sport. Positive evidence for these principles is accumulating, but a well-controlled experiment has yet to be performed.

DIETARY RATIO OF CARBOHYDRATE, FAT, AND PROTEIN

Carbohydrates. Carbohydrates are essential dietary constituents but are not the exclusive fuel for muscle. The amounts of carbohydrate used are related to the work level. The depletion of blood sugar levels below 60 mg.% results in exhaustion. A low blood sugar level may interfere with the metabolism of the central nervous system to such an extent that a mild degree of oxygen want brings on symptoms similar to those obtained under conditions of extreme hypoxia. This indicates that the fatigue of protracted, exhausting exercise has a cerebral component. Associated with the fatigue of prolonged work is a loss of mechanical efficiency because of faulty coordination. Theoretically a diet rich in carbohydrates should contribute to the maintenance of normal blood sugar concentration for longer periods during prolonged physical work. Even though this is not always actually the case and exhaustion often occurs with a high blood sugar concentration and at high R.Q.'s, the theory is supported by observations in which industrial workers are found to work more efficiently on a carbohydrate-rich than on a fat-rich diet. Evidently the blood sugar level does not always reflect the nutritional condition of the muscles, and also conditions other than the type of fuel affect the R.Q. Although the mechanisms of carbohydrate utilization are not entirely clear, there is sufficient evidence to support the principle that the athlete in training should have extra carbohydrate in his diet.

Early studies of the effects of different diets on physical performance showed that subjects working to exhaustion could work much longer after high carbohydrate meals than after mixed, high fat, or high protein meals. In these studies, the respiratory quotient (R.Q.) was used as an indirect determination of the proportion in which the various food substances were being metabolized, and mixed and protein diets give intermediate R.Q.'s.

The R.Q. gives no information about which part of the body's carbohydrate store is being utilized. Furthermore, the R.Q. shifts with the intensity of work, becoming higher at more intense workloads. This would suggest that more carbohydrate is being used, but other factors may negate this assumption. R.Q.'s greater than 1.0 are common in work of high intensity. This indicates that factors other than food metabolism, such as hyperventilation are affecting the R.Q. These vagaries make it impossible to draw conclusions regarding the role of nutrition in physical performance from R.Q. measurements.

Glycogen supercompensation. In 1966, Bergstrom and Hultman introduced a technique of needle biopsy allowing for direct measurement of muscle glycogen stores before, during, and after exercise.[2] In a series of studies of fasting, heavy endurance exercise, and dietary variation, they investigated the variation in glycogen stores. Next, in collaboration with Hermansen and Saltin, the relation of muscle glycogen content and performance of prolonged exercise was investigated.[1]

These observations showed that a depletion of glycogen stores was followed by a resupply which, in some instances, was more than double the original amount. This finding led to a manipulation of diet in order to improve performance. In events which continue for 30 minutes or more, endurance seems to be improved by the additional muscle glycogen which is available for aerobic glycolysis.

A typical 7-day protocol for glycogen supercompensation follows:

	Diet			Exercise	
Day	Carbohydrate	Fat	Protein	Type	Intensity
1	No	High	Normal	Specific to event	High
2	No	High	Normal	Specific to event	High
3	No	High	Normal	Major muscles employed in event	Exhaustive
4	High	No	Normal	Anaerobic nonspecific	Moderate

	Diet			Exercise	
Day	Carbohydrate	Fat	Protein	Type	Intensity
5	High	No	Normal	Anaerobic nonspecific	Moderate
6	High	No	Normal	Active rest	Light
7	High	No	No	Competition	

During this 7-day protocol, the muscle glycogen falls from the normal 3-4 gm./100 gm. of muscle to a very low level, about 1 gm./100 gm. at the beginning of the fourth day, and then rises to a level above 4 gm./100 gm. on the seventh day. If there are no ill effects from this severe alteration in dietary regimen, endurance performance may be markedly improved.

There are several risks of glycogen depletion and glycogen overloading. Depletion of carbohydrate stores causes an increased production of ketone bodies and an increased excretion of nitrogen.[3] Depletion of glycogen stores affects brain function since the brain uses carbohydrate almost exclusively for its metabolic processes. Symptoms of glucose deficiency in the brain are fatigue, changes in mood and disposition, irritability, slow thinking, lightheadedness, nausea, dizziness, and fainting. After the first day without carbohydrate the subject may suffer withdrawal symptoms and have an extreme craving for sweets. Athletes attempting this regimen have been observed to fight over a bottle of orange juice.

Those who are sensitive to fluctuations in blood glucose, such as diabetics and prediabetics, suffer an insulin reaction on the fourth day of the regimen because of the sudden load of carbohydrate. Insulin shock or unconsciousness may occur.

Body fluid and electrolyte balance is affected by the glycogen supercompensation regimen. For every gram of glycogen stored, 2.7 grams of water are also stored. The subject becomes waterlogged and this excess weight is a burden in events in which the body must be lifted.

The glycogen supercompensation routine should not be practiced frequently, probably not more than twice a year—and not in close succession, even by those who seem to tolerate it well. It would be foolhardy to attempt this manipulation for the first time on the week of an important competition.

Protein. Protein in the form of meat is consumed in large quantities by athletes and men doing hard physical work. The quantity of protein needed for bringing about the highest capacity for work is probably much less than the amounts ordinarily consumed by active men. A long-distance racing cyclist who was a vegetarian performed with higher gross efficiencies on a low-protein diet, but he had better endurance on a high-protein diet. Another man lived for years on a diet that provided a daily intake of only about 30 grams of protein. His physical efficiency was high, and he could perform severe exercise without increasing the nitrogen excretion.

A carefully controlled study of the effect of protein restriction on men working in the heat revealed no essential change in fitness for work in either temperate or tropical environment when dietary protein was varied from 76 to 105 and 149 grams per day, although a 4% higher work metabolism was associated with the highest protein intake.

To summarize, the dietary protein intake of an athlete may vary widely (75 to 150 grams daily) without any noticeable effect upon performance of intermittent (speed) activities. When work is prolonged (endurance), higher intakes of dietary protein comprising 12 to 15% of the daily caloric requirement may be beneficial.

Fat. Subjects maintained on a fat-rich diet showed a smaller net muscular efficiency than when they were on a carbohydrate-rich diet. By plotting R.Q. against net efficiency, extrapolation to pure fat metabolism (R.Q. of 0.70) indicated 11% greater energy expenditure per unit of work than for pure carbohydrate metabolism (R.Q. of 1).

Even though fat-rich diets are associated with reduced endurance and muscular efficiency, the exclusion of all fat from the diet is not recommended. Aside from the important vitamins and certain essential fatty acids in fats, there appears to be a factor associated with fat that is necessary for the normal metabolism of carbohydrate. A disturbed carbohydrate metabolism has been observed in rats maintained more than 1 year on a fat-deficient diet. In the light of these considerations it would seem that the amount of fat in the diet that will maintain a good nutritional condition and yet not materially reduce endurance or muscular efficiency is about 100 grams daily. Normal intake of fat should not supply more than 45% of the total Calories. The fat content of the diet during training for an athletic event in which particularly high levels of performance are desired may be reduced to 75 grams or 20% of the total Calories per day. The protein and carbohydrate content in this training diet would be approximately 15 and 65%, respectively, of the total calories per day.

VITAMINS

Vitamins in the diet are essential for good performance in work and sport. Following the principle that if a little of something is good, then a large amount of the same thing should be better, the discovery and identification of vitamins led to the administration of large doses of these substances in the hope that such a superdiet would result in superperformance. When vitamins were lacking in the diet, these superdiets did improve performance, but extra vitamins added to normal diets did not improve performance. Healthy young men expending an average of 3,700 to 4,200 Calories per day were not benefited by a daily dietary supply in excess of 1.7 mg. thiamine chloride, 2.4 mg. riboflavin, and 70 mg. ascorbic acid. Fortification of normal diets with vitamins does not improve fitness for work and exercise. This has been shown in static and dynamic work tests, muscular endurance tests, work in heavy industry, and treadmill-running tests. In neither brief, exhausting exercise nor in prolonged, severe exercise are there any indications of benefit due to dietary supplements of thiamine, riboflavin, nicotinic acid, pyridoxine, pantothenic acid, and ascorbic acid or to vitamin B complex given intravenously.

Vitamins are stored in varying amounts in the body. When diets are deficient in vitamins, the stores are depleted, and the consequent deterioration in physical condition results in a reduction in the capacity for muscular work. The effects of deficiencies of the various vitamins are discussed separately because of the specific nature of the results in each case.

Vitamin A deficiency. In men maintained for 6 months on less than 100 international units of vitamin A daily after a preliminary massive dose period of 30 days, there was no change in plasma vitamin A levels, visual thresholds, or scores in moderate and exhausting work tests. The fact that vitamin A did not disappear from the plasma in these subjects indicates that their reserves were not exhausted. The depletion of vitamin A stores in the body takes a very long time so that there is a substantial margin of safety in most cases.

Performance may be restricted by lack of vitamin A because of the effects on vision. People subsisting for long periods on diets very low in vitamin A develop night blindness. Vitamin A intake may affect color vision. The daily administration of carotene to factory workers was followed by a 75% reduction in the number of rejections for offcolor parts of stoves assembled by them. Among normal persons subsisting on diets not markedly deficient in vitamin A, there is little relation between vitamin A intake, blood vitamin A concentration, and dark adaptation.

Vitamin B deficiency. Diets containing about one-third of the recommended intake of vitamin B complex do not lead to deterioration in physical capacity within 2 weeks if the physical and environmental stresses are not great. Subjects put on a vitamin-deficient diet containing 0.16 mg. thiamine, 0.15 mg. riboflavin, and 1.8 mg. niacin per 1,000 Calories displayed no change in work capacity, psychomotor test scores, or clinical condition during the 2 weeks' deficiency period. A similar lack of effect was observed when riboflavin only was limited to 0.31 mg. per 1,000 Calories.

Thiamine is involved in carbohydrate metabolism. When thiamine is deficient, pyruvic acid accumulates in abnormal amounts and muscular activity is depressed. Ten healthy men placed on a more severe thiamine restriction, doing harder physical labor and in a colder environmental temperature, showed a clear diminution in scores in physical tests in 1

173

week. A trained subject who was fed a diet deficient in thiamine and riboflavin during a hot summer showed a significant decrease in performance on a bicycle ergometer.

Vitamin B deficiency over a long period produces a deterioration in fitness for exercise even in the absence of hard physical labor or environmental stress. The requirements for thiamine, riboflavin, and niacin are probably proportional to the intensity of the metabolism. It is justifiable to advise an increased intake of B vitamins when work is increased and when the stress of the environment is great. With a reasonably good diet this is guaranteed by simply increasing the total food intake.

Vitamin C deficiency. Low levels of vitamin C intake do not measurably reduce work performance and extra large dosages do not increase it. Men receiving only 40 mg. of ascorbic acid daily did not differ significantly in fitness for exercise nor in susceptibility to heat exhaustion from men receiving 540 mg. daily.

Vitamin E deficiency. Rats on diets deficient in vitamin E show degenerative changes in muscles and diminished capacity for treadmill running. Whether man shows similar responses to vitamin E deficiency has not yet been determined.

DISTRIBUTION OF MEALS

The effect of various distributions of meals throughout the day upon work performance indicates that frequent feeding is desirable. Three meals a day are superior to two meals a day with respect to physical efficiency. Production in industry increases when midforenoon and midafternoon snacks are provided. From the point of view of industrial efficiency, workers should be allowed a reasonable freedom of choice of what they eat and drink during the rest periods.

A breakfast of coffee alone is insufficient to support a full morning of activity. A light breakfast consisting of fruit, one slice of buttered toast, milk, and coffee, if desired, will increase the level of performance in maximal work output and choice reaction time and also will decrease the magnitude of tremor during the latter part of the morning. A heavy breakfast, consisting of fruit, cereal and cream, egg, bacon, toast and jam, milk, and coffee, if desired, is also better than coffee alone. It is doubtful that the physiological responses after a heavy breakfast are better than after a light breakfast, especially if the morning's work is not strenuous.

PREEXERCISE MEAL

Much attention has been given to the need for avoiding fatty, spiced, gas-forming, and acid-forming foods in the preexercise meal. Many athletes adhere to this rule, but others do not. Two hours before an Olympic swimmer broke the world's record in the 200 meter butterfly event she consumed a lunch consisting of two hamburgers with onions, french fried potatoes with ketchup, a root beer float, three brownies, and a candy bar.

Is it phenomenal that an athlete can achieve a world class performance after violating "common sense" rules of diet? Apparently not. Varsity athletes were studied by shifting their diet from the conventional training-table regimen to an opposite one consisting entirely of a wide variety of nonrecommended foods. A typical menu consisted of cantaloupe, chili and beans, salami sandwich with mustard, pork chop, french fried potatoes and gravy, dill pickle, cream pie, and milk. Within 2 hours after such menus the athletes performed either strenuous physical tests in the laboratory or engaged in athletic training or competition. Careful observation of their performance and well-being revealed no effect of the nonrecommended diet.

If the rule banning certain foods can be lifted, there will be one less restriction placed on the athlete.

ERGOGENIC AIDS

Attempts to increase work output by means other than training has led to many bizarre practices. The effectiveness of any substance or procedure in enhancing strength or endurance is always clouded by psychogenic factors. If the participant believes something is going to help, or hinder, performance, it will often have the predicted effect. It is then the ergogenic aid, not the belief in it, which gets the credit. Many drugs are misused and abused in the search for instant improvement.

Nutritional supplements. In previous paragraphs we have discussed the important role of vitamins, minerals, carbohydrates, fats, and proteins in supporting exercise. When used in overabundance in attempts to improve fitness or performance, the extra amounts are excreted or they may become toxic.

Vitamins. Even though vitamins are lost in the sweat during heavy exertion, exercise does not increase the body's requirement for vitamins. When taken in excess the water-soluble vitamins B complex and C are excreted in the urine. The fat-soluble vitamins can be stored, but excessive amounts may be toxic. None of the vitamins taken as supplements improve strength, endurance, efficiency, or performance.

Carbohydrates. Last-minute candy bars or other carbohydrates taken before a race do not supply extra energy or increase performance. Carbohydrate is not assimilated in such a brief time. The reserves are established by food eaten several days before the event.

Proteins. A pregame meal of steak and eggs is common among American athletes; however, such meals may increase the risk of coronary heart disease. Studies of increased protein intake have shown no beneficial effects on performance.[5] Protein is used as a major energy substrate only in malnourished subjects.[4]

DRUGS

It is probable that nearly every known drug has been used in attempts to improve performance. The most common drugs abused by athletes are amphetamines and anabolic steroids.

Amphetamines. Amphetamines, known as "pep pills," were originally developed to simulate the effects of adrenalin (epinephrine). Adrenalin, released during emotional excitement, stimulates the central nervous system, increases the strength of muscles, increases the force and rate of the heartbeat, constricts blood vessels, allays fatigue, and suppresses the appetite.

During the athletic contest, adrenalin is secreted at the appropriate moments when an extra effort is needed. At these same moments there is usually further stimulation of the central nervous system by cheering from spectators, encouragement from the coach and teammates, and shouting by the player himself.

A direct dose of adrenalin injected at these moments would probably impair judgment and possibly cause hallucinations.

Amphetamine pills cause a state of excitement which is unpredictable in individuals due to differences in sensitivity. In some, the drug is highly toxic. In using amphetamine pills there is no way to reduce their stimulating effect when it is not needed, or to apply the stimulating effect at the moments when it may be most useful. The result is unpredictable effect on performance and early exhaustion due to depletion of energy reserves.

Anabolic steroids. Androgenic anabolic steroids are compounded to resemble the male sex hormone, testosterone. When there are deficiencies in testosterone, administration of the hormone or the synthetic steroid will stimulate growth, increase body weight, increase bone density, and increase virility. In a healthy male without deficiency, the addition of the drug suppresses testosterone production, decreasing libido and fertility. Large doses diminish testicular size and function. Prolonged administration impairs liver function and may be linked with liver cancer. Anabolic steroids cause virilization in females, increasing body hair and other masculine characteristics. There is no convincing evidence that anabolic steroids can increase the strength and working capacity of normal healthy athletes.

Spokesmen for the American Medical Association state that no drug or other artificial substance can reliably or safely benefit a normal individual in endurance or strength or elicit a greater athletic performance than he already is capable of through his own natural resources or natural ability.

PHYSICAL AND MECHANICAL AIDS

Oxygen inhalation. Oxygen cannot be stored, so extra quantities inhaled *before* an event cannot improve or prolong performance. If it were practical to breathe extra oxygen *during* an exhaustive event it would probably decrease blood lactate, lower the heart rate, and delay exhaustion. Administration of oxygen *after* exertion has no demonstrable physiological effect in enhancing recovery.

Medically, the purpose of oxygen inhalation therapy is to help alleviate distress from deficient oxygen uptake in cardiac or respiratory illness.

Massage. Massage does not increase the strength of muscles. It relaxes them by means of a reflex effect mediated from the receptors in the skin to the central nervous system. There is also a reflex vasodilatation of the peripheral blood vessels. Centripetal pressures assist the return flow of blood and lymph. Such effects of massage are useful in therapy but are useless for improving performance of healthy athletes.

References

1. Bergstrom, J., and others: Diet, muscle glycogen, and physical performance, Acta Physiol. Scand. **71**:140, 1967.
2. Bergstrom, J., and Hultman, E.: The effect of exercise on muscle glycogen and electrolytes in normals, Scand. J. Clin. Lab. Invest. **18**:16, 1966.
3. Consolazio, C. F., and Johnson, H. L.: Dietary carbohydrate and work capacity, Am. J. Clin. Nutr. **25**:85, 1972.
4. Nelson, R. A., Hayles, A. B., and Wahner, H. W.: Exercise and urinary nitrogen excretion in two chronically malnourished subjects, Mayo Clin. Proc. **48**:549, 1973.
5. Rasch, P. J., and Pierson, W. R.: Effect of a protein dietary supplement on muscular strength and hypertrophy, Am. J. Clin. Nutr. **11**:530, 1962.

Suggested readings

Bourne, G.: Nutrition and exercise. In Falls, H., editor: Exercise physiology, New York, 1968, Academic Press, Inc.

Jokl, E.: Nutrition, exercise and body composition, Springfield, Ill., 1964, Charles C Thomas, Publisher.

Mayer, J., and Bullen, B.: Nutrition and athletic performance, Physiol. Rev. **40**: 369, 1960.

Morgan, W. P.: Ergogenic aids and muscular performance, New York, 1972, Academic Press, Inc.

14 EFFECTS OF EXERCISE ON BLOOD AND BODY FLUIDS

BLOOD CHANGES DURING EXERCISE

The full significance of blood changes during exercise can be appreciated only when they are considered against the background of the overall function of the blood.

The cells of the body can function normally only when they are provided with oxygen and food materials, when their waste products are removed promptly, and when their temperature and acidity are carefully regulated. The maintenance of these stable conditions is the principal function of the blood.

The normal concentration of blood glucose (about 100 mg. per 100 ml.) represents a balance between the rates at which glucose is added to the blood (from the liver and the intestines) and removed from the blood by the tissues that use it. This balance is maintained during light and moderate work, so that there is little change in the level of the blood sugar. In more strenuous exertion adrenalin is secreted in large amounts, and this hormone stimulates the delivery of larger amounts of glucose from the liver, so that the concentration of the blood glucose may rise considerably. If the exercise is both strenuous and prolonged, the level of the blood glucose may finally fall below resting levels due to exhaustion of the stores of liver glycogen that give rise to the blood glucose. In short bursts of anaerobic work, such as sprints, there is ordinarily little change in the concentration of blood glucose either during or after the exertion.

It will be recalled that contracting muscles produce lactic acid when their supply of oxygen is not adequate to meet the energy requirements. The rise in the concentration of blood lactic acid during exercise is therefore an indication of the amount of anaerobic metabolism involved. The normal resting concentration of blood lactate is about 5 to 10 mg. per 100 ml. At the beginning of exercise the concentration of blood lactate rises because the delivery of oxygen to the muscles cannot be increased immediately. If a steady state is reached, the level of blood lactate ceases to rise and may actually fall as exercise continues. If a steady state is not achieved, blood lactate rises throughout the period of exercise and may reach levels as high as 200 mg. per 100 ml. The highest blood lactate concentration reported during exercise, so far as we are aware, is 357 mg. per 100 ml. This occurred during maximal exercise of short duration on a bicycle ergometer and was associated with an arterial blood pH of 6.80 (below the value usually considered compatible with life).[2]

When a subject performs different types of exercise, the extent of the rise in blood lactate is an index of the severity of the work. When several subjects perform the same task, the rise in blood lactate is greater the less the cardiovascular fitness of the subject.

When an acid such as lactic acid is poured into the blood in increased amounts during exercise, a dangerous rise in blood acidity is prevented by the action of *buffers,* which neutralize the acids. Carbon dioxide presents little difficulty because it is readily eliminated in the lungs. Lactic acid is buffered by the blood bicarbonate, which is accordingly reduced in amount. Very strenuous exercise, especially if it is prolonged, may produce so much lactic acid that the bicarbonate buffer is greatly reduced in amount, and the blood acidity begins to increase rapidly. Exhaustion ordinarily follows soon after. Methods of determining blood lactate are described in Chapter 13 in the *Laboratory Manual.*

Effects of exercise on the blood cells. Changes in blood cell counts during exercise have been emphasized out of all proportion to their importance, perhaps because of the ease with which the studies can be carried out.

The red blood cell count is frequently increased in the early stages of exercise, probably because of simple hemoconcentration (transfer of fluid from the blood to the tissues). During more prolonged exercise, fluid passes into the blood, and the resulting dilution of course lowers the red blood cell count. Very strenuous exertion may also cause an increased rate of destruction of red blood cells due to compression of the capillaries by muscular contraction and to increased velocity of blood flow. This is especially noticeable in persons of sedentary habits who sporadically indulge in exercise.

There is a rather general belief that the number of red blood cells per unit volume of blood is increased by training, but the actual experimental evidence in man is not very convincing.

White blood cell changes during exercise. Exercise of any type increases the leukocyte count; even random activity causes a significant rise above the basal level. Following brief periods of strenuous exertion the increase in the white blood cell count is caused primarily by an increased number of lymphocytes, but if the exercise is more prolonged, the further rise in cell count is caused almost entirely by an increase in the neutrophils. The rise in the leukocyte count during exercise is remarkably rapid. Thus a count of 35,000 cells per cubic millimeter of blood (normal count, 5,000 to 8,000) has been recorded immediately following a quarter-mile race lasting less than 1 minute. The most reasonable explanation for the increases in the white blood cell count during exercise is that large numbers of the cells, which at rest are adherent to the walls of the blood vessels, are suddenly washed into the circulation by the increased volume and velocity of blood flow.

The greater the degree of stress associated with exercise, the greater is the rise in the white blood cell count, so that less fit persons show a greater rise than do athletes when the same exercise is performed by both. The reason for this is not at all clear.

Stress of any sort (strenuous exertion, excitement, anxiety) results in an increased secretion of the hormones of the adrenal cortex, and one of the results produced by these hormones is a decrease in the number of eosinophils in the blood. The maximal effect is usually reached several hours after the stress and serves as a useful index of its severity. Associated with the decrease in eosinophils, there is also a decrease in the numbers of lymphocytes and an increase in the numbers of neutrophils. The mechanism of the production of these changes in leukocytes is not well understood.

BLOOD COAGULATION AND FIBRINOLYSIS

Exercise enhances blood coagulation and could lead to an acute thrombotic event were it not counteracted by a simultaneous increase in blood fibrinolytic activity. A marked shortening of clotting time occurs immediately after exercise; clotting time returns to normal within a few hours, probably because of an increase in the antihemophilic factor activity. The effect of exercise on fibrinolysis is independent of the blood coagulation mechanism. The increase in blood fibrinolytic activity is caused by an increase in the concentration of a plasminogen activator. The degree of fibrinolytic response depends on the exercise intensity and on its duration. Brief exposures to strenuous exercise cause increased fibrinolytic activity, which disappears within an hour after exercise. Prolonged exercise increases the fibrinolytic activity for several hours.[1]

FLUID BALANCE

Fluid compartments and their measurement. The body of the average person has a water content of about 60% to 70%. The actual amount of water in a given individual (expressed as percent of body weight) varies inversely with his fat content, since fat is simply added to the body without the addition of a corresponding amount of water.

The body fluids can be considered to occupy several anatomical compartments separated by barriers and having characteristic differences in composition. The primary subdivisions are intracellular and extracellular compartments. The extracellular compartment in turn may be subdivided into vascular and interstitial compartments, the latter including all the fluids outside the cells and outside the vascular system. It includes the fluid that surrounds and bathes the tissue cells and certain localized collections of fluid such as the cerebrospinal fluid, the synovial fluid of the joints, and the intraocular fluid.

The total amount of water in the body ("total body water") can be measured by injecting intravenously a known amount of some substance that diffuses freely through all the body water. From its measured concentration in the blood plasma after distribution is complete, the "volume of distribution" (in this case the total body water) can be calculated. For example, if 5 grams of the test substance is injected, and its concentration in the blood plasma is found to be 0.1 gram per liter, the total volume of distribution is $5/0.1 = 50$ liters. Among the substances that have been used to measure total body water are isotopically labeled water, urea, antipyrine, and antipyrine derivatives.

Since the fat-free portion of the body has a reasonably constant water content (about 72%), measurement of total body water permits the calculation of the fat content of the body. For example, if the measured water content of an individual is 54% and letting X = percent fat, then

$$X = 25 \text{ or the fat content is 25% of the body weight}$$
$$(100)(0.54) = (100 - X)(0.72) + (X)(0)$$

The total extracellular fluid volume can be measured in a similar manner from the volume of distribution of a substance that diffuses throughout the extracellular compartment but does not enter the cells. Thiocyanate is a convenient (although not very accurate) test substance. Better test substances are inulin, sucrose, mannitol, thiosulfate, and radioactive sodium or chloride. The spaces measured by these different substances vary somewhat, but they usually fall within the range of 15 to 19% of body weight (except for thiocyanate, which has a "space" of about 23 to 24%). The plasma volume, measured by the volume of distribution of substances that do not leave the blood or that leave at a slow and measurable rate, is about 5% of body weight. Suitable substances for measuring plasma volume include plasma albumin labeled with ^{131}I, and the blue dye T-1824 (Evans blue), which combines with plasma albumin after intravenous injection.

The intracellular volume cannot be measured directly, but it can be calculated by subtracting the extracellular fluid volume from the total body water. Thus, if total body water is 50 liters and extracellular volume is 15 liters, the volume of the intracellular fluid is 35 liters.

The fluids in the various compartments differ in chemical composition, which indicates that free movement of chemical substances (such as electrolytes, proteins) from one compartment to another may be restricted, whereas water appears to move freely. In the extracellular fluids sodium is the most important cation, and chloride is the most important anion; in the intracellular fluids potassium is the predominant cation, and the prominent anions include phosphate and organic anions. For further details textbooks of biochemistry and physiology should be consulted.

Fluid exchange in the tissue capillaries. The exchange of fluids (including dissolved components other than proteins) between the blood and the interstitial fluid occurs in the tissue capillaries. The basic mechanisms involved in this exchange were described many years ago by the English physiologist E. H. Starling and are commonly referred to as Starling's hypothesis. According to Starling, fluid leaves the capillary at the arterial end and is reabsorbed at the venous end because of a progressive change in the balance between filtration and reabsorption forces as the blood passes through the capillary. This may be illustrated by the following example.

The blood pressure in the arterial end of the capillary, which causes fluid to pass out into the tissue spaces, is about 35 mm. Hg. It is opposed by the colloid osmotic pressure of the plasma proteins, amounting to about 25 mm. Hg, which tends to draw fluid into the capillary from the tissue spaces. The net result is a force of $35 - 25 = 10$ mm. Hg that causes fluid to leave the capillary. The blood pressure falls progressively along the capillary, reaching a level of about 15 mm. Hg at the venous end. This is less than the colloid osmotic pressure of the plasma proteins, and a force of $25 - 15 = 10$ mm. Hg is available to bring about reabsorption of fluid at the venous end of the capillary. Thus under normal conditions in resting subjects, filtration and reabsorption of fluid at the arterial and venous ends of the capillaries balance each other, and the volume of the tissue fluid is maintained constant. (This is an oversimplification that indicates the net results of opposing forces; actually the outward filtration of fluid may occur throughout the length of some capillaries, while the reabsorption of fluid occurs throughout the length of other capillaries.) If the filtration of fluid out of the capillaries exceeds its reabsorption, the volume of interstitial fluid is increased, resulting in *edema.* If reabsorption exceeds filtration, the interstitial (and eventually the intracellular) fluid is diminished and the state of *dehydration* results.

Fluid exchange between cells and interstitial fluid. The volume and composition of the intracellular fluid are carefully guarded, but if extreme changes occur in the water content of the interstitial fluid, water may pass into or out of the cells because of osmotic imbalance. This is especially likely to occur if the body gains or loses water in excess of salts or salts in excess of water. For example, as a result of excessive sweating, water is lost in excess of salt. This increases the concentration of salts in the plasma and interstitial fluid, and water is drawn from the cells.

Regulation of volume and composition of fluid compartments. The total water content of the body is determined by the balance between the intake of water (including the water content of the food and the water produced during the metabolism of foodstuffs) and the loss of water in the urine, feces, sweat, and expired air. This balance is normally maintained by appropriate adjustments among these various factors when one or more is disturbed. For example, if excessive water is lost in sweating, the excretion of water in the urine is diminished, and if water intake is excessive, the excretion of water in the urine is correspondingly increased. The two major regulatory factors in the maintenance of water balance are the voluntary intake of water controlled by the sense of thirst and the excretion of water in the urine controlled by the antidiuretic hormone of the posterior pituitary gland. The secretion of the antidiuretic hormone is thought to be regulated by the osmotic effect of changes in the salt content of the blood acting on special osmoreceptors in the hypothalamus. The hormone acts by increasing the reabsorption of water from the renal tubules and collecting ducts, thus decreasing the amount of water appearing in the urine.

Alterations in fluid balance under various conditions. Posture and acute exercise both affect fluid balance.

Posture. When a previously recumbent person stands up, the blood pressure in the lower parts of the body rises, and fluid leaves the capillaries in these regions. This results in the well-known "dependent edema" experienced by many people after long periods of standing. This is less marked if the person is able to walk about since the muscular contractions increase the reabsorption of fluid into the lymphatic vessels for eventual return to the blood.

183

Acute exercise. During a single bout of exercise fluid leaves the blood, as shown by the increased concentration of erythrocytes, hemoglobin, and plasma proteins in the blood. This condition is known as hemoconcentration, and it is a sign that plasma volume has decreased. It has been reported (van Beaumont et al., 1972), however, that the degree of change in plasma volume may be quite different from that calculated from changes in erythrocyte count (or hematocrit), or from plasma protein concentration.[4] Accordingly, it is advisable to measure plasma volume, rather than calculate it, in careful studies on dehydration in exercise. In moderate exercise the change may be no greater than that on changing from the recumbent to the standing posture, but in strenuous exercise it is more striking. The basic mechanism is the loss of fluid from the blood into the tissue spaces because of the increased blood pressure in the muscle capillaries associated with the rise in systolic blood pressure in exercise. If excessive sweating occurs during the exercise, the resulting water loss, unless balanced by decreased excretion of water by the kidney (or by voluntary intake of water), will contribute to the hemoconcentration. Finally, there is evidence that increased metabolism in the cells, by breaking down large molecules into smaller ones with consequent increase in the number of particles, may cause the osmotic absorption of fluid into the cells at the expense of the water of the interstitial and vascular compartments. As would be expected, compensatory changes in the other regulatory factors tend to restrain or correct the tendency for water to be lost from the blood during exercise. This probably accounts for the fact that, if moderate exercise is continued, there may occur a return of fluid to the blood.

During a 28-mile hike in which dehydration was prevented by the free availability of drinking water, the blood volume increased 3.9% (average). The hematocrit decreased 2.1% and there was no change in the plasma protein concentration; the calculated plasma volume increased 7.3%. Since these changes are the opposite of those taking place in short-lasting exercise, it appears that compensatory adjustments occur as exercise continues.

DEHYDRATION

Acute dehydration. Acute dehydration is an important problem in sports because of the greatly increased loss of water in the sweat and the expired air and failure to replace the water during the exercise period. Replacement may be impossible because of the nature of the activity or because of the belief of some coaches and trainers that it is harmful. Surprisingly large water losses may occur during a period of strenuous activity, especially in hot climates, and one of the results of the decreased blood volume is an elevation of the rectal temperature, sometimes to dangerous levels. Extensive laboratory and field studies stimulated by the problems of desert warfare during World War II clearly demonstrated a deterioration in performance associated with dehydration, which could be reduced by the continual replacement of water loss during the period of exercise (Figs. 24 to 26). This deterioration is manifested by a rise in rectal temperature and pulse rate (indicating additional strains on the cardiovascular and temperature-regulating adjustments required in exercise) and by the earlier onset of exhaustion. Unless the amount of sweating is extreme, as during prolonged exercise in hot environments, salt loss may be compensated by increasing the amount of salt used at meals. The use of salt tablets between meals is rarely necessary, and it may lead to gastric irritation and nausea unless accompanied by copious amounts of water.

Water and salt intake. Physical exercise depresses water intake; thirst is not a reliable guide to the need for water. During prolonged exercise in hot weather, water needs to be consumed frequently to replace body fluid lost in sweat. The body will not retain water unless there is

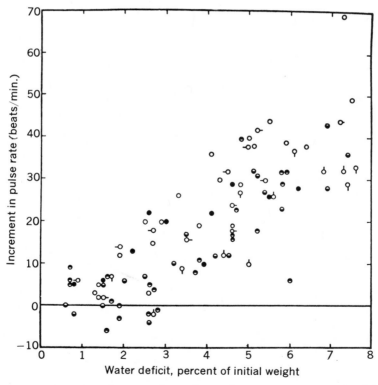

Fig. 24. Increments in pulse rate of standing subjects at various water deficits. Each symbol represents one subject. (From Adolph, E. F., and others: Physiology of man in the desert, New York, 1947, Interscience Publishers, Inc.)

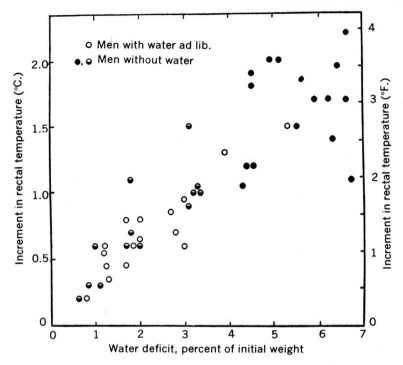

Fig. 25. Increments in rectal temperature at various water deficits induced by hiking 10 to 14 miles in the desert at air temperatures of 90° to 100° F. (From Adolph, E. F., and others: Physiology of man in the desert, New York, 1947, Interscience Publishers, Inc.)

salt to go with it. If a salt deficit is incurred, forcing water results eventually in an equal output of urine. If more than 3% of body weight is lost during exercise, salt intake needs to be increased. Water and salt losses should be replaced continuously by ingestion of salted water prepared by mixing two teaspoons of ordinary table salt in a gallon of water (a 0.1% saline solution). The salted water may be ingested at the rate of at least 1 quart per hour when sweating is extreme.

Rapid weight reduction by dehydration is often practiced by wrestlers to qualify for a lower weight classification in the hope of gaining a size and strength advantage over an opponent. This practice seems to us to be both unphysiological and unethical. At least the former criticism may be met by restoring fluid balance between weighing-in and match time. While the dehydration may have little detrimental effect on speed, strength, and reaction time, it may cause significant deterioration in cardiovascular efficiency.[3]

Chronic dehydration. Acute dehydration is usually corrected by increased water intake in the hours following the period of exercise, and compensation is ordinarily complete by the next day. If dehydration

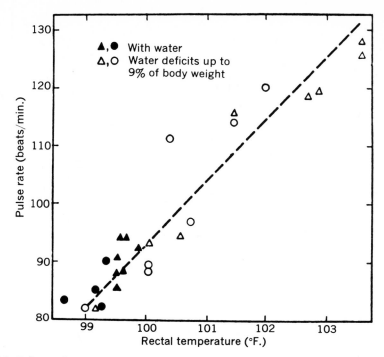

Fig. 26. Relation between pulse rate and rectal temperature of subject at work while dehydrating. (From Adolph, E. F., and others: Physiology of man in the desert, New York, 1947, Interscience Publishers, Inc.)

persists longer than 24 hours, it may be considered to be chronic. This is not a common occurrence, but it may be seen in athletes who restrict their food and water intake in order to meet weight requirements. It is occasionally enforced by coaches and trainers as part of a training regime in the belief that performance is thereby improved. The situation appears to differ in some respects from that of acute dehydration, perhaps because of more effective compensatory reactions. The decrement in work performance may be considerably lessened even though the expected effect of dehydration on pulse rate and rectal temperature is present. It is not clear whether this represents increased tolerance to dehydration or improved fitness due to training. The increased tolerance to dehydration is seen only when the dehydration is developed under cool environmental conditions and not at all in men who become dehydrated in the heat.

KIDNEY FUNCTION IN EXERCISE

The alterations in kidney function associated with exercise may be considered from two aspects: (1) the influence of exercise on kidney

187

function and (2) the contribution of the kidney to the homeostatic adjustments to exercise.

The volume of urine formed per minute depends on the balance between the rate of filtration of fluid in the glomeruli and the amount of the filtered fluid that is reabsorbed as it passes down the renal tubules. From each 100 ml. of plasma passing through the glomerular capillaries, about 20 ml. of fluid is filtered into the renal tubules. The amount of fluid thus filtered in 1 minute amounts to about 120 ml. in an average resting person. Most of this fluid is reabsorbed as it passes down the tubules, so that only about 1 or 2 ml. of urine is formed each minute under ordinary conditions, but after the ingestion of large amounts of water, the rate of urine formation may exceed 10 ml. per minute. The factor that determines the amount of water reasorbed in the kidney tubules is the action of the antidiuretic hormone (ADH) secreted by the posterior pituitary gland. This hormone causes the reabsorption of a greater proportion of the water from the fluid in the renal tubules and hence diminishes the rate of urine formation. The ingestion of large amounts of water results in a decreased rate of secretion of ADH, and a larger proportion of the water filtered in the glomeruli escapes reabsorption in the tubules. The result is a larger flow of urine and eventual elimination of the extra water ingested. In dehydration, on the other hand, the hormone secretion is increased, and a greater proportion of the filtered water is reabsorbed, thus conserving the body's water supply.

In exercise there is believed to be an increased secretion of ADH due initially to stress and emotional stimuli and perhaps later to the dehydration that may result from increased sweating. The result is a greater reabsorption of fluid from the renal tubules and a decrease in the rate of urine formation.

It is apparent that the decreased rate of urine formation commonly observed in exercise may be due to one or both of the following factors: (1) decrease in glomerular filtration rate caused by decreased renal blood flow and (2) increased tubular reabsorption of filtered fluid caused by increased secretion of antidiuretic hormone. The relative importance of these two factors has not been established.

The contribution of the kidney to the homeostatic adjustments to exercise is easy to state but difficult to explain in detail. In addition to the conservation of body water already described, the kidney plays an important role in eliminating the excess acid produced during strenuous exertion. This is readily demonstrated by measurements of the pH of the urine, which may fall dramatically during and especially following severe exercise. Since the urine is usually more acid than the blood, it is normally concerned with the excretion of acid metabolites and thus with the maintenance of a normal pH in the blood and tissues. The response to exercise probably consists largely in an exaggeration of this normal activity of the kidney with the result that the increase in acidity of the blood and tissues due to the production of lactic acid during exercise is diminished and normal acidity is more rapidly restored. The details of the mechanisms involved in the acidification of the urine are beyond the scope of this book but are described in textbooks of medical physiology.

References

1. Harold, R., and Straub, P. W.: In vivo role of factor XII (Hageman factor) in hypercoagulability and fibrinolysis, J. Lab. Clin. Med. **79**:397, 1972.
2. Osnes, J. B., and Hermansen, L.: Acid-base balance after maximal exercise of short duration, J. Appl. Physiol. **32**:59, 1972.
3. Ribisl, P. M.: Dehydration to cut weight of wrestlers "here to stay," Hospital Tribune, March 19, 1973.
4. van Beaumont, W., Greenleaf, J. E., and Juhos, L.: Disproportional changes in hematocrit, plasma volume, and proteins during exercise and bed rest, J. Appl. Physiol. **33**:55, 1972.

Suggested readings

Adolph, E. F., and others: Physiology of man in the desert, New York, 1947, Interscience Publishers, Inc.

Lichton, I. J.: Competition between sweat glands and kidneys for salt and water in man, J. Appl. Physiol. **14**:223, 1957.

Pitts, G. C., Johnson, R. E., and Consolazio, F. C.: Work in the heat as affected by intake of water, salt and glucose, Am. J. Physiol. **142**:253, 1944.

15 BODY STRUCTURE

BODY TYPE

Structure and work. There exists a mutual interrelation between body structure and heavy physical work. First, activity modifies structure. The result of many years of using a shovel or performing on a particular piece of gymnastic apparatus is a change in physique that characterizes the worker or the athlete. Second, structure modifies activity. The differences in inherent structure affect the performance of work and sport. A linear person is at a disadvantage in performing work and sport that require the carrying of heavy loads or the receiving of body blows. Persons with a lateral body build yield to those with a linear body build in the performance of activities requiring a wide range of movement.

A demonstration that activity modifies structure is provided in the asymmetry of strongly right-handed or left-handed individuals. There is a marked difference in size between the right and left upper extremities. Measurements repeated from time to time show that the superiority of the right upper extremity over the left increases with age, demonstrating the effects of development through use. Asymmetry in somatic development is induced by certain types of sports and gymnastics. Swimming gives the most symmetrical development.

Masculinization. The fear among young women that vigorous physical activity may result in masculinity of build is unfounded. Hard physical labor during youth does not tend toward the development of a significant degree of masculinity in the build of young women. Young women who already have masculine builds have some advantage in athletic ability, but muscular strength and power are of

190

much greater importance to athletic performance than is body build. Adolescent girls with broad, lateral builds possess a physical capacity superior to girls with a linear type of body build.

Among 729 Hungarian women athletes studied by Erdelyi,[3] some showed male characteristics in respect to body build and musculature, but these came originally from the less feminine, intersexual type. Those with masculine features tend to select sports requiring a high degree of muscular strength because they are stronger than women with highly feminine features.

Structural differences affecting performance. Variations in the position of the muscular attachments, the structure of the joints, and the lengths of the bony levers all affect the performance of physical activity. Usually when the anatomical structure is particularly advantageous for strength, it is disadvantageous for speed. Large joints are strong, but they also may limit motion. Long-distance runners are observed to have very flat longitudinal arches, and sprinters have smaller feet and higher arches.

Although physique plays an important part in the performance of severe exercise, it plays only a minor role in determining a person's response to moderate exercise. Endurance exercise is best performed by those with a slim body build. In general persons with thin legs have better endurance. Sprinters and discus throwers generally have the largest calf muscles.[1] Persons with a normal or stocky build have, on the average, the greatest speed, the greatest strength, and the greatest ability to sustain prolonged moderate muscular effort. Good muscular development is required for success in activities requiring speed and strength.

Size and energy exchange during work. Differences in body size affect the energy exchange during physical activity. Even at rest a large man may consume as much as 58% more oxygen than a small man. During light work (simulating operation of an airplane) a large man may require 42% more oxygen than a small man. Among 27 men the correlation coefficient between the oxygen consumption and body surface was plus 0.76 at rest and plus 0.82 at work. Because of the larger energy requirement during work, a large man accumulates heat under conditions in which a smaller man attains a heat balance. The ratio of heat production to surface area in a 218-pound man was observed to be 20% greater than in a 97-pound man.

Heart size. Heart size is related to constitutional type and thoracic circumference. Measurements of heart size in 233 athletes indicated moderate hypertrophy. Such hypertrophy is judged to be normal for athletes. If a larger than average heart is associated with a high vital capacity, an athlete usually also has a slower than average pulse rate

191

and low blood pressure and possesses a large capacity for performance of work.

HEREDITY

The way an individual is formed and is able to function is largely dependent on heredity. His genetic structure determines the form and function of (1) the sensory organs, which provide information input, (2) the intermediary nervous and endocrine systems, which control coordination and perceptual capacities, and (3) the neuromuscular effectors, which power the body's physical activities.

Genetic studies of Olympic champions show correlations of performances in various events with body type, parent-offspring pedigrees, sex chromosome components in buccal cells, and variations in the size of the Y chromosome in lymphocyte cells in blood. These studies give evidence that champion athletes in certain events possess distinct hereditary materials that permit particularly outstanding sport performance. Although the direct action of some genes on certain behavior patterns has been established, it is not possible to demonstrate the physiological effect of a single gene in determining the limits of performance of a specific activity.

RACE

There are no clear physiological differences in response to exercise or training among different ethnic or racial groups. Except for a significantly better vertical jumping ability among black as compared to white males,[4] there are few if any differences in strength and performance.

Although black Americans have a mixed heritage—African Negro, Indian, and Caucasian—their physical characteristics are generally Negroid. Their bones are usually more dense and thus they are often less buoyant than whites. Blacks tend to have shorter torsoes, a more slender pelvis, longer forearms and lower legs, longer hands, and longer and wider feet. They have, on the average, more muscle in the shoulders, upper arms, buttocks, and thighs and less in the calves and forearms.[7] These Negroid characteristics are favorable for the power events: jumping, sprinting, throwing, pole vaulting, boxing, and basketball. These anatomical advantages are important but they do not assure success in power events or failure in endurance events. Other factors, such as physiological, psychological, and cultural, influence selection of activities, training intensity, and performance capacity.[4]

BODY COMPOSITION

An increase in the amount of physical activity changes body composition. When total body weight is unchanged, there is an increase in the mass of bone and muscle and a decrease in body fat. In other words, there is an increase in lean body mass at the expense of fat.

The extent of these changes is in proportion to the intensity, duration, and frequency of exercise. In previously sedentary and slightly obese subjects the addition of 900 activity Calories/week, distributed among three 1-hour exercise sessions per week, is enough to cause fat reduction and an increase in lean body mass.[2]

The impact of exercise on body composition is not lasting. When training is discontinued there is an increase in the accumulation of body fat. Fat is laid down by the metabolic adaptation in adipose tissue. When the body remains quiet, fat cells become receptacles for the storage of more fat. During inactivity there is a reduced metabolic utilization of fatty acids and a slower release of these products from the fat depots. This results in a greater accumulation of fat.[5]

The mass of fat in obese persons constitutes an overload stress and affects other organs and systems of the body. The pelvis of an obese person is broadened to adapt to the load of excess fat. Long bones and postural (antigravity) muscles are hypertrophied and strengthened somewhat by the load of excess fat. This static type of weight lifting is not the form of exercise that enables fat metabolites to be used as fuel.

References

1. Cumming, G. R., and others: Calf x-ray measurements correlated with age, body build and physical performance in boys and girls, J. Sports Med. 13:90, 1973.
2. Ekelund, L. G.: Exercise, including weightlessness, Ann. Rev. Physiol. 31:85, 1969.
3. Erdelyi, G. J.: Gynecological survey of female athletes, J. Sports Med. Phys. Fitness 2:174, 1962.
4. Malina, R. M.: Ethnic and cultural factors in the development of motor abilities and strength in American children. In Rarick, G. L., editor: Physical activity: human growth and development, New York, 1973, Academic Press, Inc., p. 333.
5. Novak, L.: Physical activity and body composition of adolescent boys, J. A. M. A. 197:891, 1966.
6. Parizkova, J.: Body composition and exercise during growth and development. In Rarick, G. L.: Physical activity: human growth and development, New York, 1973, Academic Press, Inc., p. 97.
7. Tanner, J.: The physique of the Olympic athlete, London, 1964, Allen and Unwin Ltd.

Suggested readings

Behnke, A.: Physique and exercise. In Falls, H., editor: Exercise physiology, New York, 1968, Academic Press, Inc.

Damon, A.: Negro-white difference in pulmonary function, Human Biology 38:380, 1966.

Di Prampero, P., and Cerretelli, P.: Maximal muscular power (aerobic and anaerobic) in African natives, Ergonomics 12:51, 1969.

Levine, L.: The biology of the gene, ed. 2, St. Louis, 1973, The C. V. Mosby Co.

Ponthieux, H. A., and Barker, D. G.: Relationships between race and physical fitness, Res. Quart. 36:468, 1965.

Thompson, R.: Race and sport, London, 1964, Oxford Press.

Wyndham, C. H., and others: Differences between ethnic groups in physical working capacity, J. Appl. Physiol. 18:361, 1963.

PART FIVE

ENVIRONMENTAL FACTORS

16 HEAT AND COLD

CONCEPT OF "BODY TEMPERATURE"

If the oral or rectal temperatures of a group of resting subjects are measured at the same time, a range of values is obtained. For example, the oral temperatures of a group of 276 medical students measured between 8 and 9 A.M., ranged from 96.5° to 99.3° F.[3] There is also a diurnal variation of several degrees in the oral or rectal temperatures in the same individual, being highest in the late afternoon and lowest during the early morning hours. Finally, the rectal temperature is usually about 1° F. higher than the oral temperature, and even in the rectum there are variations of from 0.1° to 1.5° F., depending on the depth of insertion of the thermometer or other measuring device. The need for careful standardization of procedures in experiments involving measurement of "body temperature" is obvious.

A rectal temperature of 99.6° F. does not mean that all parts of the body are at this temperature; for example, the skin temperature may be 10° to 15° F. lower than the rectal temperature, and if a needle thermistor is inserted into the subcutaneous tissue, temperatures intermediate between those of the skin and the rectum are recorded. From the standpoint of temperature regulation, it is convenient to consider that the body is composed of two compartments, a central core and a peripheral shell. The core consists of the contents of the cranial, thoracic, abdominal, and pelvic cavities and the deeper portions of the muscle masses of the extremities. The shell includes the skin, subcutaneous tissues, and the superficial portions of the muscle masses. It is of variable thickness, depending on the environmental temperature; it increases in thickness during exposure to cold and decreases in thickness in response to environmental heat or to exercise. The shell may be thought of as a layer of insulation

197

surrounding the core and helping to maintain a constant core temperature. The temperature of the shell is not only lower than that of the core under nearly all conditions, but there is a gradient of temperature of the shell, from core temperature in its deepest portion to skin temperature at the periphery. In general, the temperature-regulating mechanisms operate in such a way that the temperature of the core is protected, whereas the temperature of the shell may vary considerably. Oral and rectal temperatures, if carefully measured, reflect the temperature of the core. Shell temperature may be measured by thermocouples or thermistors mounted in contact with the skin and by needle thermistors inserted to various depths beneath the skin.

NATURE OF THE REGULATION OF BODY TEMPERATURE

The core temperature represents a balance between the rates at which heat is added to the body and lost from the body. When these two rates are equal, the temperature remains constant. Ordinarily the major source of heat gain is from metabolism, but under certain conditions the body may also gain heat from the environment. Heat is lost from the body by the physical processes of radiation, conduction, convection, and the vaporization of water. These are aided by two physiological factors—variations in the blood flow through the skin (which determine the amount of heat transported from the core to the surface) and the secretion of sweat (which provides water for cooling the skin by vaporization). Ordinarily the regulation of body temperature is achieved by adjustments in the rate of heat loss; the capacity for altering heat production is limited to such activities as shivering and voluntary muscular activity during exposure to cold. Variations in the rates of heat production and of heat loss that are necessary for the maintenance of a constant core temperature are controlled by temperature-regulating centers in the hypothalamus.

CHANNELS OF HEAT LOSS

Heat loss by *conduction* occurs when the body is in direct contact with something that is colder than the skin. The rate at which heat is lost by conduction depends both on the difference in temperature between the skin and the medium in contact with the skin and on the heat conductivity of the medium. For example, water is a much better conductor of heat than is air, and for this reason the body loses heat much more rapidly in cold water than in air at the same temperature. Conductive heat loss is ordinarily of minor importance.

Heat loss by *convection* involves movement of the medium (air or water) in contact with the body surface. Cooler air or water is brought into contact with the skin, where it is warmed by conduction and then moves on, carrying with it the heat gained from the body. This is the principle of the cooling effect of fans.

Heat loss by *radiation* is the result of the fact that all warm bodies emit electromagnetic heat waves; this is the way in which the earth is warmed by the sun. The human body is constantly gaining and losing heat by radiation, but under normal environmental conditions the loss exceeds the gain, and this constitutes the most important channel of heat loss in resting men in moderate climates. When men are directly exposed to the sun in hot deserts, there may be a net gain of heat by radiation.

Heat loss by *vaporization* is due to the fact that the evaporation of water, that is, conversion from liquid to gas state, requires the absorption of 0.58 kilocalorie per gram of water vaporized. The vaporization of sweat on the skin cools the skin by abstracting from it the necessary heat to vaporize the water of the sweat (the abstraction of heat from the surrounding air is negligible because of the low heat content of the air). It should be emphasized that sweating cools the skin only if the sweat is vaporized. Under conditions of high relative humidity the sweat may simply drip from the skin without cooling it.

SOURCES OF HEAT GAIN

In a resting subject exposed to a comfortable environmental temperature, the heat gain is due entirely to metabolism. Metabolic heat production is increased in exercise; in very strenuous exercise it may increase as much as thirtyfold. Metabolic heat production is also increased during exposure to cold by the type of muscle contractions known as shivering. Finally, if the body is exposed to intense, direct sunlight or to warming devices such as stoves, it may gain heat by radiation, and if it is exposed to a medium having a high temperature (for example, very hot water), it may gain heat by conduction. The physiological adjustments of heat production are quantitatively much less important than are those of heat loss, and the regulation of body temperature is largely a matter of appropriate adjustments of heat loss.

PHYSIOLOGICAL ADJUSTMENTS THAT DETERMINE HEAT LOSS

Although the actual loss of heat from the body is the result of the physical processes of conduction, convection, radiation, and vaporization of water, the operation of these physical processes is conditioned by physiological mechanisms that determine the amount of heat brought to the skin and the amount of sweat available for vaporization.

Heat is transported from the core to the skin primarily by the blood; only a small amount reaches the skin by conduction through the shell. Thus an increase in the blood flow to the skin increases the heat loss by conduction, convection, and radiation. The amount of skin blood flow is determined by the degree of constriction of the skin blood vessels, and this is regulated by the vasoconstrictor nerve fibers that supply these vessels. When vasoconstriction is increased, the blood flow through the skin and the heat loss from the skin are diminished; this occurs when the body is exposed to a cold environment, preventing excessive loss of heat. When vasoconstriction of the skin blood vessels is diminished, the increased flow of blood through the skin increases the heat loss; this occurs in response to greater heat production, as in exercise, or to an elevation of the environmental temperature.

The second physiological factor that determines heat loss from the skin is variation in the activity of the sweat glands. When heat load is increased, more sweat is secreted and evaporative heat loss is greater; this occurs in response to increased heat production (exercise) or to elevated environmental temperature. Exposure to cold, on the other hand, results in the cessation of sweating.

The adjustment of the amount of skin blood flow and of the amount of sweat secreted to meet changing requirements for heat loss or heat conservation is under the control of the temperature-regulating center located in the preoptic-anterior hypothalamus. If small thermodes (heating or cooling probes) are inserted bilaterally in this area and perfused with warm or cool water, marked thermoregulatory responses are evoked. This indicates that neurons sensitive to heating or cooling are intermingled in this area. Presumably these thermally sensitive neurons respond both to changes in blood temperature and to afferent nerve impulses from thermal receptors in the skin and elsewhere. The relative importance of these two sources of stimulation is uncertain, and it may vary according to whether the heat stress is of metabolic or environmental origin.

The regulation of sweating in exercise has been studied intensively in recent years, and conflicting points of view are not yet completely reconciled. It appears that when work intensity is varied while environmental temperature is maintained constant, the rate of sweating is determined by the deep body temperature. When, on the other hand, work of constant intensity is performed at different environmental temperatures, the sweat rate varies with the skin temperature.[4,5] Furthermore, since for comparable values of rectal and skin temperatures both sweat secretion and skin circulation are much higher during work than during rest, it has been suggested that neuromuscular reflexes take part in temperature regulation as they do in the regulation of respiration.[7] The reflexes probably originate in thermoreceptors in the working muscles or in contact with veins draining the working muscles. Direct evidence has been obtained for a neurogenic stimulation of sweating in exercise. Isometric contractions of the arm muscles performed in a warm environment while the circulation to and from the working muscles was arrested by an inflated arm cuff resulted in a prompt increase in sweating (within 1.5 to 2.0 seconds after beginning the exercises). In these experiments warmed blood from the exercising muscles could not have reached the heat-regulating centers in the hypothalamus.

The operation of the temperature-regulating system may be illustrated by a description of the response to changing from a thermally neutral environment to a hot or a cold environment. On changing to a hot environment, the skin temperature rises and heat receptors in the skin are stimulated. Afferent impulses from these receptors are transmitted to the heat-sensitive neurons in the hypothalamus, which respond by decreasing the discharge of vasoconstrictor nerve impulses to the skin blood vessels and by sending impulses along the secretory nerve fibers to the sweat glands. The result is an increased capacity for dissipating heat from the skin, which balances hindrance to heat loss due to the increased environmental temperature, and body temperature is prevented from rising. Exposure to cold, on the other hand, stimulates cold receptors in the skin, and impulses are transmitted to the cool-sensitive neurons in the hypothalamus, which respond by increasing the constriction of the skin blood vessels and by inhibiting the activity of the sweat glands. The result is a diminished rate of heat loss from the skin and a conservation of body heat.

TEMPERATURE REGULATION IN EXERCISE

When exercise is performed under comfortable environmental conditions, the only problem is the elimination of the excess heat of metabolism. The additional problems that result from the performance of exercise in the heat will be discussed later.

The amount of excess heat produced in most types of exercise is known only approximately because of the difficulty of making the necessary measurements. Laboratory studies indicate that the rate of heat production may easily rise to 10 to 20 times that of the resting subject, and it may be as high as 30 times the resting level in extreme cases. This obviously imposes a severe burden on the temperature-regulating mechanisms, and the failure to prevent an excessive rise in core temperature may contribute to the earlier onset of exhaustion.

Saltin and associates observed that subjects performing exhaustive work were forced to quit before the rectal and esophageal temperatures reached the higher levels observed in extended submaximal exercise.

They concluded that storage of body heat per se is not a factor limiting performance in exhaustive exercise, and stated, "The one internal body temperature with a consistent value at the end of exhaustive exercise is a muscle temperature of around 40° C., which temperature could conceivably be a key factor that determines the limit of performance."[8]

As the body temperature rises during exercise, there occurs an increase in the rate of sweating and in the amount of skin blood flow, the stimulus to the hypothalamic centers being an increase in blood temperature. In the case of the circulatory adjustment, however, there is a conflict of interests since there is a requirement for increased blood flow both to the skin and to the active muscles. The result is a compromise in which each requirement suffers, especially in very strenuous exercise performed in the heat. It has long been known that the deep body temperature rises during exercise and that the amount of rise is proportional to the severity of the exercise. This does not indicate that temperature regulation is inadequate, however, since for any level of exercise the temperature rises to a plateau that is then maintained without further increase.[6] When a plateau is not achieved, the situation is abnormal; this will be discussed later.

It appears that the rise in body temperature in exercise is the result of a "resetting" of the hypothalamic "thermostat" at a higher level just as in clinical fever. In fact, Haight and Keatinge have suggested that the elevation of the set point for body temperature regulation after prolonged exercise is due to the liberation of pyrogens from damaged cells, especially in the muscles and kidneys.[2] The mobilization of neutrophilic leukocytes into the circulation (well known to occur in exercise) would make these cells available for phagocytosis of damaged tissue cells with release of pyrogens, so that heat loss balances heat production at a higher body temperature. Furthermore, since most of the excess heat is produced in the active muscles, their temperature rise is certainly greater than that of the whole body, as reflected in the oral and rectal temperatures. A rise in body temperature that is well tolerated by an exercising man may cause great distress in a resting man, and in fact, athletic performance is actually improved by a moderate rise in body temperature. The increased tolerance to hyperthermia in exercising persons is due to the fact that increased cardiac output permits the maintenance of an adequate cerebral blood flow, whereas exposure to heat without exercise is associated with a decreased cerebral blood flow (because of decreased cardiac output and cerebral vasoconstriction resulting from respiratory alkalosis). The beneficial effects of an elevated muscle temperature during exercise may perhaps be attributed to the resulting increase in the breakdown of oxyhemoglobin and delivery of oxygen to the muscle fibers and to the decreased internal viscosity of the muscle protoplasm. If the structural rearrangements that take place during contraction and relaxation of muscle fibers are facilitated by the elevated temperature, greater tension might be developed before the state of excitation of the fiber is over.

EXERCISE IN THE HEAT

When exercise is performed in a hot environment, especially by a person who is not heat acclimatized, the increased requirement for blood flow to the active muscles and to the skin for thermal regulation may exceed the capacity of the heart to increase the cardiac output. The situation then resembles the incipient circulatory shock of a person who has lost blood by hemorrhage, and fainting may occur, terminating a potentially dangerous activity. The circulatory inadequacy also results in impaired temperature regulation, and if the warning signs of dizziness and faintness are ignored, the extremely serious condition of heat stroke may result. The high rectal temperatures and pulse rates and the dizziness and nausea associated with exercise in the heat may be dramatically reduced by heat acclimatization, which is achieved by daily periods of work in the heat.

The following statement on exercise in the heat has been developed by the American College of Sports Medicine.*

ACSM position statement on
prevention of heat injuries during distance running

Based on research findings and current rules governing distance running competition, it is the position of the American College of Sports Medicine that:
1. Distance races (>16 km or 10 miles) should **not** be conducted when the wet bulb temperature—globe temperature† exceeds 28° C (82.4° F).
2. During periods of the year, when the daylight dry bulb temperature often exceeds 27° C (80° F), distance races should be conducted before 9:00 A.M. or after 4:00 P.M.
3. It is the responsibility of the race sponsors to provide fluids which contain small amounts of sugar (less than 2.5 g glucose per 100 ml of water) and electrolytes (less than 10 mEq sodium and 5 mEq potassium per liter of solution.)
4. Runners should be encouraged to frequently ingest fluids during competition and to consume 400-500 ml (13-17 oz.) of fluid 10-15 minutes before competition.
5. Rules prohibiting the administration of fluids during the first 10 kilometers (6.2 miles) of a marathon race should be amended to permit fluid ingestion at frequent intervals along the race course. In light of the high sweat rates and body temperatures during distance running in the heat,

---

*From Sports Medicine Bulletin **10**:1, July 1975.
†Adapted from Minard, D.: Prevention of heat casualties in Marine Corps Recruits, Milit. Med. **126**:261, 1961. WB-GT = 0.7 (WBT) + 0.2 (GT) + 0.1 (DBT)

race sponsors should provide "water stations" at 3-4 kilometer (2-2.5 mile) intervals for all races of 16 kilometers (10 miles) or more.

6. Runners should be instructed in how to recognize the early warning symptoms that precede heat injury. Recognition of symptoms, cessation of running, and proper treatment can prevent heat injury. Early warning symptoms include the following: piloerection on chest and upper arms, chilling, throbbing pressure in the head, unsteadiness, nausea, and dry skin.

7. Race sponsors should make prior arrangements with medical personnel for the care of cases of heat injury. Responsible and informed personnel should supervise each "feeding station." Organizational personnel should reserve the right to stop runners who exhibit clear signs of heat stroke or heat exhaustion.

It is the position of the American College of Sports Medicine that policies established by local, national, and international sponsors of distance running events should adhere to these guidelines. Failure to adhere to these guidelines may jeopardize the health of competitors through heat injury.

ACCLIMATIZATION TO HEAT

The heat-acclimatized person is able to work in the heat with a lower rectal temperature and heart rate, a better regulation of body temperature, and fewer unpleasant symptoms than a nonacclimatized person. There appear to be two major factors in the development of heat acclimatization: an earlier onset and greater volume of sweating, and the development of a greater capacity for cutaneous vasodilatation. The circulation is improved by an increase in plasma volume and interstitial fluid volume, together with an improved venous return to the heart. Stroke volume increases and cardiac output is maintained at a lower heart rate. The process of acclimatization is rapid, being completed in a period of 4 to 7 days, and can be achieved by short intermittent periods (2 to 4 hours daily) of work in the heat; exposure to heat without exercise results in only slight acclimatization. Heat acclimatization is retained for several weeks after the cessation of exposure and then disappears slowly during a period of several months.

While it is true that heat acclimatization is developed most rapidly by work in the heat, it has been reported that a degree of heat acclimatization can also be developed by interval training in a cool environment.[1] In this case, however, the efficiency of heat acclimatization was less, and the time required for its development (8 weeks) was considerably longer than that resulting from work in the heat. Of greater importance is the clear understanding of the potential danger of exhausting work in the heat by men who are not heat acclimatized; the results may be serious or even fatal although usually exhaustion terminates the activity before this point is reached.

A final practical point concerns the proper clothing for work in the heat. Uniforms and equipment that are of a dark color and restrict the ventilation of air and retard the loss of heat from the skin add to the dangers of the situation. There is need for a more scientific approach to the designing of such equipment, based on the requirement for adequate protection without undue hindrance to heat loss.

DISTURBANCES OF HEAT REGULATION

When the total heat load of the body exceeds the capacity of the compensatory mechanisms, various incapacities occur. In the order of increasing severity, they are heat cramp, heat fatigue, heat exhaustion, and heat stroke. The first three are temporarily disabling, but not dangerous if they are recognized and if the activity is terminated; heat stroke, on the other hand, is an acute medical emergency and may be fatal if treatment is not rapid and vigorous. The pertinent facts about these four conditions may be summarized as follows.

Heat cramp is an indirect effect of exposure to heat, and the body temperature is usually normal. The muscle pain and spasms are the result of depletion of electrolytes due to excessive loss of salt in the sweat, and the condition is relieved by rest and the administration of salt and water. Drinking water temporarily relieves dehydration but lowers the concentration of salt in extracellular fluid, giving rise eventually to heat cramp. *Heat fatigue* is also caused by a depletion of salt and water due to sweating. The body falls behind in its ability to dispose of excess internal heat. Alertness is dulled and work capacity is diminished. Symptoms may include sluggishness, headache, nausea, hallucinations, and weak and rapid pulse. This condition is also relieved by replacement of salt and water and a period of rest in a cool place. *Heat exhaustion* characteristically occurs during heat waves, especially those occurring early in the summer, or when athletes who are not heat acclimatized engage in strenuous sports on a hot day. It is a form of circulatory inadequacy caused by pooling of blood in the dilated skin vessels or by marked dehydration. The symptoms include weakness, headache, dizziness, and vomiting. The body temperature is usually only slightly elevated, sweating is profuse, and the pulse is weak and rapid. Treatment consists of rest in the shade in a recumbent position and replacement of fluids and salt by sips of diluted salt water. *Heat stroke* is a serious condition that can result in death; it requires the care of a physician. There is prostration and often coma. The pulse is rapid and weak. The skin is usually hot, and it may be dry or moist; occasionally it is cold and clammy, suggestive of shock. Whether a failure of the sweating mechanism occurs, because of central nervous system damage, has not been established. Dehydration is not a necessary condition, since heat stroke has been

205

observed in well-hydrated subjects. Body temperature may rise to very high levels, approaching 110° F. in extreme cases. To make the situation even more complex, heat stroke occasionally (though not usually) appears to commence some hours after the cessation of heat stress. From a practical standpoint, immediate steps should be taken to lower the body temperature (immersion in cold water, ice packs, alcohol spray) while awaiting medical care.

The cause of heat stroke remains unknown. The temperature regulatory center in the hypothalamus may be involved in some manner, although lowering the body temperature by appropriate treatment often fails to prevent death. A feature emphasized in the current medical literature is the widespread occurrence of intravascular coagulation, often followed by hemorrhages into the tissues caused by exhaustion of the supplies of clotting factors in the blood. It has been suggested that the intravascular coagulation is triggered by heat damage to the endothelial cells of the small blood vessels, causing clumping of platelets and the formation of multiple thrombi.[10]

The practice of withholding water from athletes during workouts is a dangerous one. Such restriction coupled with copious sweating causes a rapid depletion of water and electrolytes and can lead to serious heat illness. During exercise in the heat it is essential to replace sweat water loss. It is helpful, in anticipation of exercise in the heat, to drink water a few minutes before the start of exercise.

Salt needs to be replaced daily, preferably by extra salting of food within the bounds of taste. Salt tablets are poorly absorbed, especially when the stomach is empty, and can be irritating to the stomach.

HOT ENVIRONMENTS

During exercise in a comfortable environment the deep body temperature rises to a new level that is proportional to the severity of the exertion. This rise in body temperature is not due to a failure of the mechanisms that rid the body of excess heat, but to a higher "setting" of the hypothalamic thermostat. An interesting point is that the final body temperature reached during exercise does not depend on the absolute magnitude of the energy expenditure, but on the level of metabolism relative to the individual's maximal aerobic power. This means, for example, that the rise in body temperature will be the same in a nontrained and a trained person when each is exercising at a level of 50% of his maximal aerobic power, even though the absolute rate of energy expenditure is much greater in the trained person. This appears to be a definite training effect, but its mechanism is obscure.

When a subject performs a standard exercise at different environmental temperatures, the increase in rectal temperature is the same in each case. Since the heat production is the same at each environmental temperature, the heat loss from the body must also be the same. It is observed, however, that as the external temperature rises, the heat loss by conduction, convection, and radiation decreases, while the heat loss by the evaporation of sweat increases. It is obvious that the ability to maintain a constant body temperature during exercise at increasing environmental temperatures may fail if the rate of evaporative heat loss becomes inadequate, as it might in a very humid environment. If the exercise is continued for long periods at a high environmental temperature, without periodic replacement of the water lost in the sweat, the resulting dehydration also disturbs the regulation of body temperature. Subjects acclimatized to intermittent exposure to heat walked at a fixed rate up a constant slope in an environmental temperature of 100° F. and a relative humidity of 35 to 45% (Fig. 27). When water was not taken, their body temperatures rose steadily to 102° F., and they tired easily and worked inefficiently. When they were allowed to drink as much water as they wished, their temperatures did not rise to as high a level and they finished the walk in much better condition. When they were required to drink enough water to replace their sweat loss, performance improved still further, and the body temperatures rose either very little or not at all.

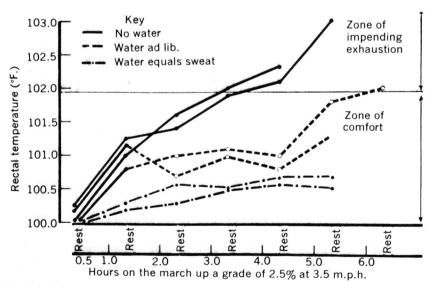

Fig. 27. Effect of water consumption on subjects marching in the heat. Six experiments on subject at temperature 100° F. and relative humidity 35 to 45%. (From Pitts, G. C., Johnson, R. E., and Consolazio, F. C.: Work in the heat as affected by the intake of water, salt, and glucose, Amer. J. Physiol. **142:**254, 1944.)

Work in dry heat. The capacity for working in dry heat depends not only on the environmental temperature, but also on whether there is direct exposure to the sun. During exercise in dry heat in the shade, the body may gain heat by conduction and convection from the surrounding air. This heat gain is usually modest because of the low heat capacity and thermal conductivity of air, and is balanced by evaporative heat loss. If, however, the work is performed during direct exposure to the sun, additional heat is gained by radiation, and evaporative heat loss must accordingly be increased. Performance under this condition is improved by the wearing of loose, lightweight clothing that allows evaporation of sweat to continue while protecting against heat gain by radiation.

Work in humid heat. High humidity has a marked influence on the ability to perform prolonged moderate work in the heat, because of interference with the evaporation of sweat. In one experiment, resting subjects tolerated a 60-minute exposure to an environmental temperature of 145° F. when the relative humidity was 10%, but they could not tolerate an environmental temperature above 104° F. when the relative humidity was 90%. These differences are exaggerated if the subjects are performing work.

An unusual syndrome is sometimes observed in men working in a hot, humid environment. More water is lost in the sweat than can be absorbed from the gastrointestinal tract no matter how much water is drunk, and the subjects become obviously ill (nausea, vomiting, cramps).

Very high rates of sweating, with little cooling effect, may characterize work in humid heat. Loss of water and salt may be excessive, and water loss is seldom balanced by voluntary water intake, so that dehydration is not uncommon, and a temporary salt deficit may be incurred. Performance is improved by the wearing of minimal clothing unless direct exposure to the sun requires protection against heat gain by radiation.

Water should be given in more frequent and smaller amounts in hot, dry climates. A hot, dry atmosphere is not tolerated as well as a hot, wet atmosphere when water losses are not replaced. When ample water is given, the same effect is obtained in a hot, dry (109° F., 38% humidity) atmosphere as in a hot, wet atmosphere at the same effective temperature (87.5° F., 87% humidity).

Sweating. Sweating provides the water to wet the skin surface and the evaporation of this water cools the skin. Sweating, if excessive, also robs the body of water and salt and these losses may impair performance if they are not compensated by prompt and adequate replacement.

The regulation of sweat secretion by the sweat glands is discussed earlier in this chapter. To that discussion we may add two interesting facts. First, sweat glands appear to suffer "fatigue" after prolonged periods of sweating, with a corresponding decrease in the rate of sweating. Second, acclimatization to heat includes alterations in sweat gland activity: these include a more prompt onset of sweating on exposure to heat, and the formation of larger amounts of sweat with a lower salt concentration. The beneficial effects of these adaptations is clear, but the mechanisms responsible for them are not. One of the factors in heat acclimatization may be an actual increase in the number of active sweat glands in the skin surface. There is also evidence that the salt content of the sweat is decreased by an increased secretion of aldosterone, the sodium-conserving hormone of the adrenal cortex. Another explanation is that acclimatization results in a smaller body temperature rise in response to a standard heat stress, and that this is responsible for the decreased secretion of salt in the sweat.

The rate of sweating of the whole body can be estimated from the weight loss during the period of heat exposure. The rate of sweat secretion on different skin areas is measured by a simple procedure. A metal ring about 3 inches in diameter and 1 inch deep, with a tightly-fitting lid to prevent evaporation is lightly pressed on the skin area. After 2 minutes the lid is removed, and during the next 30 seconds the sweat collected within the ring is absorbed by a previously weighed cotton pledget. The gain in weight of the pledget is the weight of the sweat formed. Using this technique, investigators have observed that during work in a hot humid environment, about 50% of the total sweat secretion occurs on the trunk, 25% on the lower extremities, and the remaining 25% on the head and upper extremities. The total amount of sweat secreted during hard work in the heat may amount to as much as 8 liters (nearly 20 pounds) in one day.

Cooling to suppress sweating. If environmental temperatures are low enough, sweating is not needed to dissipate the extra metabolic heat of work. When the environmental temperature is lowered by lowering air-wall temperature or by wearing a water-cooled garment, sweating can be suppressed during a work level of 900 Cal./hr. Heart rate and rectal temperature increase as a function of work level, while skin temperature becomes lower. After 30 to 60 minutes of the work period there is gradual heat storage, followed by a steady state. During the steady state the cooling required to suppress sweating is calculated to be about 80% of the heat production. Presumably the remaining 20% leaves the system as external physical work.

Salt. A daily intake of 20 grams of salt appears to be sufficient for most men in most environments. A sodium chloride intake of about 15 grams per day was adequate for 49 men working in dry heat (120° F.). When the salt intake was reduced to 6 grams daily, they lost more than twice as much body weight (water), drank less water, and sweated less. They had higher pulse rates and rectal temperatures and poorer cardio-vascular adjustments. Dehydration, nausea, vomiting, tachycardia, hypo-tension, vertigo, and collapse occurred in 25% of the men on the low sodium chloride intake and in only 2.5% of those on the 15 grams daily intake. The subjects on the 6 grams daily salt intake suffered an average net deficit of 13 grams of salt for 3 days in the heat (8.39 grams on the first day). The volume of sweat lost varied between 5 and 8 liters (11 and 17.6 pounds) daily. There was no advantage when the daily salt intake was raised to 30 grams.

Salt given without water produces gastrointestinal discomfort without improvement in heat tolerance. Given with water, both bring improved performance. Extra salt added to the hourly supply of water in hot environments is not indicated in persons receiving meals containing ade-quate salt.

The final stages of acclimatization to heat are marked by increased sweat loss and reduced salt concentration in the sweat. A more rapid onset of sweating promotes evaporative loss before the body temperature rises markedly. In this condition of adaptation men are able to remain in sodium chloride balance and retain their physical fitness on a salt intake as low as 5 grams per day while performing heavy work in a hot, wet climate and producing 4 to 9 liters of sweat in 24 hours. This adjustment is due to a sharp fall in the urinary excretion of sodium chloride and to the ability of the sweat glands to produce a fluid con-taining lower concentrations of salt when the supply is diminished.

Vitamin C. Vitamin C (ascorbic acid) is present in sweat to the extent of 0.55 to 0.64 mg. per 100 ml. Because of this loss coal miners who sweat heavily may develop scurvy on what would otherwise be an adequate diet. The diet of men working in the heat should include larger amounts of foods containing vitamin C than are included in ordinary diets.

Protein. Alteration in the dietary ratio of fat, carbohydrate, and protein has little influence upon the ability to work in the heat. Theoretically, the specific dynamic action of a high-protein diet in hot weather places undue stress on the heat-dissipating mechanisms. Experimentally, altering the protein content of the diet from 76 to 105 to 149 grams per day had no demonstrable effect upon the feelings or work performance of human subjects under temperate, hot dry, or hot humid conditions. The 4% higher work metabolism associated with the high protein intake was a negligible factor under the conditions of the experiments where the heat exposure was intermittent. In any event, if an active person is able to maintain heat balance at all, any extra heat load due to protein is physiologically insignificant in comparison with his caloric expenditure.

Clothing. No matter how lightweight it is, clothing definitely hinders the regulation of temperature in hot, humid environments because it limits the vaporization of water. As a result of this limitation, a clothed subject cannot tolerate work at as high a temperature as can a nude subject. A coverall of herringbone twill reduced by 2 degrees the temperature at which a standard work load could be performed. In hot, dry environments, evaporation of sweat is, in the daytime, the sole avenue of heat loss because the gradients for radiation, conduction, and convection are small or actually reversed. Loose, lightweight clothing allows evaporation to proceed effectively and yet protects against heat absorption by radiation.

Body size and body composition. Body size is not an important factor affecting the performance of work in the heat. When clothing is worn which prevents the evaporation of sweat, the big man is at a disadvantage because he usually has a smaller ratio of body surface to weight and therefore, has more difficulty in eliminating the excess heat resulting from exercise.[9]

It is generally believed that a thick layer of subcutaneous fat also imposes a limitation on heat elimination during work because of an insulating effect of the fat. This may not be very important, however, since heat from the body core is brought to the surface mostly by the blood, rather than by conduction through the insulating shell.

COLD

Heat conservation involves hemodynamic and insulative phenomena. Vasoconstriction and adipose tissue are the major factors.

The body protects itself from exposure to cold by peripheral vasoconstriction, which conserves body heat by reducing blood circulation through skin blood vessels. Under the direction of the hypothalamus the temperature of the skin is thus permitted to fall, thereby decreasing heat loss by reducing radiation and conduction. Cooling of deeper tissues is resisted by increasing heat production through increases in metabolic rate by means of voluntary exercise or shivering. High humidity and air movement increase the rate of loss of body heat during exposure to cold. When fatigue from work or shivering has been reached, heat production will fall but heat loss will continue, resulting in a drop in body temperature.

Diet. Subjects exposed to cold maintain heat balance best when the proportion of fat in the diet is high and least well when the proportion of protein is high. In addition they are better off with many small meals than with a few large ones.

Clothing. Clothing can become a handicap in the temperature regulation of men working in the cold. Excessive sweating occurs when men fully clothed in standard Arctic uniforms work hard at 0° F. The sweat is condensed in the clothing and does not achieve skin cooling. During rest periods the moisture gradually evaporates and robs the body of heat that it can ill afford to lose at that time. When men working hard at 0° F. wore light clothing, their sweating was reduced from between 350 and 400 to 50 grams per hours. Men working in the cold should be provided with sufficient layers of easily removable, loose clothing so that the amount of clothing can be adjusted to the rate of work and so that the moisture-laden air can be circulated away from the body in order to keep the clothing dry.

The hands and feet are first to cool when the entire body is cooled. Until the body is warmed, it is very difficult to rewarm the extremities. If the body is heated while the hands and feet are exposed to cold, constricted blood vessels will be reopened and temperatures in the hands and feet will rise. These observations indicate the importance of keeping the whole body warm.

Drying effect of respiration on oral mucosa. The drying effect of respiration on the oral mucosa is a function of the absolute vapor pressure of the inspired air. Marked drying of the mucosa occurs at air temperatures below 53° F. with any moisture content, at a temperature of 60° F. with less than 77% relative humidity, and at a temperature of 70° F. with less than 39% relative humidity. The drying effect is particularly marked during ice skating, skiing, snowshoeing, and tobogganing in the outdoor winter air. If the drying effect is to be controlled under normal conditions (70° F.), over 50% relative humidity of the inspired air must be maintained.

Influence of cold on efficiency. Data on performance as affected by extreme cold are not clear-cut because of difficulties in controlling shivering and because of difficulty in describing the cold environment due to variable water vapor and air currents between layers of clothing and outside the clothing. Reported deterioration of finger dexterity and hand strength probably results from a lack of adequate local insulation by subcutaneous fat. This lack of fatty tissue may explain the apparent greater susceptibility of the hands to extremes of temperature.

AQUATIC THERMAL ENVIRONMENTS

The warmth of swimming-pool water is a critical factor in the function of the swimmer's temperature-regulating mechanisms. Bathers and other nonswimmers who perform only light exercise seem to be most comfortable in water warmed to 85° to 90° F. Learning to swim may take place faster in warm water than in cold because shivering and discomfort interfere with coordination and concentration.

Competitive sprint swimmers whose exposure to water lasts only a few seconds, as in the 50-yard dash, perform best in water between 84° and 94° F. Prolonged races are best performed in water between 74° and 79° F. Since it is usually not feasible to change swimming-pool temperature for each race or to use separate pools for different events, a cool temperature (about 75° F.) is selected to accommodate the distance swimmers whose exposure is longer. Even at this temperature heat exchange is a problem, and acclimatization of distance swimmers is an important training objective. Shifting the blood to peripheral vessels for conductive and convective cooling during vigorous exercise in water may deprive the working muscles of the extra blood supply they need to support the heavy metabolic load.

Should survivors of shipwrecks in cold waters exercise in the water or remain quiet to preserve their body temperature? Exercise produces body heat but causes peripheral vasodilatation, which brings the blood to the surface where the heat is more quickly dissipated. Resting quietly in cold water conserves energy fuels and permits the body to warm the water immediately next to the skin, providing a protective envelope. If the water is in motion, this advantage is lost.

Marathon swimmers who are exposed to cold water for prolonged periods accumulate fat subcutaneously, rather than in the deep fat deposits. The effectiveness of body fat in protecting channel swimmers from cold exposure is subject to question. As long as the fat tissue is warm it delays heat loss. When the fat becomes cold, however, it may be compared to an ice pack. The continued fall in deep temperature of the body following removal from cold environments may, at least in part, be explained on the basis of the continued loss of heat to the chilled inactive fat.

References

1. Gisolfi, C. V.: Work-heat tolerance derived from interval training, J. Appl. Physiol. 35:349, 1973.
2. Haight, J. S. J., and Keatinge, W. R.: Elevation in set point for body temperature regulation after prolonged exercise, J. Physiol. 229:77, 1973.
3. Ivy, A. C.: What is normal or normality? Quart. Bull. Northwestern Univ. Med. School. 18:22, 1944.
4. Nielsen, B., and Nielsen, M.: On the regulation of sweat secretion in exercise, Acta Physiol. Scand. 64: 314, 1965.
5. Nielsen, B., and Nielsen, M.: Influence of passive and active heating on the temperature of man, Acta Physiol. Scand. 64:323, 1965.
6. Nielsen, M.: Die Regulation der Körpertemperatur bei Muskelarbeit, Scand. Arch. Physiol. 79:193, 1938.
7. Robinson, S.: The regulation of sweating in exercise, Adv. Biol. Skin 3:152, 1962 .
8. Saltin, B., and others: Body tem-

peratures and sweating during exhaustive exercise, J. Appl. Physiol. **32:**635, 1972.

9. Shwartz, E., Saar, E., and Benor, D.: Physique and heat tolerance in hot-dry and hot-humid environments, J. Appl. Physiol. **34:**799, 1973.

10. Sohal, R. S., and others: Heatstroke, Arch. Intern. Med. **122:**43, 1968.

Suggested readings

Adolph, E., and others: Physiology of man in the desert, New York, 1969, Hafner Publishing Co.

Burton, A., and Edholm, O.: Man in a cold environment, London, 1955, Edward Arnold.

Dill, D. B., editor: Handbook of physiology. Section 4, Adaptation to the environment, Washington, D. C., 1964, American Physiological Society.

Edholm, O., and Bacharach, A.: The physiology of human survival, New York, 1966, Academic Press, Inc.

Epstein, S., and others: Effects of a reduction in environmental temperature on the circulatory response to exercise in man, N. Engl. J. Med. **280:**7, 1969.

Hammel, H.: Regulation of internal body temperature, Ann. Rev. Physiol. **30:** 301, 1968.

Hardy, J.: The "set-point" concept in physiological temperature regulation. In Yamamote, W., and Brobeck, J., editors: Physiological controls and regulation, Philadelphia, 1965, W. B. Saunders Co.

Keatinge, W.: Survival in cold water—the physiology and treatment of immersion hypothermia and drowning, Philadelphia, 1969, F. A. Davis Co.

Webb, P., and Annis, J.: Cooling required to suppress sweating during work, J. Appl. Physiol. **25:**489, 1968.

Wyndham, C. H., and others: Changes in central circulation and body fluid spaces during acclimatization to heat, J. Appl. Physiol. **25:**586, 1968.

17 ATMOSPHERE AND GRAVITY

HIGH ALTITUDES

There is increasing interest in the effect of high altitude on work performance. In addition to the approximately 10 million people who live and work at high altitudes, there are many who climb mountains for sport, athletic events are often held at medium altitudes (the 1968 Olympic Games in Mexico City, elevation 7,600 feet), and military personnel must sometimes be transported rapidly to high altitudes and there required to lead an active life.

The physiologically most important feature of high altitude is the diminished pressure of oxygen in the atmosphere, and most of this discussion will be concerned with the effect of low oxygen pressure on work performance. There are, however, additional features of the high altitude environment that must be mentioned. The *reduced density of the air* affects the mechanics of breathing. The diminished resistance to air flow in the respiratory tract decreases the work required to move a given volume of air into and out of the lungs. Another effect of the decreased air density is a diminished air resistance to movement of the body that may result in improved performance in sprint-type activities, and in other events in which air resistance is a factor (jumping, discus, javelin). The *air is cooler and dryer* at altitude; this makes exertion more pleasant but it also increases the water loss from the respiratory tract, and this may contribute to the dehydration of exercise, as well as giving rise to a sensation of soreness and dryness of the throat. *Solar radiation* is more intense at high altitude than at sea level and care must be exercised to avoid sunburn and snow blindness. The *force of gravity* is slightly less at altitude so that the work required to lift the body (as in the high jump and pole vault) is decreased. The practical effect on performance is probably quite small.

Effect of high altitude on performance. It has been mentioned that performance may actually be improved at high altitude in certain types of activity that are of short duration, because of the reduced air resistance. The reason for this is that sprint activities are powered largely by anaerobic metabolism and hence are not greatly affected by the reduction in oxygen availability. Aerobic power (maximal oxygen uptake) is, on the other hand, reduced at high altitude. This means that the intensity of work that can be performed in a steady state (such as distance running events) is reduced, and anaerobic metabolism must be called on to supplement aerobic metabolism at a lower level of exertion. In the Mexico City Olympics, there was either improvement or no impairment of performance in running events up to 400 meters. There was an impairment of about 3% in the 800 meter run and of 10% in the 5,000 and 10,000 meter events. It was also observed that the time required for recovery after events was much greater in Mexico City than at sea level. Exercises of strength (for example, weight lifting) are, like sprint activities, powered largely by anaerobic metabolism and are therefore not appreciably affected by high altitude.

Effect of high altitude on aerobic capacity. When maximal oxygen uptake is reduced due to the lowered oxygen tension at altitude, the maximal work rate is decreased proportionately. Other physiological responses are reduced in relation to the decreased intensity of the stress. The proportional contribution of anaerobic glycolysis and the resultant appearance of lactate during exercise at altitude is similar to that during an equivalent intensity of work at sea level. Muscle high-energy phosphate concentrations are reduced in amounts proportional to the lowered oxygen uptake and work rate at altitude. Apparently, it is the reduced availability of oxygen which is the major factor affecting physiological responses to exercise at altitude.

The maximal values reported for heart rate, stroke volume, and cardiac output are not reduced during an acute exposure to altitudes up to 14,000 feet, indicating that the efficiency of the heart in pumping blood is not impaired. This is supported by the absence of electrocardiographic evidence of myocardial ischemia (deficient blood supply) during maximal exertion at altitude. With a normal maximal cardiac output at altitude, the reduction in maximal oxygen uptake must be due entirely to the decrease in the oxygen content of the arterial blood. In a study of subjects performing maximal work at a simulated altitude of 4,000 meters (13,200 feet), the maximal oxygen uptake and arterial oxygen content were 72 and 74%, respectively, of the sea level values, while maximal cardiac output was 100% of the sea level value. After sojourns of several months at very high altitudes, the maximal cardiac output may be markedly reduced below sea level values, because of reduction in both heart rate and stroke volume, especially the latter. This suggests that the contractile power of the heart muscle may be limited by its reduced oxygen supply during exercise at very high altitude.

Respiration. Newcomers to altitude often have difficulty in adjusting respiratory volumes to decreased air density and hypoxia. In medium altitudes some hypoventilate and others hyperventilate. At high altitudes, above 5,000 meters, almost everyone hyperventilates.

After about a week at high altitude the buffer capacity of the blood is reduced, and with it the ability to tolerate high blood lactic acid levels. The reduced blood buffer capacity results from the increased excretion of bicarbonate in the urine, which compensates the respiratory alkalosis caused by hyperventilation. The reduction in blood buffer concentration means that anaerobic capacity, which is normal on first exposure to high altitude, is gradually lowered during continued sojourn.

With prolonged stay at altitude, acclimatization occurs and performance improves. The important features of altitude acclimatization are increased hemoglobin concentration in the blood, growth of new capillaries in many organs, and increase in the myoglobin concentration of the heart and skeletal muscles. The initial alkalosis resulting from hyperventilation is compensated by the excretion of bicarbonate. The blood pH and cerebral blood flow return to nearly normal levels. These alterations improve the capacity for the transport and utilization of oxygen, and hence increase the aerobic power toward the normal sea level value.

Altitude training. If athletic events lasting more than 2 minutes are to be performed at altitude, a period of training at altitude is essential for optimal performance. At the altitude of Mexico City (7,600 feet), a 2- or 3-week period of training was found to be adequate for most events. Many experts recommend rather light work intensity during the first week at altitude, followed by a gradual increase to the maximum. The intensity of training exercise should be as high as possible in order to minimize the detraining effects that result from the fact that maximal exercise intensity at altitude is usually lower than that at sea level. There seems to be no advantage in training at a higher altitude than that at which the competition will take place, because the detraining effect increases with altitude. A period of altitude training longer than necessary may also be detrimental to performance, because of a slight muscular detraining effect and a diminution of plasma volume and stroke volume.

While training at altitude improves performance at altitude, there is little evidence that it improves performance at sea level (more than would training at sea level). In fact, some of the changes resulting from altitude training may be detrimental to sea level performance (for example, the reduction in blood bicarbonate that occurs at altitude). Similarly,

217

breathing low oxygen mixtures during sea level training affords no advantage to performance at sea level.[2]

EXERCISE IN SPACE

Neuromuscular adjustment to weightlessness in space is almost immediate. There is a kinesthetic awareness of the lack of weight of body segments, clothing, and objects. Crewmen soon learn to send objects to each other at minimal velocity, or to "park" them in space. Locomotion and changes in posture are accomplished by easy swimming motions, and by rolling, tumbling, and spinning. The energy cost of movement is less than under earth gravity conditions.

Sensory adaptation to weightlessness takes a day or two. A feeling of fullness in the head accompanies the escape from earth gravity, and gradually disappears after the first day in space. Movements of the head must be made cautiously during the first two days to avoid stomach awareness, nausea, and vomiting. Until adaptation occurs there seems to be an enhancement of sensory inputs from the semicircular canals to the central nervous system during head movements in space.

Other changes are taking place in the body that are not noticed by the astronaut until gravity loading during reentry deceleration and return to earth gravity conditions.

During the first few hours on earth after a week or more in space, any posture change speeds the heart rate. There is a tendency toward fainting on sudden standing.

The effort of standing and moving about is difficult. The astronaut feels heavy, with sensations similar to those under stress of 2 g. in a centrifuge. As a consequence he prefers to lie down and, by doing so, return to the ease of weightlessness.

Tests of orthostatic hypotension bear out the sensations of circulatory difficulties. Under lower body negative pressure (LBNP) of 50 mm. Hg, the heart rate accelerates to 160 per minute; it stays below 100 before the flight. During vertical passive standing for 5 minutes after remaining supine for 5 minutes, the heart rate after space flight accelerates above 110 per minute as compared with a stabilized preflight heart rate of 80.

There is other objective evidence of cardiovascular deconditioning caused by space flight. While riding a bicycle ergometer at a controlled heart rate after space flight the subject produces less physical work. Evidence that this decrement in work performance is due to lessened cardiovascular efficiency is a reduced oxygen pulse (cost in heart rate to deliver a unit of oxygen) during the test exercise postflight.[1] There is also a loss of red cell mass, up to 20% in pure oxygen cabin atmosphere, and 4.4% when a nitrogen-oxygen mixture is used. There is a loss of bone minerals, up to 15% in some areas of the body such as the calcaneus, which receives little stress in space compared with the heel strike jolts it customarily receives in walking on earth. Blood and bone losses are not sensed, but they could seriously limit performance under emergency conditions.

After being on earth for 24 to 36 hours, red cell mass, cardiovascular function, and exercise response return to preflight states. Bone density is restored shortly thereafter. Longer flights require a longer recovery time. After an 18-day space flight, the cosmonauts took 10 days for normal function to return at ground level.

The deconditioning effect of space flight demonstrates the impermanence of our adjustment to earth gravity. Whether weightlessness is a more "natural" environment for man than earth gravity remains to be discovered in longer space flights. If red cell mass, bone density, and other body substances stabilize at an acceptable level rather than continuing to decrease during weightlessness, it may be that man has found an environment more suitable to him, at least in terms of gravity. With reduced gravity he may even live longer away from earth because of decreased physiological deterioration, since orthostatic stress is reduced.

Astronauts easily perform useful work on the surface of the moon and readily adjust to the ⅙ gravity of the lunar environment. There is a temptation, because of the feeling of lightness, to use hopping and jumping forms of locomotion. The energy cost of lunar locomotion, estimated by monitoring oxygen usage and liquid-cooled garment temperatures, is about 30 Calories per hour. Peak heart rates above 140 per minute during collection of lunar rock samples revealed that astronauts do heavy work during their exploration of the moon.

The slight deconditioning of the cardiovascular system and diminished exercise capacity incurred during the 3-day flight to the moon do not significantly affect work performance on the moon. However, the men who will work for several months on orbiting space stations and travel in space for more than a year to explore Mars, Venus, and other planets will need improved methods of on-board exercise to aid in the preservation of performance capacity.

TIME ZONE CHANGES

The increasing speed of air travel to distant points of the world results in quick time shifts and changes in normal daily rhythms of darkness-light cycles, low and high temperatures, activity and inactivity, sleep and wakefulness, meal routines, and psychological estimation of time. Such asynchrony disturbs the metabolic and circulatory functions, which usually have peak levels in the afternoon or early evening. These disruptions in circadian rhythms may delay the adaptive processes in acclimatization of travelers to high altitude and hot climates.

ECOLOGICAL FATIGUE

The combined effects of rapidly changing time zones, altitudes, climates, foods and waters, and sights, sounds, and smells encountered on extended travel tours can gradually erode the individual's adaptability to these changes. The declining performance of athletes that often occurs on world tours may be due to such "travel sickness" or ecological fatigue. Preventive measures include the allowance of at least a 4-day adjustment period in each new environment before high performance is demanded, and duplication as much as possible of "home" conditions every day during travel.

References

1. Rummell, T. A., Michel, E. L., and Berry, C. A.: Physiological response to exercise after space flight—Apollo 7 to Apollo 11, Aerospace Med. **44:** 235, 1973.
2. Shephard, R. J.: The athlete at high altitude, Canad. Med. Assoc. J. **109:** 207, 1973.

Suggested readings

Faulkner, J. A.: Maximum exercise at medium altitude. In Shephard, R. J., editor: Frontiers of fitness, Springfield, Ill., 1971, Charles C Thomas, Publisher, p. 360.

Goddard, R., editor: The effects of altitude on athletic performance, Chicago, 1967, Athletic Institute.

Weike, W. H., editor: Physiological effects of high altitude, Oxford, 1964, Pergamon Press.

PART SIX

EXERCISE TRAINING

18 FITNESS AND TRAINING

ADAPTATION

Use and disuse. Unlike machines, which wear out more rapidly when they are used, living organisms generally develop an adaptive increase in functional capacity in response to increased use and undergo a decrease in functional capacity when they are not used. With use enlargement and reorganization of tissue structures also occur, and with disuse the tissues become smaller.

Just as the capacity of an individual to perform a task depends on the demands which he has met in the preceding period, so the capacity of each organ to function is adjusted to its demands. Physical activity engages every organ and system of the body and promotes adaptation to use. An organism will deteriorate with lack of exercise.

Specific adaptation to imposed demands. Adaptation to physical activity varies in accordance with the type of exercise. The organism adapts specifically to the demands imposed upon it. This is the SAID principle of exercise: Specific Adaptation to *I*mposed *D*emands.

The effects of frequent and regular physical activity are seen most dramatically when exercise is stopped. The muscles of an arm or leg immobilized in a plaster cast atrophy and lose strength in a few days. A week of complete bed rest causes orthostatic hypotension and ataxia. These abnormalities are corrected when activity is resumed. The degree of restoration is generally proportional to the degree of activity, and within this process several laws seem to be operating.

Exercise increases the capacity for more exercise, by stimulating morphological, physiological, and behavioral changes in the organism. Lamarck's expression, "Use makes the organ" is a concise description of the phenomenon. As Hippocrates explained, "That which is used develops and that which is not used wastes away." In this chapter we shall explore the phenomena of repeated muscular activity in an attempt to explain the physiological laws and principles of exercise training.

Law of overcompensation. Growth, development, and further improvement by training take place, in some way, by a process involving both destruction and repair. In the process of repair there is an overproduction of lost materials. The callus on the palm of the hand is an overproduction of skin in response to the loss of skin due to friction. Muscle fibrils are splintered during strong contractions, and these develop into additional units. The fatigue of acute exercise is more than overcome, giving the organism a greater capacity to resist further fatigue. The body develops an immunity to the stress of exercise when given small doses of exercise, just as it develops an immunity to a toxin when small doses of the toxin are given.

PHYSICAL FITNESS

Physical fitness is the quality of the whole body in terms of its state of adaptation to physical activity. A physically fit person is not overly fat, has a strong skeleton, has neuromuscular strength, has strong connective tissues, and has good circulorespiratory endurance. Being physically fit does not necessarily mean being healthy or being able to perform a highly skilled event. Health and performance are separate qualities: one can suffer from cancer yet be fit for strenuous exercise; one can be unfit for hard work and unhealthy and be a superior performer in skill events.

Being physically fit means, in general terms, more than having strong legs, having a high oxygen uptake, or having a powerful heart. These discrete qualities are termed leg strength fitness, aerobic fitness, and cardiac fitness.

An unfit person is one who has deadapted to physical activity because of a lack of exercise. His proportion of fat to other tissues is often high, his skeleton is fragile, he is weak, and he has poor stamina. His body quality has deteriorated so that he has a poor ability to perform movement functions.

The term "fitness" implies a relation between the task to be performed and the individual's capability to perform it. If the task is a specific one, such as lifting a heavy weight, a person's fitness for it can be easily demonstrated by an attempt to lift it. If he is successful, it can be said that his fitness for that task is adequate. If he fails to lift it, he can be judged unfit. A simple test such as this, however, does not reflect the individual's *degree* of fitness; perhaps the weight was just barely too heavy for him. Neither does it tell his *capacity;* perhaps a few weeks of training would enable him to lift it. Furthermore, it is not known why he failed; perhaps it was because of a fear of injuring himself.

If the task is nonspecific, such as the carrying out of normal daily life activities, fitness implies that the individual accomplishes these with a reasonable degree of efficiency, without undue fatigue, and with complete recovery before the next day's activities are begun. He is unfit if any of the activities are performed unsatisfactorily, if he is overly fatigued by them, or if his recovery is too slow. In this circumstance one can always become more "fit" by reducing the intensity of his daily life activities or by improving his efficiency, increasing his resistance to fatigue, and adopting more effective recovery procedures.

Fitness relates to a task; it does not describe a state of health. Diabetic persons have been tennis champions. Individuals with heart disease have become successful distance runners. Victims of cancer continue to perform well in the early stages of the disease. In such instances the pathological condition has not become a limiting factor in the performance of work. It is not until the disease becomes debilitating that it affects fitness.

ASPECTS OF FITNESS

An individual's state of fitness for exercise is dependent upon the suitability of his body structure for the work to be performed, the effectiveness with which his organs and systems support the effort, and the view that the individual takes of the task as he approaches it and carries it through to completion.

Anatomical fitness. In order to be fit, the individual must possess all of the body parts essential to the performance of the task and must possess the appropriate body size and shape for the task. Genetic imperfections in organs and tissues are responsible for weakness in structure and function. These limit the individual's capacity for strength, endurance, and skill.

Slight individual differences in the points of attachment of tendons to bones and differences in lengths of bones result in different mechanical leverage advantages or disadvantages for various events. Thus one person is fit for weight lifting, another for sprint running, and another for jumping. If a person enters a competition for which he is anatomically unfit, he does so with a distinct disadvantage compared to his opponents who possess anatomical features more fit to the event.

Physiological fitness. For the physiological systems of the body to be fit they must function well enough to support the particular activity that the individual is performing. Since different activities make different demands upon the organism with respect to neurological, respiratory, circulatory, metabolic, and temperature-regulating functions, physiological fitness is specific to the activity. Physiological systems are highly adaptable to exercise, as has been shown in preceding chapters. The response of each system is discrete; hard work in the heat is necessary to improve the fitness of the temperature-regulation mechanism. Each task has its major physiological components, and fitness for the task requires effective functioning of the appropriate systems.

Psychological fitness. If the individual possesses the necessary perceptions, emotional stability, motivation, intelligence, and educability to accomplish the task, he is psychologically fit for it. Anxiety can become a barrier to performance by contributing tension, elevated heart rate and blood pressure, and endocrine disturbances that add to the stress of the task and therefore contribute to the individual's unfitness for it. No one is without anxieties, but some are better able to adapt to the stress of anxiety in their lives, and these persons are more psychologically fit for arduous work.

ASSESSMENT OF GENERAL FITNESS

General fitness implies more than one task and is usually meant to include not only the activities of everyday life but also emergencies in which a person is unexpectedly called upon to perform activities demanding unusual expenditures of strength, energy, and adaptive ability under extremely unfavorable environments. Examples of these are motor vehicle accidents, home fires, floods and mudslides, shipwrecks, falls, and physical attacks.

It would be unrealistic to expect that the person in a sedentary occupation would prepare himself by regular exercise to meet all of these emergencies. The demands of this spectrum of emergencies are so widespread that the person trained to meet them adequately would have to spend several hours every day in preparation. Only an exercise addict would do this.

A more rational goal that would keep the individual prepared to cope to some extent with emergencies and also to enjoy physical recreations would be at that level represented by an hour of vigorous tennis or an afternoon of moderately heavy yard work every other day.

PHYSIOLOGICAL FACTORS IN FITNESS

Homeodynamics. Physiological fitness for exertion is dependent for the most part upon nervous system coordination of muscular activity, respiration, circulation, and temperature regulation. This coordination, which ultimately regulates behavior, is crucially dependent upon effective functioning of homeostatic mechanisms that have been established for survival in and adaptation to situations involving stress. It is the function of these homeostatic mechanisms to maintain the internal environment of the organism within the range of limitations necessary for the normal activity of the cells.

When an individual exerts himself, the internal environment is upset, and the stress, which occurs as a result of the upset, stimulates the mechanisms that reestablish homeostasis. If the activity is sustained and a steady state is established in the internal environment, a new level of metabolic, respiratory, circulatory, and temperature-regulatory balance may be achieved. In a sense the internal environment is "at rest" during activity; the processes are in balance at an elevated level. The process of establishing a steady state at elevated levels of physical activity may be termed *homeodynamics*. The ability to establish and maintain a steady state at elevated levels of physical activity is a measure of a person's *homeodynamic fitness*. The highest level of activity at which a person can maintain a steady state represents his *homeodynamic capacity*.

Limiting factors in homeodynamic capacity are the maintenance of adequate blood sugar levels, the preservation of optimal hydrogen ion concentration, and the provision of adequate oxygen supply. The proper function of the nervous system depends on each of these. The first sign of failure of any of them is a lightheaded or dazed sensation followed by fatigue and dizziness and, in extreme failure, collapse and coma. In the fit person coordination, strength, and other characteristics of performance are affected less in early stages of homeodynamic breakdown. In advanced stages both fit and unfit behave alike; they reel, stumble, and fall.

Maintenance of blood sugar level. Heavy physical activity causes fluctuations in the blood sugar level above and below the 60 to 90 mg. per 100 ml. normal level. Blood sugar levels above the 90 mg. upper limit (*hyperglycemia*) are reached in heavy physical exercise in which exhaustion occurs after 10 to 40 minutes. Activity that results in exhaustion in less than 10 minutes usually raises blood sugar somewhat but not beyond the normal range. If exhaustion occurs in less than 3 minutes, there is usually only a small elevation in the blood sugar level. Although fit individuals tend to experience less hyperglycemia than those less fit for exertion, the elevated blood sugar during this temporary period seems to have neither beneficial nor detrimental effects.

If hard work is continued for over an hour, as in marathon running, and no food is taken, the blood sugar level falls below 60 mg. per 100 ml. and *hypoglycemia* occurs. In the fit individual regulatory mechanisms that cause the liver to maintain normal blood sugar levels operate more effectively, so that activity can proceed longer before hypoglycemia occurs. The fall in blood sugar concentration after an hour of hard work is greater in unfit than in fit persons. The smaller fluctuations in blood sugar levels in the fit individuals in both brief and prolonged exhausting exercise are a measure of the superiority of their homeodynamic mechanisms.

Preservation of hydrogen ion concentration. The pH of the blood is usually about 7.4, with a normal range of 7.3 to 7.5 and an extreme range of from 6.8 to 7.8. The acid residues of heavy work almost never change the blood from slightly alkaline to acid. The catabolic acids are reduced by the buffers in the blood, acid excretion from the kidneys, and elimination of carbon dioxide through the lungs. As a result, 30 minutes of moderately heavy work followed by a sprint to exhaustion reduces the pH only to 7.25. Fit individuals are only slightly better able to maintain normal pH than are those unfit for exertion.

Provision of oxygen. Continuous muscular work depends upon an adequate supply of oxygen. Although fuels for energy may be present and some of them can be used without oxygen, without sufficient oxygen energy production soon fails to support physical activity. The relation between oxygen consumption and the production of work is linear, and this linearity has been widely used as a basis for determining fitness for exertion.

A major factor limiting the working capacity of an individual is the maximal oxygen supply to the working muscles. The required oxygen is supplied by a chain of processes in series as follows:

1. Transport of oxygen from the atmosphere into the alveoli through pulmonary ventilation. As discussed in Chapter 8 pulmonary ventilation is usually sufficient and does not limit oxygen uptake.
2. The diffusion of oxygen from the alveoli into the pulmonary capillary blood, including its combination with hemoglobin. Diffusion limitation in the lungs occurs during heavy exercise at high altitude, but not at sea level.
3. The transport of oxygen by the blood from the pulmonary capillaries to the muscle capillaries, including cardiac output and blood flow to the working muscles. As shown before, cardiac output is the principal limiting factor for oxygen supply.
4. The diffusion of oxygen from the muscle capillary blood into the muscle cells.

Maximal oxygen consumption is an index of aerobic power and is also the best measure of fitness for continuous exercise. The estimation of oxygen consumption requires special apparatus and is time consuming. It is usually necessary to repeat the maximal work several times, otherwise maximal values for oxygen uptake and heart rate may not be obtained. Therefore, classifying the fitness of individuals using this method is impractical if many subjects are to be tested.

Fortunately, however, pulse rate, which is easy to measure, correlates significantly with oxygen consumption during exercise. This correlation has been employed successfully in a number of fitness tests. (See Chapters 8, 14, and 17 in the *Laboratory Manual*.)

BED REST—DETRIMENTAL EFFECTS ON FITNESS

Prolonged bed rest has drastic—but fortunately, reversible—effects on a number of physiological functions, including the calcium metabolism of the bones, muscle strength, the cardiovascular response to standing, and the maximal oxygen uptake.

Prolonged bed rest may cause a twofold increase in urinary calcium excretion. This is not due to lack of exercise, since it is not prevented by bicycle ergometer exercise in the supine position. It appears to be due to the absence of weight-bearing stress in the long bones, since it is prevented by 3 hours quiet standing in addition to the supine bed rest. This loss of calcium from the bones is a matter of concern for astronauts during prolonged periods of weightlessness.

The decreased muscle power associated with bed rest is caused by disuse, and it can be prevented (if the condition of the patient allows it) by subjecting the muscles, for a few seconds each day, to submaximal contractions of more than one-third the maximal strength. Isometric contractions are suitable for this purpose.

Prolonged bed rest produces a marked deterioration in the cardiovascular response to standing (excessive rise in heart rate and fall in blood pressure). This reduced tolerance develops after only a few days of bed rest, especially in older persons, but it disappears after a few days of ambulation. It may be largely prevented by a few hours ambulation each day or by the application of intermittent negative pressure to the lower part of the body during recumbent posture.

There is a striking decrease in maximal oxygen uptake in supine exercise after a few weeks in bed. Despite an increase in the heart rate there is a decreased cardiac output, because of a reduction in the stroke volume. The arteriovenous oxygen difference is increased in submaximal exercise, indicating a less adequate blood flow through the working muscles. The major deterioration in oxygen transport capacity is the result of the reduction in maximal stroke volume, suggesting that the contractile power of the heart muscle has been impaired.

TRAINING

Diminishing returns from maximal training. If a person in poor condition starts an intensive training program and exercises as hard and as long as he can every day without injuring himself or becoming overfatigued, his rate of training will resemble that charted in Fig. 28. Gains will come most rapidly at first. Nearly half of the improvement which can be expected from point A to point E will occur in the time period from point A to point B.

The very slight gains beyond point E are made at great expense of time and energy in training. This prospect is discouraging to all but the dedicated athlete or the fitness fanatic.

Achievement of training benefits at point B is relatively easy and rewarding, a reasonable goal of any physical fitness program. In a young adult, if point A represents a deconditioned state following months of

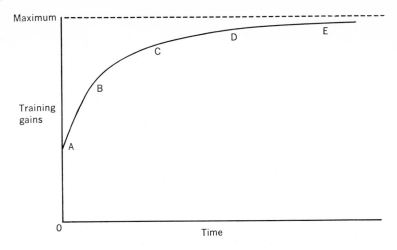

Fig. 28. Chart of decreasing gains in progressive training. See text for reference to letters *A* through *E*.

sedentary living, point B would represent a training level achieved by a moderate fitness program. To maintain this B level the participant would need to be physically active for only a short time each day equivalent to about 300 extra activity Calories—to lift something moderately heavy at least once; to climb stairs or other similar exertion to elevate the pulse rate above 110 for a few minutes; and to twist, turn, and stretch the joints to their full range of motion.

Diminishing gains in continuous training. A person in poor condition who starts progressive training at point A can be expected to improve to point B in about 2 weeks—a considerable gain. During the second 2 weeks the improvement from point B to point C will be only half of that gained during the first 2 weeks. The returns from training diminish gradually until about the sixth week, point D, beyond which gains are less and less noticeable.

Effect of starting condition on training gains. Gains in strength, endurance, or other qualities of function are greatest during the early period of training and in participants who were most severely deconditioned at the start of training. A person who starts at point A will make nearly twice the gain in the first 2 weeks of training as will the person in better condition starting at point B. A third person in D condition will make only barely perceptible gains in 2 weeks of training.

Again referring to our training chart in Fig. 28, let level B represent the fitness needed for an event—strength required for tennis, as an example. It is advantageous to train to level C in order to acquire an adequate reserve. But, the time and effort required to advance to level D in strength would be wasteful. That much strength is not needed for the power requirements of tennis. The time and effort would be better spent on the development of more essential qualities, such as skill.

The advantages of reserve strength and endurance are appreciated on occasions when unusually strenuous effort is required, when the event is carried into extra time periods, or when the climate is oppressive (too hot, too humid, high altitude). The presence of a reserve of training also gives the contestant a feeling of confidence. He feels superior to the demands he is likely to meet and is able to focus on strategy and tactics, rather than worrying whether he can apply sufficient force. As a pilot once reminded us when he saw the rigorous physical training program we had designed for his groups, "I don't have to be able to lift the aircraft in order to fly it!" He was right.

Training intensity. Physiological changes resulting from training are generally related to the intensity of the exercise. Intensity is expressed in terms of effort relative to the subject's initial capacity. The enhancement of capacity is greatest when loads of 90 to 100% of the individual's capacity are imposed. Maximal loads are potentially injurious and painful, and are utilized mainly by athletes in their final training for championship performance.

Significant training changes occur at levels of intensity as low as 25% of maximal. Cardiovascular function of middle-aged men improves identically at the intensities of 80 and 92% of the individual's maximum heart rate, equal to 70 and 87% of his maximal oxygen uptake.[7] The lower levels are safer and much better tolerated by nonathletes.

In deconditioned subjects the initial training exercise can safely and effectively start at an intensity of 65% maximal heart rate or its equivalent, 50% maximal oxygen uptake. Training intensities above 80% maximal heart rate and 70% maximal oxygen uptake are restricted to healthy young subjects and athletes, and to exercise testing of others under carefully supervised and controlled laboratory conditions.

When trained at the same relative intensity, greater improvement will occur in less fit subjects than in more fit subjects. Intensity levels below 65% of maximal heart rate (or 50% maximal oxygen uptake) may be too low to induce further training in young subjects who are already moderately fit.

Arbitrary heart rates should be used with caution in monitoring physical training activities. A heart rate of 120 represents 60 and 71% of the age-predicted maximal heart rate of persons age 20 and 50, respectively.
number of lifts, is even more imprecise in defining the intensity of effort.

Use of physical work units, such as time and distance or weights and
The same physical work may require twice the effort in a poorly conditioned person than in a well-conditioned one, and four times as much in

a postcoronary patient. Use of a physiological unit such as heart rate is safer because the effort is controlled and changes in efficiency due to training, illness, fatigue, and climate are automatically adjusted; less physical work is required to produce a heart rate of 120 on a cool day than on a hot, humid one.

Indices of intensity of effort. The main factor that influences the response to a training regimen is the *intensity* of effort relative to the subject's initial capacity.

The index of intensity of muscular effort is the tension which the muscle develops during contraction. Tension is proportional to the resistance to the contraction, or the load placed upon the muscle.

There are several indices of the intensity of circulorespiratory effort. The most direct one is the rate of oxygen uptake.

Indirect indices of circulorespiratory effort are heart rate, blood pressure, pulmonary ventilation volume, blood lactate, and electrocardiographic changes. Heart rate is the most convenient and reliable indirect index of circulorespiratory effort.

Heart rate has an additional value in measuring the intensity of exercise in that it expresses the degree of cardiac stress. Heart rate, expressed as percent of maximal heart rate, bears significant relationships to coronary blood flow, myocardial oxygen uptake as a percent of maximal oxygen uptake, respiratory exchange ratio, lactate production, and catecholamine excretion.[4]

CONTROL OF INTENSITY

Energy cost and point systems. Physiological responses to physical activities vary from session to session because of the vigor applied, emotional states, fatigue, and variations in climate. Therefore the use of tables of energy cost of activities or other estimations of the intensity of activities (see p. 123), such as point systems,[2] to regulate the intensity of exercise are erroneous. Thus there can be no pharmacopoeia of activities.

Monitoring physical work versus physiological effort. Training protocols may be controlled by monitoring either the *physical work* or the *physiological effort* during the activity.

Physical work is expressed in terms of distance and time (rate), load (resistance or mass), and number of contractions (repetitions). In the physical mode of control, the work is defined and the performer attempts to follow the schedule. Other than exhaustion, the degree of physiological effort is not considered. Exhaustion may or may not occur, and the work may be too light to stimulate physiological development. Monitoring the physical work does not take into account the day-to-day variations in physiological efficiency, nor does it adjust for the daily changes in climate.

Physiological effort is expressed in terms of heart rate, which is easily monitored (see p. 88), or the degree of perceived exertion, which is a reliable estimate of the energy expended during steady state work (see p. 161). In the physiological mode of control the heart rate or degree of perceived exertion, together with the time the effort is to be applied, are defined. In following this schedule the performer's exertion is controlled at the level that stimulates development. Exhaustion can be avoided by scheduling the effort within tolerance limits. Physiological monitoring provides a continuous adjustment for transient changes in the organism and for environmental influences, since the body responses to the effort are proportionately greater the greater the degree of fatigue, body heat storage, and other factors which add to the effort of performance. By holding the physiological effort constant in a training protocol, the performer will automatically adjust his intensity or rate of work to the changing internal physiological and the external environmental conditions from moment to moment. The following is an example of a training protocol based on physiological effort.

Time (min.)	Activity	Physiological effort	
		Perceived exertion	*Heart rate*
0-3	Walking, limbering, and stretching	9-10	90-100
3-8	Walking briskly uphill	13-14	130-140
8-10	Walking slowly	10-11	100-110
10-12	Sitting at rest	8-9	80-90

Original prescription. It is always prudent to commence a regimen of exercise at a low intensity and very gradually work up toward a maximal level. The practice of establishing an exercise prescription on the basis of a test of maximal work or aerobic capacity is dangerous except for young athletes in proven good health. It is safer and more effective to use a starting point based on the subject's estimated capacity. This can be done in terms of either heart rate or oxygen uptake. A safe starting level in adult subjects who are deconditioned is at 65% of the age-adjusted estimated maximal heart rate. This is equivalent to 50% of maximal oxygen uptake.

Mode of exercise. Improvement in physical fitness is similar whether the group of skeletal muscles is exercised in one or another form of activity. Use of the leg muscles in walking, running, and cycling may produce equal increases in maximal oxygen uptake, equal decreases in resting heart rate, and equal weight loss from a reduction in fat.[7]

There is no cross-adaptation, however. Training of the leg muscles does not produce training of the arm muscles, and vice-versa. Because of this lack of cross-adaptation, training of leg muscles improves cardiac response to exercise when the legs are used. Cardiac response to arm exercise is not improved by leg exercise training. A physical fitness program should thus include a variety of exercises which use all major muscles in the body.

Progressive overload. The main factor influencing the extent of training produced by a training program is the *intensity* of the training effort, with *frequency* and *duration* exerting lesser effects. Fitness is best improved by high-intensity, high-frequency, and long-duration exercise sessions. Similar, but not as high level, benefits can be obtained by less intense, less frequent, and shorter periods of exercise.

PROGRESSION

The principle of overload was illustrated by the legendary Milo of Crotona, who became able to carry a 4-year-old bull because he had practiced lifting it from the time it was a calf. By today's standards of man and beast, either it must have been a small bull or Milo was a superman. Today's bull calves gain over 500 pounds a year. Nevertheless, the principle of training by loading oneself a little more heavily each session is a sound one.

If the load on the organism is constant from day to day, the body will at first gradually adapt to that load. Eventually, when adaptation is complete, the load will no longer stimulate the training processes and there will be no further improvement. Finally, some deterioration in condition will occur as the body systems become refractory to the unchanging stimulus. Suppose, for example, a person who is sedentary but otherwise healthy starts jogging a mile in exactly 10 minutes once every day. His physiological responses to that exercise will improve rapidly during the first 3 weeks, gradually taper off the second 3 weeks, show little further gain during the third 3-week portion, and will probably begin to deteriorate somewhat during the fourth 3-week period. Eventually, a new level of dynamic homeostasis will be reached as he becomes totally adjusted to the jogging stimulus. This final condition will be somewhat less than it was at the peak of training, but it will be well above his original sedentary state. In terms of fitness, he will now be fit for his new lifestyle; sedentary living plus the mile in 10 minutes—no more, no less.

There are many ways to progressively overload, as summarized below, and the most effective training regimens employ several in systematic order.

Intensity. Milo's method of increasing the *weight* lifted every session is limited, as we have seen. Adding even a very small increment of weight to one's exercise every session eventually leads to failure, exhaustion, or injury long before maximal capacity for training has been reached.

The same is true in methods of intensifying load employing *speed,* such as attempting to run a distance a little faster every day. The day soon comes when speed cannot be increased, so that is the end of that training regimen.

Instead of adding heavier weights, overload in successive sessions can be achieved by increasing the number of *repetitions* of submaximal loads. Or, the duration of the exercise can be increased—gradually increasing the distance of jogging, for example, without increasing the speed. Progression in intensity is achieved by rotating the order of additions of weight, speed, and duration.

Frequency. The gain in aerobic power decreases from 19.5 to 16.0% when the frequency of training is decreased from five to three sessions per week.[8] Cardiovascular fitness is retained nearly as effectively by three sessions per week as by four sessions per week.[1] Lesser degrees of improvement occur with two or one sessions per week, but if the training is intensive the improvement is significant. The notion that one workout a week is worse than none at all is invalid.

Duration. Duration is the least sensitive parameter of the intensity-frequency-duration triad of training. In general, high-intensity, high-frequency, short-duration exercise sessions are as effective as those of longer duration. An interval training program of four periods of bicycle ergometer exercise each lasting 3 minutes, interrupted by 3-minute rest periods, produces significant improvements.[9] Longer training sessions allow for more variety in exercises and provide time for recreational activities when groups are involved. This greater diversity leads to better adherence and may account for the superiority of group over individual training.

Time taken for warming up, preparations and instructions for exercise, and cooling off are usually included in experimental training protocols, so the actual minimal duration of intensive exercise required to produce and maintain physiological training effects is probably about 30 minutes per week.

	Methods of monitoring	
Methods of progressive overload	*Physiological effort*	*Physical work*
Load	Perceived exertion (degree of heaviness)	Mass, or weight to be lifted, or resistance to be overcome
Rate	Exercise heart rate	Speed
Duration	Time	Time
Repetition	Exercise heart rate	Counts per set

Methods of progressive overload	Methods of monitoring	
	Physiological effort	*Physical work*
Sets per session	Count	Count
Recovery between sets	Recovery heart rate	Time
Frequency	Sessions per week	Sessions per week

Persistence of training. When training is halted, the physiological systems return to the pretrained state. The changes may not be perceptible in the first week if training has been maintained for several months. When all training is discontinued, about 50% of the gain in aerobic power is lost in 5 weeks, and most circulatory parameters return to pretraining levels after 10 weeks of detraining.[5]

At the cessation of an exercise regimen there is a period of 2 or 3 days during which the level of training persists if the participant remains fairly active. (In bed rest, strength diminishes about 5% every 3 days.) This persistence of training allows for an occasional layoff for a day or two without a loss in performance capacity.

After the second or third day of diminished activity, there is a perceptible decline in strength and endurance. If training is discontinued further, there is a sharp decline for a week or two. After 2 weeks, decline begins to level off and a new plateau of training is reached in about a month.

Warming up. Performance is improved if the muscles have been slightly warmed up just before the activity. Most baseball pitchers, for example, work better on warm days. Failure to warm up before vigorous activity may lead to an actual tearing loose of muscle fibers from their tendinous attachments.

Observations on the contraction of isolated muscles provide a clue to the nature of the warming up process. If the muscle is slightly warmed, the speed with which it contracts and relaxes and the force of contraction are increased. If a previously inactive muscle is stimulated repeatedly, the first few contractions are often small and irregular, and relaxation is incomplete. After this the contractions become stronger and relaxation is complete. It is probable that warming up is due in part to these changes in the muscle itself, involving a local rise in temperature and the accumulation of metabolic products. It is possible that the viscosity of the muscle is thereby decreased, allowing contraction and relaxation to occur with greater promptness. In the body these same factors also increase the local blood flow through the muscle by dilating the small blood vessels. This improves the functional condition of the muscle by increasing its oxygen supply.

The muscles most frequently torn during strenuous activity that has not been preceded by a warming up period are the antagonists to the contracting muscles. These "cold" antagonistic muscles relax slowly and incompletely when the agonists contract and thus retard free movement and accurate coordination. At the same time the force of contraction of the agonists and the momentum of the moving part exert a strain on the unyielding antagonists, with consequent tearing of the muscle fibers or their tendinous attachments.

Warm-up activities preliminary to a performance may be of two types: (1) general or (2) specific. *General warm-up* activities are unrelated to the performance and are for the purpose of an overall preparation of the body for optimal function during strenuous effort. Typical activities for a general warm-up are calisthenic stretching and body movement exercises. It may also include a body massage, but such passive warm-up is not as effective as active warm-up.

The physiological mechanisms of general warm-up consist of a slight rise in body temperature and a slight increase in metabolic rate. Blood circulation and respiratory function are augmented. At the cellular level oxygen transport is increased and hemoglobin is better able to release its oxygen. Vascular resistance is lessened and oxygen is more accessible to the cells.

The slight rise in body temperature facilitates a faster speed of nerve impulses, and warm muscles contract and relax faster. The viscosity of the muscles decreases, making contraction and relaxation easier. The oxygen attached to myoglobin is released more readily in the warmed muscle.

General warm-up delays the onset of muscle soreness and may extend exercise capacity. By decreasing the viscosity of tissues, general warm-up may reduce the susceptibility to musculotendinous injury.

Specific warm-up activities are related to the actions and skills used in the actual event or contest. Swinging the bat or golf club, throwing the baseball, or passing and shooting the basketball in modes simulating conditions of play are examples of specific warm-up.

Specific warm-up rehearses the reflex nervous system which controls movement. By regaining familiarity prior to a contest, complex skills become better integrated.

If the process of warming up is carried to the point at which body temperature is measurably raised, work capacity will be lowered. As was shown in Chapter 16, removal of excess body heat storage requires considerable increase in skin blood flow; this blood is withdrawn from the supply available for physical work.

Carrying the warm-up to the point of fatigue is obviously deleterious to performance, but activity short of this point may also make inroads on working capacity. Warm-up activities at high oxygen consumption rates not only deplete the oxygen from capillaries at the site of the working muscles; if continued too long, they can deplete the reserve of oxygen in the venous system (see Chapter 9). These considerations suggest that the warm-up should be a brief, mild rehearsal of specific body movements just sufficient to warm the tissues involved and to open the blood vessels that feed them and to increase the acidity in the contracting muscles. The main objectives of warm-up for an endurance performance are to increase the oxygen utilization capacity without depleting the oxygen supply and without jeopardizing the oxygen supply for the sake of removal of excess body heat.

A warm-up for a brief violent effort, such as a javelin throw or a rope climb, would be more extensive in order to increase muscle heat to the degree that viscosity is lowered and to rehearse the movements so that coordination is perfected. Working up to a sweat is probably justified, but not to the extent that fatigue develops, because this would reduce power and coordination—lowering performance and increasing the risk of injury. In all events, a moderate warm-up is superior to a heavy one.

References

1. Brynteson, F., and Sinning, W. E.: The effects of training frequencies on the retention of cardiovascular fitness, Med. Sci. Sports 5:29, 1973.
2. Cooper, K.: The new aerobics, New York, 1970, Bantam Books.
3. Donald, K. W., and others: Cardiovascular responses to sustained (static) contractions, Circulat. Res. 20:1-15, 1967.
4. Kotchen, T. A., and others: Renin, norepinephrine, and epinephrine responses to graded exercise, J. Appl. Physiol. 31:178, 1971.
5. Michael, E., Evert, J., and Jeffers, K.: Physiological changes of teenage girls during months of detraining, Med. Sci. Sports 4:214, 1972.
6. Naughton, J. P., Hellerstein, H. K., and Mohler, J. C., editors: Exercise testing and exercise training in coronary heart disease, New York, 1973, Academic Press, Inc.
7. Pollock, M. L., and others: Effects of training two days per week at different intensities on middle-aged men, Med. Sci. Sports 4:192, 1972.
8. Shephard, R. J.: Intensity, duration and frequency of exercise as determinants of the response to a training regime, Int. Z. angew. Physiol. 26:272, 1968.
9. Siegel, W., Blomqvist, G., and Mitchell, J. H.: Effects of a quantitated physical training program on middle-aged sedentary males, Circulation 41:19, 1970.

Suggested readings

Alderman, R., and Howell, M.: The generality and specificity of human motor performance on the evaluation of physical fitness, J. Sports. Med. Phys. Fitness 9:31, 1969.
Cureton, T.: The physiological effects of exercise programs on adults, Springfield, Ill., 1969, Charles C Thomas, Publisher.
Edholm, O.: Fitness for what? Proc. Roy. Soc. Med. 62:617, 1969.
Larson, L., editor: International guide to fitness and health, New York, 1973, Crown Publishers.
Rifenberick, D. H., Gamble, J. G., and Max, S. R.: Response of mitochondrial enzymes to decreased muscular activity, Am. J. Physiol. 225:1295, 1973.
Shephard, R. J.: Endurance fitness, Toronto, 1969, Toronto Press.
Shephard, R. J., editor: Frontiers of fitness, Springfield, Ill., 1971, Charles C Thomas, Publisher.
Thomas, V.: Science and sport. How to measure and improve athletic performance, Boston, 1970, Little, Brown and Co.

19 MUSCULAR DEVELOPMENT

When muscles are atrophied and weak the development of some degree of muscular hypertrophy, muscular strength, and muscular endurance occurs as the result of any form of muscular exercise. As training progresses, development of each of these characteristics becomes specific and further hypertrophy can be achieved with but little gain in strength and practically no gain in endurance; strength in a muscle of normal size can be increased without significant further increase in size, and the type of training required to develop muscular endurance is entirely different from that designed to produce hypertrophy or to strengthen muscle.

In training for sports in which the body is moved or supported, such as jumping or running, it is advantageous to increase strength and endurance without hypertrophy. Muscles that are too heavy can be as much burden to movement as too much fat. The objective is to give the muscles as much strength and stamina as possible while keeping the mass of muscle tissue at a minimum. In other sports in which body mass can be an advantage, such as weight lifting, shot putting, and football line play, on the other hand, it is advantageous to induce as much hypertrophy as possible.

The development of hypertrophy is brought about by an increase in the number and size of the myofibrils, and in the contractile proteins in muscle. The development of strength is accomplished through the reconstitution of muscle tissue into predominantly white fibers and the more concerted activation of these fibers by the nervous system. The development of muscular endurance is brought about by an increase in numbers of capillaries, together with reconstitution of muscle tissue into red fibers (more myoglobin) and an attendant increase in oxygen uptake and nutrient supply capacity. In this chapter we shall study the physiological processes by which these changes are achieved.

239

GENERAL MUSCULAR DEVELOPMENT

Muscular weakness and atrophy following injury and immobilization can be corrected by a program of *progressive resistance exercises* (PRE). In the PRE program, originally defined by Delorme and Watkins,[3] the patient exercises muscles to be trained by lifting progressively heavier weights. During each set of exercises the weight is lifted ten times. After a period of rest for 2 or 3 minutes, the set is repeated. Each exercise session consists of three such sets of ten lifts each. Prescriptions of three sessions of exercise per week, on alternate days, are apparently as effective—and are better tolerated by the patient—as daily sessions.

In the PRE program the load to be lifted is very light at the start, and very small weights are added at each session to provide an overload stimulus. Eventually the load becomes so heavy that the patient can barely complete the ten repetitions. This limit load is termed *repetitions maximum* or RM. The PRE program is then continued by adjusting the weight to be lifted to the 10 RM capacity of the patient. If necessary, the weight is reduced in the second and third set, so that the patient can complete the full three sets at 10 RM.

After a month of PRE training noticeable gains in muscle girth, muscle tone, and muscle strength are registered in the trained areas. Within three months the muscles are restored to a near-normal state. Thus, for therapeutic or low fitness application, the PRE program of weight training is an effective one for restoring normal muscle structure and function.

8-12 repetition rule. The 8-12 repetition rule used in therapeutic weight training is a method of PRE in which load and repetitions are varied. The rule states that if it is not possible to complete the exercise eight times the weight should be reduced. And if it is possible to complete more than twelve repetitions the weight should be increased. In weight training the procedure is to "load to 8 and train to 12."

Injury. A word of caution is necessary in the interpretation of studies of muscular development during progressive rehabilitation following injury. Initial measurements of muscular strength may not be valid, especially when the force is transmitted through the site of the injury. Fried and Shepard, in their assessment of a lower extremity training program, concluded that the apparent improvement in isometric strength of 13% in measurements above the site of injury and a gain of 34% in measurements below the injury were due mainly to an initial voluntary limitation of effort because of apprehension and an initial lack of skill in those not accustomed to using a dynamometer.[5] Since there was little or no increase in muscle mass they concluded that much of the functional loss might have been regained without specific therapy.

Therapists follow three rules in applying resistance exercise to injured or atrophied muscles: (1) rhythmical, smooth, even pressure is applied from the beginning to the end of each movement to prevent injury from sudden, unexpected strains; (2) the force applied in the starting position at full extension of a muscle is gradually diminished during shortening to comply with the loss of strength in a muscle as it moves from a stretched to a slack position; and (3) a period of complete relaxation follows each muscular effort to avoid fatigue.

Isometric (static) versus isotonic (dynamic) muscle training. Isometric and isotonic exercises differ in their training effects. Isometric contractions of sufficient power to have any training value derive their energy from anaerobic sources, since blood flow through the contracting muscle is greatly reduced or abolished entirely. For this reason, isometric exercises are without training value with respect to the oxygen transport capacity. They do, however, increase the strength of the muscles that take part in the exercise.

In previously untrained muscles, isometric contractions induce nearly 100% increase in strength and 25% increase in cross-sectional area of arm flexors after 100 days of 10-second contractions (6 days per week, three times a day). A 30% increase in strength is found in the muscles that are not exercised.

Isotonic or dynamic exercises, by subjecting the oxygen transport system to stress, may increase endurance (as explained in an earlier section) while having little effect on the strength of the muscles involved.

It is apparent that the value of isometric exercises is limited to the strengthening of individual weak muscles; for example, the strengthening of sagging abdominal muscles as an aid to better posture.

Persistence of training effects. So far as is known, all the effects of training are reversible, and they gradually disappear when training ceases. The apparent persistence of certain of the characteristics associated with training long after the termination of training probably reflects the superior natural endowments of the subjects rather than retention of the effects of training. Motor skills, though impaired by the absence of practice, may persist in some degree for many years. This emphasizes that the training of neuromuscular activity has unique features not shared by other types of training.

It is an unsettled question whether training effects once lost by disuse are regained more quickly than they were gained initially. One difficulty is that the condition of the subjects usually differs in the initial training and retraining experiences (an example is that of age).

241

BIOLOGICAL LONG-TERM EFFECTS OF TRAINING

"Biological long-term effects of training" is the expression used by Åstrand and Rodahl to describe the structural and functional changes in the organs and systems of the body (as opposed to the improvements in performance) resulting from training.[1] These are the changes that are responsible for the improved performance and their scientific study is one of the major preoccupations of exercise physiologists.

The biological effects of training may conveniently be considered under two main categories—the effects on muscles and the effects on the oxygen transport capacity. As we shall see, the biological effects of training on muscles include not only increase in muscle strength, but also vascular and metabolic alterations in the muscles that are important in increasing endurance.

EFFECTS OF TRAINING ON MUSCLES

It is necessary to recall certain facts about muscles that were discussed in Chapters 1 to 5. A muscle is composed of a large number of muscle fibers, and each fiber is supplied with blood by one or more capillaries that course along the surface of the fiber. When the size of a muscle is increased by training, the increase is due to an enlargement of the individual muscle fibers (hypertrophy); there is no increase in the number of muscle fibers (hyperplasia).

A muscle fiber contains a fluid matrix, the sarcoplasm, in which are embedded the contractile elements, the myofibrils. The sarcoplasm contains the energy-generating enzyme systems and the red pigment, myoglobin.

Increase in the strength of a muscle resulting from training is due to an increase in the contractile power of the individual muscle fibers. It is not clear whether the increase in size of the muscle fibers makes highly significant contributions to strength, nor is it clear whether the increase in size is due to increase in the amount of sarcoplasm, or in the number and size of the myofibrils, or both.

Increase in the endurance of a muscle due to training involves several separate factors, including increases in vascularity, in myoglobin concentration, and in the activities of the enzyme systems involved in the production of energy for sustained muscular activity.

After this preliminary survey, we may proceed to examine the evidence for the occurrence of these various effects of training on the muscles.

The increase in muscle endurance resulting from training apparently involves all the steps in the transport of oxygen to the muscles, and the utilization of oxygen in the muscles. There is a greater maximal cardiac output as a result of training, and also an increase in the vascularity of the muscles. The latter change not only allows the muscles to accept a larger blood flow, but it also means that the average muscle fiber may receive oxygen from a greater number of capillaries, with the result that the oxygen tension within the muscle fibers is increased. The increase in the number of capillaries in trained muscles may be due partly to the opening of previously unused capillaries and partly to the actual formation of new capillaries. The cause of the increased vascularity of trained muscles is not known; among the possibilities are local hypoxia and the mechanical effect of an increased flow of blood into muscle capillaries through the dilated muscle arterioles during the training exercise.

The increased cardiac output and muscle vascularity together result in a considerable augmentation in the maximal blood flow (and delivery of oxygen) to trained muscles. Within the muscle fibers, a second effect of training is an increase in the concentration of myoglobin in the sarcoplasm. Myoglobin plays a dual role in the intracellular utilization of oxygen. First, it combines with oxygen reaching it from the blood when oxygen is abundant, and releases it to the mitochondria when the intracellular oxygen tension is lowered. Second, it probably serves as a mechanism for the rapid transport of oxygen within the cell. It is apparent that the increased concentration of myoglobin, together with the increased transport of oxygen to the muscles, favors the delivery of adequate amounts of oxygen to the muscle mitochondria even during high levels of muscular activity. These changes in muscle blood flow and myoglobin concentration are the most important effects of training on endurance in exercise.

Training increases not only the maximal capacity for the transport of oxygen to the mitochondria in the muscle fibers, but also the capacity of the metabolic machinery that utilizes the oxygen (the mitochondria and the enzymes they contain). It has been observed, for example, that rats trained by forced running on a motor-driven treadmill have more mitochondria in their leg muscles and that the individual mitochondria are larger and more densely packed with cristae. Direct measurements of the amounts of the mitochondrial enzymes indicate that some of them are increased by training. This suggests that the rate of formation of ATP is more likely to keep pace with the rate of its breakdown during exercise in trained muscles.

SPECIFIC MUSCULAR DEVELOPMENT

Development of muscle to supernormal conditions requires a more specific regimen of exercise than the PRE program. Athletes and others needing maximal or near-maximal strength would achieve some gains using the PRE program in early training, but relatively greater results

243

can be expected by what we shall term a *specific muscular development* program, which progresses in three phases: (1) development of muscular hypertrophy; (2) development of explosive strength; and (3) development of strength endurance. During each phase some development of all three characteristics will occur, but the major purpose during each phase is to develop each characteristic to the desired level one at a time.

In training for power events such as the shot put or weight lifting, hypertrophy of muscle tissue is carried to an advanced degree. If hypertrophy is needed, it is developed first because, in a real sense, the objective is to obtain a larger "engine" which will deliver the force in muscular work. For endurance and speed events such as distance running or tennis an excess of muscular hypertrophy would be a burden.

Explosive strength development is concomitant with hypertrophy development because it is the intensity of contraction that induces hypertrophy. However, final development of explosive strength, if such is needed, will require a slightly different training protocol than the one which is optimal for hypertrophy. Again, limit of explosive strength is not needed in activities with a low to moderate strength component, as in badminton or baseball.

Development of strength endurance will occur to some degree during the development of muscular hypertrophy and strength, but these exercises are essentially anaerobic. To develop muscular endurance, both anaerobic and aerobic mechanisms must be enhanced.

We shall now proceed to an examination of the physiological basis for the development of these aspects of muscular development.

DEVELOPMENT OF MUSCULAR HYPERTROPHY

In accordance with the principle of Specific Adaptation to Imposed Demands (SAID), skeletal muscle reacts to frequent demands for forceful contractions by muscular enlargement (hypertrophy) and an increase in contractile strength.

When high-resistance loads are combined with moderate frequency, the resistance must be reduced well below the maximal load. As a result, hypertrophy is induced but muscular strength or muscular endurance is not developed to maximum.[2]

Thus when muscles are atrophied and development of muscle tissue mass is desired, the type of exercise selected is one involving repeated muscular exertions of moderate frequency against moderately heavy resistance.

The enlargement of muscles beyond their normal size is accomplished by the application of the law of overcompensation. Tissues adapt to nondestructive stress by increasing their size and improving their function.

Muscle hypertrophy occurs only in the fibers that are overloaded.

During a single mode of exercise, such as arm flexion, there is a selective enlargement of the fibers which are stressed, rather than a slight change in all of the fibers of the muscles involved.

It is probable that every element in muscle and its associated tissues—contractile protein, capillary, and connective tissue fiber—is increased in the process of muscular hypertrophy. Thus hypertrophy is induced by applying nondestructive overloads to all elements.

Measurement of muscular hypertrophy must be made in terms of the cross-sectional area of the muscle fiber. There may be a 30% increase in mean fiber diameter without a noticeable increase in the girth of the limb. Tape measurements of girth areas are influenced also by changes in fat, dehydration, amount of vasodilatation, and the length of muscle. Girth measurements of flexed and contracted muscles are less descriptive of hypertrophy changes than measurements taken with the limb extended and the muscles relaxed. Tape measurements of girth areas should reflect significant changes in muscular hypertrophy in adults if the measurement conditions are duplicated and if there has been no change in body composition. Often in early stages of training there is a decrease in body fat while the muscle size increases, resulting in unchanged girth area measurements and unchanged body weight measurements.

Techniques of measuring muscular strength and muscular endurance are presented in Chapter 3 in the *Laboratory Manual.*

It would seem from our studies of myofibril dynamics and contractile energy in early chapters that the limit of the ability of muscle to be trained to perform brief maximal work (strength) or prolonged maximal work (endurance) would depend on the quantity of contractile protein available. We shall see in this chapter that, although a reduction of contractile protein (atrophy) does lower the capacity for muscular strength or endurance, an addition of contractile protein above normal amounts (hypertrophy) may not increase the capacity. Factors in addition to hypertrophy are apparently responsible for the effects of muscular training.

Endurance training exercise, such as long-distance running, has a different effect on skeletal muscle. Such training utilizes red fibers whose cross-section diameters do not increase as much as do those of white fibers. Within trained red fibers there is an increase in the concentration of myoglobin, and the red and intermediate pink fibers become more red. There is also in trained red fibers an increased concentration of enzymes involved in the synthesis of ATP and an increase in the numbers of mitochondria, the organelles in which oxidation of substrates occurs and ATP is synthesized.

The increase in the numbers of capillaries which supply the exercised fibers may occur in two ways; an opening of unused vessels by a relaxation of precapillary sphincters, and formation of entirely new vessels. Capillarization occurs at a much higher rate in the red fibers, enhancing their endurance properties.

The site of fiber hypertrophy training may be in the nervous system. Diameters of nerves to white muscle fibers are larger than those to red fibers, which may account for the faster action of white fibers. Speed work against high resistance stimulates the development of larger nerve fibers, which in turn would stimulate the development of white fibers.

The intensive type of training that causes hypertrophy of white fibers also causes hypertrophy of the extracellular substances of connective tissue. The volume of tendons and ligaments is increased, enhancing their tensile strength.

Hypertrophy of muscle in response to exercise occurs in three types of tissues: the enclosed, force-producing contractile muscle tissue, the myofibrils; the enclosing, force-transmitting connective tissue; and the capillaries which supply oxygen and nutrients to the connective and muscle tissues.

Forceful, fast contractions cause greater hypertrophy in the connective tissue and in the white muscle fibers. Submaximal, slower, continuous contractions utilize the myoglobin-rich red fibers and increase the demand for oxygen from the surrounding capillaries.

Weight training exercises which employ rapid contractions of high intensities for short periods of time increase the requirement of white fiber cells for actin, myosin, and tropomyosin. These proteins are synthesized on large polyribosome aggregates in the fiber sarcomere. They then apparently polymerize into filaments and attach in some way between the fiber sarcomeres. It is this synthesis of filaments, or myofibrils, that causes a thickening of white muscle fiber and resulting hypertrophy.[4] The difference in hypertrophy in the different fiber types is thus possibly due to the reaction of these fiber types to different types of stimulation.

These considerations point to the logic of developing muscle in three phases: first, the development of hypertrophy of the force-transmitting connective tissue and force-producing white muscle fibers to provide the machinery for strength; second, the development of muscular strength by the use of this improved muscle machinery; and finally, the development of muscular endurance, which is usually achieved together with improved strength.

An example of an exercise program meeting these requirements for forceful, fast contractions would be circuit training using heavy weights at each station to develop hypertrophy in desired areas. Each set of exercises would be of an isotonic nature and would be executed at high speed, using a full range of motion. The exercise would be continued for 30 to 40 seconds, or until fifteen to twenty repetitions had been completed. Body builders who rely mainly on this type of exercise to produce massive muscular development with clear definition of each muscle call this type of exercise "pumping." Using a dumbbell or pulley weight, they "pump up" the biceps by elbow flexions, then they rest the biceps and "pump up" the triceps by elbow extensions. After a series of two to three sets each, a total of four to six sets for the two muscle groups, they progress to other groups of muscles, such as knee flexors and extensors.

Increases in strength and muscular endurance are minor by-products of this type of exercise. Increases in circumference after this type of weight training correlate with increases in strength by only $r = 0.422$.[8]

If the load lifted is less than 60% of maximum, hypertrophy can occur without a significant gain in strength. Initial training may be commenced at this low intensity in order to avoid fatigue or injury, but the load should be gradually increased to 80% of maximum and higher in order to start the development of strength while building muscular mass.

Development of muscular hypertrophy should not proceed at too rapid a pace, particularly if the exercise is performed in a hot, humid climate. A syndrome of heaviness in the legs and loss of power which football players know as "dead legs" occurs in intensive early season physical conditioning. Track runners speak of a "tear and repair" mechanism of early training in which muscles are "broken down and rebuilt." Such breakdowns have been experienced also in military basic training. This syndrome has been investigated by Nichols and co-workers, and the phenomenon appears to be related to a doubling (from 43.8 to 89.1 gm./kg.) of myofibrillar nitrogen in hypertrophied muscles without concomitant changes in muscle electrolyte composition.[7] This imbalance caused by extra protein may somehow affect the energetic mechanisms of muscle strength.

In a typical training program using weights to develop hypertrophy, the regimen is started with weights so light that four sets of twenty repetitions each can be performed with ease. Before each exercise session the weight is increased slightly until only fifteen contractions can be accomplished. Practice with this load is then continued until twenty repetitions can be completed. The weight is again increased each session until only fifteen repetitions (15 RM) can be completed. This mode of training leads to the expression "load to 15 and train to 20."

The following activities are the types which lead to the development of hypertrophy if they are performed at a fast rate and at high intensity: isometrics (pull, push, twist); weight training (barbells, dumbbells, wall pulleys); chinning (pull-ups); dipping (on parallel bars); gymnastics; wrestling; punching heavy bag; pick and shovel work; and surfboard paddling.

DEVELOPMENT OF EXPLOSIVE STRENGTH

Once the desired degree of hypertrophy is reached, it can be maintained by the same process by which explosive strength is being developed. Explosive strength is the force which can be applied by a brief maximal effort. (Methods of measurement are found in Chapter 3 in the *Laboratory Manual.*) Explosive strength is an anaerobic effort since it is usually completed within 10 seconds. The muscular "engine" is quickly driven to maximal acceleration. The quick energy substrates such as ATP and creatine phosphate furnish the fuel for the sudden contraction. Not more than five such explosive maximal contractions can be performed without fatigue. If more contractions are desired, they must be at submaximal effort and spaced so that the active fibers can be rested and aerobic metabolism can occur. This slower submaximal work is used to develop muscular endurance, as we shall see later. The submaximal effort does not develop explosive strength to its limit.

Brief maximal effort depletes anaerobic fuels and thereby induces overcompensation. It is probably not this adaptive buildup of anaerobic fuel which is the major cause of increased explosive strength. It is more likely the recruitment of more fibers and the better coordination of the teams of fibers that contribute most to the development of greater explosive strength when such efforts are practiced. How such "learning" takes place is not yet understood. The effort to provide a maximal training stimulus must be a maximal one, not extended beyond a period of 10 seconds. Such an effort has a profound effect on the strengthening of muscular contraction ability. One such brief maximal effort three times a week—for a total of 30 seconds of effort per week—is sufficient to increase explosive strength. Once achieved, explosive strength can be maintained by a single brief maximal contraction once a week in addition to moderate daily physical activity. In the absence of such activity, explosive strength is lost at the rate of about 3% per day.

The explosive strength training stimulus is well defined: a single brief maximal contraction (1 RM) which evokes a large, general neuromuscular response. Practice beyond five such repetitive isotonic efforts, or isometric contractions held beyond 10 seconds, are not as stimulating as shorter exertions because the tension produced tends to be less than maximal.

During the specific muscular development program in which the explosive strength development exercises follow the hypertrophy development series, the load for the first explosive strength practice session is the same as that finally used for the hypertrophy series. For the transition to explosive strength development the load is increased slightly each session until it is possible to execute only one lift (1 RM). Training with that load is practiced until it is possible to execute the lift five times. The load is then increased slightly each session until once more only one lift (1 RM) can be accomplished: "load to 1 lift, train to 5 lifts." If an isometric mode is used, time is the controlling factor: "load to 5 seconds, train to 10 seconds."

On days when, because of fatigue or other factors, the accustomed load cannot be lifted (or resistance cannot be overcome as in isometric exercise), a lighter load is applied. *It is the physiological effort which stimulates training, not the external physical work.* The external load merely provides a resistance against which the organism can struggle. It is the degree of struggle, not the size of the load, which induces the adaptive changes that we call training.

When adequate explosive strength is achieved—a fairly high level for a swimmer, and a peak capacity level for a shot putter—the desired level is maintained by single maximal contractions three times a week.

Muscle strength increase during training probably results from two factors: (1) a gradual increase in the ability of the contractile elements in each fiber to contract more strongly, and (2) a gradual recruitment of a higher proportion of the total available fibers in each contraction. Both qualities are achieved by gradually increasing the degree of tension developed in the muscle.

STRENGTH TRAINING

Tension is the key to muscle strength development. A thousand contractions a day will not increase strength unless sufficient tension is developed in the muscle. If tension is above two-thirds of maximal capacity, a single contraction of only 6 seconds duration once a day will strengthen weak muscles.[6] As muscles become stronger, either the tension must be increased or the duration and frequency of the application of tension must be increased in order to stimulate further strength development.

Duration and frequency cannot, however, be extended to a degree of fatigue that would require a reduction in tension. Since tension is the primary stimulus to strength development, fatigue must be kept out of the picture. This is accomplished by resting after a set of about six repetitions and repeating the sets three or more times in each training session. If the day's session is fatiguing, different groups of muscles should be exercised on alternate days.

The state of training of the explosive strength characteristic of muscle function is expressed as a percentage of its *limiting strength,* which Müller has defined as the maximal strength that can be achieved by maximal exercise.[6] In severely deconditioned individuals and in patients recovering from injury, Müller has observed the rate of increase of strength with maximal exercise to be approximately 12% per week, increasing linearly up to 75% of limiting strength. With no exercise other than a return to ordinary daily life activity the rate of increase would be considerably slower, and the 75% level would probably not be attained without more aggressive exercise.

Above 75% the rate of increase of strength with aggressive exercise diminishes progressively to become zero at limiting strength. Variation in training responses is often due to exercise at different degrees of stretched length of the muscles.

Muscular training is highly specific; high-resistance, explosive type strength is poorly related to unloaded limb speed. While high resistance training would benefit a football lineman, it would not help the quarterback who is trying to throw the ball faster. For the quarterback training should consist of light resistance and high-speed exercises.

Furthermore, although some cross-education may occur, strengthening one group of muscles does not develop strength in other groups. Muscular development in the legs due to a running program may not affect arm development. In designing a program the specific areas of need for muscular development must be defined, and the specific type of training related to the performance requirements must be applied. As muscular condition improves the training program must become more and more highly specific to produce continued gains in performance.

In a deconditioned state a single brief maximal contraction has a prolonged stimulating effect on the development of muscular tissue. Müller has observed this effect to last for a week, and he notes that this stimulus is reinforced very little by repetition of a maximal contraction within the next 24 hours.[6]

This sensitivity to training stimulus makes muscles equally susceptible to lack of exercise. Müller finds that strength decreases about 5% per day in the absence of any contraction of a muscle and 1.0 to 1.5% per day during bed rest.[6] He also notes that one contraction a day at half the maximal strength is enough to prevent such decreases. Since a maximal contraction triggers such a prolonged developmental stimulus, only one maximal contraction a week in addition to the usual daily physical activities is sufficient to maintain strength.

Utilizing degree of tension (load), number of contractions, and rate of contractions as variables, a 6-week training program of daily exercise to develop muscular strength, followed by a prolonged maintenance period, might resemble the following schedule.

	First two weeks	Second two weeks	Third two weeks	Maintenance
Degree of tension (% of maximal)	65-75%	75-90%	90-100%	95%
Number of contractions	15-20	10-15	5-10	5
Rate of contractions (% of maximal)	75-85%	85-95%	95-100%	95%
Sets	5-6	4-5	3-4	3

The ideal method of training would be to monitor the electromyogram using an oscilloscope to project the maximal and estimate the desired percentage of tension. Without such physiological monitoring equipment, during the first week the objective would be to find the resistance (load) which can be repeated just twenty times before fatigue occurs. If the resistance first selected is too light, contractions will exceed twenty without fatigue. If too heavy, fatigue will occur before twenty contractions are completed. In succeeding sessions after twenty contractions maximum have been established, the number of contractions per set is gradually reduced to fifteen by the end of the first 2-week period, while the degree of tension (load) is gradually increased so that fatigue occurs at fifteen, not at a higher or lower number of contractions. The same pattern could be continued during the remaining weeks as charted, gradually increasing the rate of the contractions and the number of sets in each daily session.

The type of exercise which improves muscular strength—repetitious contractions of a few seconds' duration against heavy resistance—does not improve cardiovascular function. Athletes who train only in this manner do not have the enlarged hearts, low resting and exercise heart rates, and high maximal oxygen uptakes of endurance athletes.[1]

The following types of activities lead to the development of explosive strength if they are performed occasionally at maximal force: isometrics, weight training, archery, sailing, throwing, tennis, jumping, tumbling, field events (shot put, etc.), and sprinting up stairs or steep grade.

MUSCULAR ENDURANCE DEVELOPMENT

Adaptive changes which occur in skeletal muscles in endurance activities such as distance running or swimming are quite different from the changes we have described previously. There is no hypertrophy, little or no change in strength and, as we shall see later, very little change in skill. Instead there is an increase in the capacity for prolonged aerobic metabolism which is made possible by adaptations in muscle blood flow and in the energy metabolism systems within the cells, as introduced in Chapters 1 and 2. As a result of these adaptive changes there is an increased capacity of the involved muscles for aerobic metabolism.

Again, these endurance adaptations are specific to the muscles used. Distance swimming does not improve endurance for distance running because the arm and shoulder muscles are primarily involved in swimming while muscles of the legs do the major work in running.

Increasing strength may increase muscular endurance, but muscular endurance exercise does not increase strength. Müller reports a study in which hand cranking daily for 40 minutes at a load of about 40% of maximal strength improved cranking endurance, while muscular strength dropped at the same time.[6]

Repeated submaximal contractions against low resistance cause the white muscle fibers to become redder because of an increase in myoglobin. This change causes an increased ability to maintain tension over a longer period of time or to extend the capacity for repeating the contractions. It may, in early stages of training, increase the size of the muscle. It does not, however, increase the capacity for maximal tension.

The ability to continue repeated contractions for a prolonged period, or to maintain a contraction for a long time, requires both anaerobic and aerobic metabolism and involves the circulatory and respiratory adjustments that supply oxygen to the muscles. There is a strong link between aerobic metabolism in skeletal muscles and the uptake of oxygen. The utilization of oxygen by contracting muscles and the transport of oxygen by the circulating blood are probably the two key factors in endurance work. It is the muscular aspect of endurance training that will concern us here. We shall take up the training of the circulorespiratory systems in Chapter 20.

The aerobic component of muscular work increases as the duration of maximal work is increased. From a ratio of 85% anaerobic to 15% aerobic in 10 seconds of explosive strength effort as discussed above, to a ratio of 15% anaerobic and 85% aerobic in endurance muscular work for 10 minutes, there is a gradually changing dependence on anaerobic and aerobic systems as maximal work time increases. During maximal work of 2 minutes' duration, the anaerobic and aerobic production of energy is about equal.

The specific strength development program for muscular endurance improvement thus consists of a combination of anaerobic and aerobic conditioning. This is best accomplished by a series of brief spurts of highly intensive muscular effort interrupted by intervals of effort at a moderate level.

The purposes of such anaerobic-aerobic interval training are (1) to repeat contractions more rapidly, thus increasing the speed of continuous movement, and (2) to perform contractions for a longer period of time, thus increasing the endurance for prolonged work.

Circuit training. The circuit training method of developing muscular endurance and cardiorespiratory endurance is usually employed for preseason conditioning. It is an exhausting procedure and so is scheduled at the end of the daily workout.

A series of exercises is performed nonstop at several stations. The stations, usually 6 to 10 in number, are arranged in a closed path. At each station the special equipment and instructions for exercising a certain muscle group are provided. The performer progresses from station to station, exercising each muscle group at the intensity and duration needed to increase muscular endurance.

The intensity is adjusted to be low enough so that at least forty contractions can be performed before fatigue occurs, and yet high enough so that no more than fifty contractions can be accomplished before the intensity of effort starts to fall.

The rate of contractions simulates the speed of movement of the event for which the performer is training. A baseball pitcher exercises arm extensions at throwing speed.

The exercises at each station are chosen after an analysis of the major muscle groups employed in the performer's event. An exercise to develop each muscle group is set up at each station. Special stations may be established to exercise minor muscle groups which appear to be limiting a player's performance.

The participant circulates rapidly from station to station without rest. Local fatigue is avoided by exercising a remote muscle group at succeeding stations. Each muscle group is given a chance to rest while the others are being exercised.

Typical circuit training exercises are listed below:

Station	Area	Exercise
1	Thigh	Bench squat
2	Fingers	Wrist rolling
3	Abdomen	Inclined sit-up
4	Back and shoulder	Rowing
5	Arm flexion	Front curls
6	Arm extension	Bent arm pullovers

Progression in training is accomplished by gradually increasing the number of circuits around the stations, and by gradually reducing the time allowed to complete each circuit.

Cardiorespiratory development may be gained from circuit training by programming the heart rate (see Chapter 20). The heart rate is counted and recorded at the final station. At the start of training the target heart rate may be set at 140 per minute. Each week the desired heart rate can be advanced 5 or 10 beats per minute so that a target heart rate of 180 is set during the final week of preseason conditioning. At the end of each circuit (at the last station) the participant compares his heart rate with his target for the day. If the rate is lower, the next circuit is conducted at a more intensive and more rapid level in an attempt to match the target rate at the next reading. If the rate is above the target heart rate, the pace is lowered to readjust the heart rate to the target level.

After the final set at target rate the participant performs one more circuit at a very easy pace in order to prevent muscle stiffness.

Development of muscular endurance results from activities of low resistance and high frequency, such as the following: walking (brisk), carpentry, sawing, chopping wood, fencing, water skiing, jumping rope (fast), half squats, and sprinting.

METHODS OF OVERLOADING FOR MUSCULAR DEVELOPMENT

The training system used by the legendary Milo of Crotona, in which the youth lifted a bull calf once daily from its day of birth until it became full grown, employs only one mode of overload, that of weight. Milo's system would fail unless the final weight of the bull matched the lifter's final strength limit, and unless the daily weight gain of the animal matched the lifter's rate of training.

Even so, weight increments alone are an incomplete method of overloading to induce training. As mentioned in Chapter 18, overloading can be made infinitely progressive by employing numerous means of applying graded stress. For muscular development, training protocols can be constructed using the following means of overloading:

1. Increasing the weight, resistance, or effort
2. Increasing the speed or rate of movement
3. Increasing the range of movement
4. Increasing the isolation of a muscle by postural adjustment; making the muscle work more strongly by eliminating the assistance of synergistic muscles
5. Increasing the dependence on a muscle in a movement by eliminating accessory motions; reducing preparatory accelerations such as swinging or rocking
6. Increasing the duration of the effort
7. Increasing the repetitions of the effort
8. Increasing the number of sets of exercises
9. Decreasing the rest intervals between sets
10. Decreasing the duration of each set of exercises by shortening the pause between each movement
11. Increasing the level of activity during the rest period between sets; shifting from quiet rest to active rest
12. Adding new movements to exercise sessions
13. Increasing the frequency of exercise sessions; adding more sessions per week

Selection of the above elements for progressive overloading is made on the basis of the specific goal of exercise, to induce hypertrophy, to gain explosive strength, or to increase muscular endurance.

Methods of overload which increase the intensity of effort are the most productive, but they are also potentially the most injurious. Additions in intensity should follow additions in duration and frequency, and the increase in intensity should be very slight.

A theoretical model for weight training to induce specific muscular development is presented in Table 12. The seven variables are the ones commonly employed by body builders and weight lifters. The table could be expanded to include some of the six other variables listed above. A range of values is presented for each developmental goal. The low values represent an initial setting for a phase of training during the middle to final period of a developmental program. As training progresses one of the values at a time is intensified, i.e., one more repetition is added or the rest period between sets is reduced a few seconds. Manipulation of the intensity of these variables permits an infinitely graded progression.

The shift from development of hypertrophy to strength to endurance is ideally a graded, overlapping process. During a 4- to 8-week program, depending on initial muscular condition, the number of repetitions (or duration of exercise) is decreased while the intensity of contractions is very gradually increased toward maximum in order to add strength to hypertrophying muscles. Then, when limiting strength (no further increase in subsequent maximal exercise sessions) is reached, it is maintained by a single maximal contraction two or three times a week, while on alternate days during the week a program of muscular endurance exercise with moderate load and high repetitions is instituted.

At the end of the developmental period, hypertrophy, strength and endurance of muscles can be maintained indefinitely by twice weekly

Table 12. Theoretical weight training model for specific muscular development

Variable	Hypertrophy	Explosive strength	Muscular endurance
1. Load (% of maximal)	70-80	90-100	60-70
2. Duration (seconds)	30-40	5-10	90-120
3. Repetitions	15-20	1-5	40-50
4. Sets	4-6	3-4	2-4
5. Period of rest between sets (minutes)	4-5	3-4	1-2
6. Frequency (sessions/week)	5-6	3-4	10-14
7. Speed (% of maximal)	80-90	90-100	70-80

maximal intensity, short duration "speed" workouts, and alternate three times weekly high-intensity, long-duration "endurance" workouts.

CONTRIBUTION OF MUSCULAR DEVELOPMENT TO SKILL

As we shall discuss further in Chapter 21, repetition of movements against heavy resistance improves the precision and the economy of the movements. With practice, unnecessary contractions are progressively reduced and the tension in antagonistic muscles is lowered. Movement is simplified and becomes automatic as voluntary actions are replaced by reflex actions. As a result the energy cost of an exercise is reduced and the stress on the circulorespiratory systems is diminished.

With the adding of resistance to a movement there is an increase in sensory stimuli, particularly from muscle spindles. Feedback from these kinesthetic proprioceptors acts to produce corrective changes in movement and posture, and thus the coordination of a motor act is facilitated. Adding weights to the limbs during performance thus activates more strongly the autogenic governors of the muscle machines.

For this reason, the motions during resistance training should duplicate as closely as possible the activity to which the training is directed. Training movements should duplicate activity movements in posture, direction and range of motion, and speed of motion. Only force of motion should be increased during the period of muscular skill development.

Basic rules. Experienced weight lifters practice certain rules which have been found to contribute to muscular development and help to avoid injury.

1. Never lift maximally every day using the same muscle contractors. It takes 36 to 48 hours for a muscle fiber to recuperate after a maximal lift.
2. Always warm up with stretching exercise and lifting light weights before practicing lifts at maximal effort. Follow each lifting period with warm-down exercise.
3. Lift with the back flat to avoid injury.
4. Never hold the breath. Breathe normally, if possible, or inhale through the nose on exerting pressure and exhale through the mouth on release. Do not take rapid breaths during or prior to lifting.
5. Never walk near or talk to a person who is in the act of lifting.
6. Never lower a weight faster than you can control the movement.
7. Use exercise specific to the activity for which you are training, concentrating on the major muscles employed and their position of greatest strain.
8. Use isometric (static) exercise to develop muscles which perform isometrically (e.g., abdominal muscles) and isotonic (dynamic)

exercises to develop muscles which perform isotonically (e.g., limb muscles).

9. Keep limb speed as close to maximum as possible, never less than one-fourth of the speed of actual performance.

10. Train, don't strain. A slight muscle pull or ligamentous strain can undo weeks of hard training.

References

1. Åstrand, P.-O., and Rodahl, K.: Textbook of work physiology, New York, 1970, McGraw-Hill Book Co.
2. Barnard, R. J., Edgerton, V. R., and Peter, J. B.: Effect of exercise on skeletal muscle, II. Contractile properties, J. Appl. Physiol. 28:767, 1970.
3. Delorme, T. L., and Watkins, A. L.: Technics of progressive resistance exercise, Arch. Phys. Med. 29:263, 1948.
4. Edgerton, V. R.: Exercise and growth and development of muscle tissue. In Rarick, G. L., editor: Physical activity in human growth and development, New York, 1973, Academic Press, Inc., pp. 1-31.
5. Fried, T., and Shephard, R. J.: Assessment of a lower extremity training program, Canad. Med. Assoc. J. 103:260, 1970.
6. Müller, E. A.: Influence of training and of inactivity on muscle strength, Arch. Phys. Med. Rehab. 41:449, 1970.
7. Nichols, B. L., and others: Syndrome characterized by loss of muscle strength experienced by athletes during intensive training program, Metabolism 21:187, 1972.
8. Rasch, P. J., and Morehouse, L. E.: Effect of static and dynamic exercises on muscular strength and hypertrophy, J. Appl. Physiol. 11:29, 1957.

Suggested readings

Clarke, D. H.: Adaptations in strength and muscular endurance resulting from exercise. In Wilmore, J. H., editor: Exercise and sport sciences reviews, Vol. 1, New York, 1973, Academic Press, Inc.

Falls, H. B., Wallis, E. J., and Logan, G. A.: Foundations of conditioning, New York, 1970, Academic Press, Inc.

Hettinger, T.: Physiology of strength, Springfield, Ill., 1961, Charles C Thomas, Publisher.

Noble, L.: Effect of resistive exercise on muscle size, a review, Am. Corrective Therapy J. 24:199, 1971.

Rasch, P. J., and Burke, R. K.: Kinesiology and applied conditioning, Philadelphia, 1971, Lea & Febiger.

Shephard, R. J.: Endurance fitness, Toronto, 1969, University of Toronto Press.

Taylor, A. W.: Training—scientific basis and application, Springfield, Ill., 1971, Charles C Thomas, Publisher.

20 CIRCULORESPIRATORY DEVELOPMENT

Development of endurance for exercise of moderate duration (1 to 60 minutes) involves some of the same processes as development of muscular endurance of short duration (less than 60 seconds). As discussed in Chapter 19, there are increases in muscle mitochondria and in enzyme concentrations, enhancement of strength and skill, and improvement in anaerobic and aerobic power—the aerobic power being improved by the increase in local oxygen transport capacity in the contracting muscle. In addition to these processes, development of endurance for exercise of moderate duration requires an increase in maximal cardiac output.

Development of endurance for more prolonged efforts, lasting for more than an hour, involves yet another set of qualities such as muscle glycogen and other food resources, fluid reserves, and thermal balance.

The duration of effort is only one of three factors necessary to overload the circulorespiratory systems; the second factor is the amount of muscle tissue involved in the effort, and the third is the pumping action provided by rhythmic contractions and relaxations of the muscles. Exercising a small amount of muscle tissue for several minutes will stress the local oxygen transport mechanisms without overloading the circulorespiratory systems. When near-total body musculature is involved in sustained effort, large demands are made on the oxygen transport mechanism. Unless the third factor is present—the rhythmic alternating contraction and relaxation of the working muscles—the circulorespiratory systems may not be overloaded because of the blockage of venous return by the contracting muscles.

Thus, development of circulorespiratory endurance is best achieved by sustained efforts which involve near-total musculature in rhythmic activity; walking, running, swimming, and cycling. It is this type of activity which is most effective in reducing excess body fat (see Chapter 22) and protecting the heart against coronary disease (see Chapter 23).

Adaptive changes that improve circulorespiratory endurance are central and peripheral, the peripheral ones being dominant. The central change is the efficiency with which the heart increases its output and the lungs exchange respiratory gases. Peripheral changes are many, such as an improved distribution of arterial blood and an improved venous return, an increased extraction of oxygen, and increased myoglobin and mitochondria in trained muscle cells.

It is because these peripheral changes are so dominant that endurance exercises using the legs will not show the adaptive changes present in endurance exercises using the arms.

Function of the heart and lungs are not the limiting factors in circulorespiratory endurance unless they are severely incapacitated. Patients with certain heart defects often run well in marathon races, as do patients with one lung removed.

As we shall see later (Chapter 24), the main benefit of endurance exercise in cardiac patients is the improvement of peripheral mechanisms that reduce the load on the damaged heart.

Anaerobic capacity is necessary for short activities of high intensity, or for activities that require more energy than is available from the oxygen transporting system. As discussed in Chapter 10, this energy is derived from high-energy phosphate compounds, resulting from the breakdown of glycogen to lactic acid without requirement for oxygen. Sprinters and other athletes whose events are of short duration (less than 60 seconds), and who do not train for longer periods of intensive exercise, show little or no improvement in endurance or cardiovascular function. They do not have the enlarged hearts, the low resting and exercise heart rates, or the high maximal oxygen uptakes typical of endurance athletes.

EFFECTS OF TRAINING ON OXYGEN TRANSPORT CAPACITY

The oxygen transport capacity is determined by the interrelations of a number of physiological functions, including pulmonary ventilation, cardiac output, total body hemoglobin, and local vascular adjustments. The experimental evidence indicates that the most important effects of training are those involving the cardiac output and the local circulation in the muscles. The importance of adaptive changes in respiration and blood volume (including total body hemoglobin) is not firmly established.

Since the objective of oxygen transport training is to increase endurance, the training exercise must involve dynamic (isotonic) muscle contractions. Interval training has been found to be superior to continuous training for the development of increased oxygen transport capacity. The load on the oxygen transport system should be maximal; however, since maximal oxygen uptake can be reached at a submaximal running speed, the lower speed may be sufficient as a training stimulus. A final consideration concerning the appropriate exercise for endurance training is that it must involve the use of large muscle masses. The intensive use of small muscle groups elevates the arterial blood pressure (sometimes with dangerous results), but it does little to improve the cardiac output and the efficiency of the circulatory adjustments in the muscles.

Effect of training on maximal oxygen uptake. The maximal oxygen uptake is increased by training, due mainly to two factors: (1) increased maximal cardiac output, and (2) increased extraction of oxygen from the blood flowing through the muscles. According to Åstrand and Rodahl these two factors appear to contribute about equally to increasing the maximal oxygen uptake.[1] They will be discussed separately in subsequent sections of this chapter.

The magnitude of the increase in maximal oxygen uptake resulting from training varies widely in different reports, indicating the difficulty in controlling all the variables in longitudinal studies of training effects. In nine studies reviewed by Åstrand and Rodahl, the increase in maximal oxygen uptake produced by training varied from 7 to 33%.[1] In two subjects studied by Ekblom the increase in maximal oxygen uptake was 27% in one subject (after 18 months training) and 44% in the other subject (after 51 months training).[4] Maximal oxygen uptake in skiers and cross-country runners has been reported to be nearly twice that in sedentary subjects.

Maximal oxygen uptake (VO_2 max. L./min.) is highest in running and walking uphill, and slightly (6 to 12%) lower in cycling and swimming.[6] The differences may be due to the degree of training, the size of muscle mass involved, body position, and conditions for heat exchange. The benefits of running for training carry over into other activities more than do those of bicycle training.

The gain in maximal oxygen uptake is greatest when training is done on a bicycle exerciser. The extent of this gain is not apparent when a treadmill is used for testing. When treadmill running is used for training, the gains in oxygen uptake are shown in both bicycle and treadmill testing.[9]

Higher values of maximal oxygen uptake in running and walking uphill on a treadmill are obtained in discontinuous graded exercise (3-minute progressive work periods interrupted by 5-minute rest periods) than in continuous graded exercise (stepwise work not interrupted by rest periods).[5] Continuous exercise appears to generate an increased heat load resulting in an increase in skin blood flow. The resulting shunting of blood to the skin lowers the rate of muscle oxygen consumption that can be achieved during exercise.

The maximal oxygen uptake (ml./kg./min.) of Canadian athletes in various sports was measured at the 1967 Pan American Games.[3] The average scores listed below show the probable effect of training on aerobic fitness.

Cycling	71	Sprinting	53
Distance running	66	Basketball	53
Water polo	58	Volleyball	52
Swimming	57	Paddling	52
Weight lifting	56	Field hockey	52
Tennis	55	Soccer	51
Boxing	55	Judo	49
Diving	54	Gymnastics	42
Wrestling	54	Throwing	38

The relatively high scores of anaerobic performers such as weight lifters and divers undoubtedly indicate the extent to which they include running and other aerobic exercises in their training regimens.

Effects of training on cardiac output. The cardiac output for a given intensity of submaximal exercise is probably not affected by seasonal training. According to some reports, it may actually be lowered; this is attributed to a decrease in the amount of blood flow required because of the greater efficiency of the muscles in extracting oxygen from the blood (see discussion of local vascular adjustments below). The maximal cardiac output that can be achieved is significantly higher in trained athletes than in nontrained persons of the same body size. It should not be concluded, however, that this difference is due entirely to the effects of training, since the reported increase in maximal cardiac output after training is often rather modest. The superior natural endowment of athletes should be considered in all cross-sectional studies of training effects. Training does, however, increase the maximal stroke volume of the heart, so that a given cardiac output can be achieved with a slower heart rate, and this increases the efficiency of the heart as a pump. It is believed that the greater maximal stroke volume of the highly trained athlete is made possible by an increase in the strength of the heart muscle resulting from increased work load, comparable to the increase in strength of skeletal muscles after appropriate training exercise. It is claimed by some that the maximal heart rate that can be attained in exhausting exercise may actually be reduced by training, perhaps because of increased vagal restraint on the heart.

The exercise bradycardia induced by training is operative only when the skeletal muscles that have been trained are used.[2] This is another demonstration of the specific response to training discussed in Chapter 18. Clausen trained two groups on a cycle ergometer; one group used their arms and the other their legs.[2] After training, the heart rate during a test exercise was lower only when the trained limbs were used. The mechanism of this response was not investigated, but the findings suggest either that the exercise bradycardia was due to an improved work efficiency (explained in Chapter 11) or that training somehow induced a neural signal or vascular response in the periphery that modified the chronotropic or inotropic control of the heart during exercise.

Effect of training on extraction of oxygen from blood flowing through muscles. It is often stated that training results in the extraction of a greater proportion of the oxygen from the blood flowing through the working muscles. This is attributed to an increase in the vascularity of the muscles and to a more efficient shunting of the blood into the nutrient capillaries as opposed to the non-nutrient vessels. It is difficult, however, to find evidence supporting this claim, based on actual measurements of the oxygen content of the blood entering and leaving the muscles involved in the exercise. In a study of twelve athletes and fourteen nonathletes the femoral venous oxygen tension measured during bicycle ergometer exercise was almost identical in the two groups. It can be argued that it is desirable that a smaller proportion of the oxygen be extracted from the blood, since this would maintain the venous (and hence the tissue) oxygen tension at a higher level. This important topic requires additional study.

Effect of training on heart size and coronary blood supply. The heart volume (per kilogram of body weight) is larger in athletes trained for endurance than in athletes trained for strength or in sedentary subjects, but there are considerable variations within each group. A contribution of the increase in heart size to the greater maximal stroke volume of athletes is suggested by the high correlation between heart size and maximal oxygen uptake.

An important influence of age on the response of the heart to training is suggested by experiments on rats. Young (1 month of age), young adult (3 to 4 months of age), and middle-aged (12 months of age) rats were subjected to daily or intermittent (twice weekly) swimming exercise. In the young animals cardiac hypertrophy was produced by both daily and intermittent exercise; in the young adult animals, only the daily exercise increased the heart size; in the middle-aged animals, exercise caused an unexplained decrease in cardiac muscle mass. Comparable experiments on human subjects would be of great interest. Coronary blood flow per gram of heart was increased by training in all three age groups of rats. In the younger animals this was due to an increased total number of capillaries, but in the older animals to a loss of cardiac muscle tissue. Again, comparable data on human subjects would have obvious relevance to the question of the beneficial effects of jogging.

The heart muscle of a deconditioned subject remains somewhat trained because it continues to beat while the skeletal muscles are at rest. The resting heart rate, and thus the resting work of the heart which determines its demand for oxygen, is actually increased during a period of sedentary living. Perhaps because of the maintenance of some degree of training by the continuously beating heart, it—in contrast to skeletal muscle—does not undergo an adaptive increase in mitochondrial content or respiratory capacity in response to endurance exercise.[7]

The percentage of energy derived from the oxidation of fatty acids, the rate of muscle glycogen depletion, and the rate of accumulation of lactate are not observed to change in heart muscle during training.[8]

When the untrained heart is exercised by strenuous endurance activities, it increases in size. This hypertrophy of the trained myocardium apparently increases its output capacity by increasing the force of ventricular contraction. The increased systolic power causes a more nearly complete emptying of the ventricles during each systole. Systolic power is also improved due to more nearly synchronous contractions of the myocardial fibers. The improved coordination of myocardial fibers which occurs during training increases the efficiency of the heart action, thus the myocardium requires less oxygen and nutrients to support the demands of exercise.

Cardiac hypertrophy commonly seen in endurance runners is a healthy condition formerly known as "athlete's heart." The heart, like any other muscle of the body, becomes larger and stronger as the result of increased physical activity. A healthy heart is never damaged by progressive endurance training.

The walls of hearts weakened by disease are dilated or ballooned out, but this type of enlargement has no relation to the athlete's heart. In contrast, the walls of the athlete's heart are thickened and made stronger by exercise. Hearts are damaged by disease, not by physical exercise.

To develop cardiovascular hypertrophy, multiple muscles should be exercised in a continuous rhythmic activity such as rowing, cycling, brisk walking, hill climbing, or stair climbing.

Effect of training on blood volume and total body hemoglobin. The total blood volume is increased slightly by training. This appears to be caused entirely by an increase in plasma volume, and its influence on maximal oxygen transport is uncertain. The increase in plasma volume without a corresponding increase in total red cell volume causes a decrease in the proportions of cells to plasma in the circulating blood. The result is that each volume of blood can carry less oxygen, but the decreased viscosity of the more dilute blood reduces the cardiac work required to force the blood through the small blood vessels.

Total body hemoglobin and maximal oxygen uptake are highly correlated, probably because of the correlation of each with body size. There is no evidence that an increase in total body hemoglobin above the normal amount for the body size would in itself increase the maximal oxygen uptake, but of course a decrease below normal in the total body hemoglobin would decrease the maximal oxygen uptake.

Effect of training on pulmonary ventilation and gas exchange. The effect of training on respiration appears to be much less important than the effect on the circulation. The vital capacity is probably not increased by training, although the breathing pattern (greater depth and slower rate) may reduce the work of breathing. Perhaps the best index of the efficiency of respiration is the volume of pulmonary ventilation required for the uptake of 1 liter of oxygen. This is not affected by training in the performance of submaximal work, but the volume of ventilation required in heavy work is reduced by training, perhaps because of the more effective ventilation of the alveoli with the deeper breathing. The diffusing capacity of the lung for oxygen (milliliters of oxygen diffusing from alveoli to blood in 1 minute for each mm. Hg difference in alveolar and pulmonary capillary oxygen tensions) is generally thought to be unchanged by training; the high values reported for champion swimmers may reflect natural endowment rather than training effect.

Heat acclimatization in exercise training. The training of heat-regulating mechanisms is an important part of increasing the circulorespiratory endurance for strenuous exercise. Under the combined demands for circulating blood for muscular contractions and for heat dissipation through the skin, the total blood volume may become inadequate. The capacity of the heart to recirculate the blood is taxed. Some contribution to the volume of available blood, about one liter per minute,[10] is made by the partial shutdown of the perfusion of the kidneys and liver during heavy exercise, but the muscles and skin may need more than this.

In the untrained person, intensive prolonged exercise causes a sudden large increase in cutaneous circulation (about six liters per minute) and the skin flushes a bright pink.[11] This lavish adjustment for the maintenance of core temperature soon causes a shortage of blood for the muscles, and the cardiac output capacity is exceeded. The skin begins to become cyanotic (blue). Now the competition for blood by the skin is lost to the muscles in their last desperate search for oxygen and the flow is diverted from the skin to the muscles. The skin then becomes ashen grey.

Training, either by repeated intensive sustained exercise, or by less intensive exercise in a warm climate, causes a more modest adjustment of the circulation of blood to the skin, an increased cardiac output, and improved ability to dissipate heat through earlier onset of sweating (see Chapter 16).

Continuous versus intermittent exercise. Is training more effective when the exercise is continuous or when it is intermittent—when periods of very severe exercise are interspersed with periods of mild exercise or rest? It is not easy to answer this question and, in fact, the answer depends to some degree on the objectives of the training. There are, however, some general principles that are relevant. One of these is that for maximal training effect the system being trained must be subjected to maximal stress. For example, in endurance training the objective is improvement in the capacity for oxygen transport and this is best achieved by training that extends the systems involved in oxygen transport to the limit of their capacity. If the training period is, for example, about 1 hour in length, the exercise must be performed in a steady state in order to avoid the accumulation of lactic acid and the early onset of exhaustion. It has been observed that in untrained persons only about 50% of the maximal aerobic power (maximal oxygen uptake) can be utilized in steady state exercise, so that the oxygen transport system is not maximally stressed. If, on the other hand, periods of very strenuous exercise, but of brief duration, are alternated with periods of rest, the oxygen transport system can be taxed to its maximal capacity without the occurrence of exhaustion or the accumulation of high levels of lactic acid. On theoretical grounds, such a program should be more effective in endurance training than one based on continuous work of lesser severity. This is the scientific basis of "interval training."

Interval training. Interval training is not an entirely novel method of exercise. Children ordinarily play hard for a short period and then become inactive for a while before starting another period of hard play. In most team sports, such as basketball or football, players alternately shift from spurts of intense play to intervals of easier effort.

However, when the aim of exercise is to condition for maximal performance, the intervals of effort and recovery are measured in terms of intensity and duration. The objectives are to deliver a precise amount of stimulus to the muscular, anaerobic, aerobic, circulatory, and respiratory systems, and to permit a precise degree of recovery between a planned number of bouts of effort.

There are five basic variables in interval training:
1. The duration of the work interval
2. The intensity of activity during the work interval
3. The duration of the recovery interval
4. The intensity of activity during the recovery interval
5. The number of times the work intervals are repeated

The duration of the work interval is measured in terms of the time period during which effort is sustained at high intensity. As a convenient alternative a distance to be run is prescribed, such as 200 meters. The period should be short enough to permit the repetition of high intensity effort for a great number of times. It should, however, be long enough, 90 seconds or more, to overload muscular, circulatory, and respiratory systems sufficiently to improve aerobic capacity.

The intensity of activity during the work interval is measured either in physical terms such as the speed or work, or in terms of physiological effort such as the heart rate. Speed or effort should be carefully graded in order to prevent injury and should progress to near maximal intensity in order to deliver a strong training stimulus. This is the most important of the five basic variables in inducing training. During the final phase of training, the exercise heart rate of young adult athletes should exceed 170 beats per minute during work intervals.

The duration of the recovery interval can be measured in physical terms such as a period of time during which work rate is lessened, or a distance which is to be traversed at a reduced rate of speed. In physiological terms, recovery time is determined by the time elapsed before the pulse rate returns to a desired level. The recovery period should be short (no longer than 2 minutes) in order to stress aerobic systems.

The intensity of activity during the recovery interval is measured in terms of speed or pulse rate. Complete rest in the reclining or quiet standing position is contraindicated because of blood pooling. Continued motion aids venous return and preserves circulatory adjustments to the work. Activity during recovery should be light to permit removal of anaerobic metabolites such as lactic acid, and to allow partial repayment of oxygen debt, thus permitting more intensive effort during the work interval. One method of adjusting the intensity of activity during recovery is to compute one-third of the difference between the pulse at rest and the pulse during exertion and subtract the quotient from the maximal pulse during exertion. An athlete with a resting pulse of 55 and an immediate postexercise pulse of 170 is allowed to recuperate at a level of light activity until his pulse is reduced to 132 beats per minute. The intensity of activity during the recovery interval can be adjusted so that the athlete's recuperation pulse rate reaches the computed value at the end of the desired period. The intensity should never be so light as to permit the pulse rate to drop below 120 beats per minute, the minimal level of stimulus for aerobic and cardiovascular training.

The number of times the work is to be repeated depends on the state of training. If work intervals are sufficiently short and recovery intervals sufficiently long, the athlete in early training should be able to repeat the work at least 10 times. Another method of adjusting the number of repetitions is to set the length of the exercise session (to 30 minutes, for example). Within the total time limit, adjustments in all five basic variables are made so that the participant completes the session before exhaustion occurs.

As training progresses, the total number of work units per week should gradually increase. Use of this measure of total work as a guide is called *volume training.*

Using the acronym D-I-R-T-Y, runners train by adjusting the following variables: D = distance run, I = interval of recovery, R = repetitions, T = time of each run, and Y = "your" activity during the recovery interval.

In training for the mile run a typical regimen for a midseason workout follows this pattern:

D = 220-yard distances to be run
I = 2-minute recovery intervals
R = 8 repetitions
T =

Lap	Seconds
1	31.5
2	31.0
3	30.5
4	30.0
5	29.5
6	29.0
7	28.5
8	28.0

Y = Brisk walking during recovery to maintain pulse rate above 120/minute

Progressive overload is applied in interval training by increasing one variable while the other four remain constant. Specificity of training is achieved by gradually adjusting the duration and intensity of the intervals to coincide more closely with the duration and intensity of a particular event.

Strict adherence to this system is called *formula interval training.* Some athletes can adhere to this rigid system with ease, and derive adequate satisfaction from improvements in condition demonstrated by advances in the basic training variables. Others find formula interval training too mechanistic and would lose motivation to train if some less rigid modes of exercise were not introduced.

There is a wide variety of alternatives to formula interval training.

Hill running. Gravity overload by running uphill to increase endurance, alternating with running downhill using momentum to facilitate speed.

Sand running. Running on soft sand alternating with running on hard sand.

Load running. Running while pushing, pulling, or carrying various amounts of weight.

Recovery cooling. Cold applications (shower bath) between bouts of work to drive cooled blood into working muscles, reduce

stored heat, and decrease sweat rate. However, cold-induced cutaneous vasodilatation may limit this objective.

Breath holding. Holding breath while walking or running to increase
tolerance to pain.

Resistance breathing. Breathing through a small mouthpiece or pursed
lips to increase effort of inhalation and exhalation.

Progression in the *physical work mode* of interval training is achieved
by lengthening the distance, increasing the load of work, increasing the
rate of work, increasing the frequency of work, or shortening the rest
periods. In the *physiological effort mode* of interval training, progression
is achieved by increasing the heart rate or degree of perceived exertion,
increasing the duration of the effort, or shortening the rest periods.

Various forms of interval training have been devised to increase the
speed and endurance in middle distance (2- to 30-minute) events. All
follow the basic protocol: (1) cover a distance shorter than the event
distance at a very fast, anaerobic pace, (2) rest until recovery is partially
complete, and (3) repeat the distance. Some types of interval training
are:

Repetition runs. The pace of the run is precisely determined to duplicate racing speed and the rest period is long enough to allow
nearly complete recovery.

Tempolauf. The run is at top speed for a short period, 20 seconds
or less. The rest period is very short, 5 to 10 seconds. Physiological systems are stressed to near maximum and exhaustion
occurs in about 5 minutes. After long recovery periods the effort
is repeated.

Fartlek, "Speed-play." Long periods of moderate effort, such as cross-
country running interspersed with peak efforts in an informal
manner. On a track the pace is varied every 400 meters or so, alternating slow and fast running according to the subject's feeling
at the moment.

Pyramid. Gradually decreasing the intensity and duration of effort
and increasing the duration of rest intervals to coincide with the
progressive fatigue state of the performer.

Resistance running. The effort is intensified at intervals by running
against greater than normal resistance, such as running up sand
hills, pulling heavy rollers, or running through water.

Paarlauf. A team of two or more runners does a continuous relay, with
one running while the others rest. In competition, the teams run for
a set time, usually an hour, selecting their own interval distances,
usually a quarter of a mile.

Rabbit running. Team of 5 to 10 runners jogs in single file. Last in line runs ahead to take lead position, followed by next to become last in line, and so on. Runner temporarily in lead position sets the jogging pace.

Vita Parcours. A Swiss physical fitness program translated as "life course," a 1- to 2-mile trail through a wooded area with one to twenty exercise stations at intervals along the way. The participant jogs or runs from station to station and performs the prescribed exercise at each. At the initial stations are light warm-up exercises. Exercises are progressively more intensive at middle stations, and become lighter at the final stations.

Circuit training. If sustained exercises are included in the stations described in the previous chapter, cardiovascular endurance can be increased. The exercises at each station are selected in accordance with the specific muscular and cardiovascular elements to be developed. To develop endurance the performer gradually increases the number of times he traverses the circuit and then progressively increases the speed at which he completes the circuit. As a target, the individual notes the time taken to complete three laps of the circuit at maximal speed, and then attempts to halve this time by training. When the target time is reached the individual advances to a more difficult circuit and the whole process is repeated.

An example of a weekly training schedule for a middle distance runner who is exercising two sessions every day in the latter part of pre-season is as follows:

	Session 1	*Session 2*
Monday	Circuit training, repetition runs	Resistance run
Tuesday	Paarlauf, tempolauf	Long run
Wednesday	Circuit training, repetition runs	Resistance run
Thursday	Paarlauf, tempolauf	Long run
Friday	Circuit training, repetition runs	
Saturday	Paarlauf or club competition	Long run
Sunday	Fartlek run	

The following activities, if performed vigorously for 3 minutes or more, either continuously or in intervals, will contribute to circulorespiratory endurance: walking, stationary bicycling, road bicycling, golf (walk 18 holes), hiking, hand mowing, jogging in place, jogging, running for distance, mountain climbing, stair climbing (more than three flights), running in place, running, orienteering, dancing, step exercise, interval training, hill climbing, jumping rope (prolonged), skating, skiing (cross-country), canoeing, rowing, kayaking, swimming, handball, squash, ping pong, badminton, tennis (singles), basketball, soccer, speedball, and volleyball.

RESPIRATORY TRAINING IN HEALTH AND DISEASE

In individuals with normal lungs, exercise training has but little effect on pulmonary ventilation. Vital capacity and air flow rates may increase slightly because of an increased strength and flexibility of the thoracic musculature and diaphragm, but hardly enough to improve endurance capacity. Improved efficiency of the mechanics of breathing due to training may make an energy cost saving of about 5%, which may enhance endurance and maximal working capacity somewhat.

Involuntary versus voluntary control of breathing in exercise. The involuntary increased rate and depth of breathing during continuous intensive exercise seem to be as effective as any form of voluntary control in producing the training effects on pulmonary ventilation and efficiency of breathing. During running and other rhythmic forms of activity, breathing rate becomes synchronous with limb movements. Voluntary attempts to speed or slow the rate of breathing, or to breathe more deeply, do not usually augment respiratory function during exercise. One exception may be the voluntary control over the tendency in novice performers to hyperventilate early in exercise, especially at altitude. Dizziness and "spots before the eyes" may be abolished if the performer deliberately quiets his respiratory response to exertion by reducing his rate and depth of breathing.

Exercise therapy in respiratory disease. The problems of vigorous exercise in lung patients are hypoxia and hypercapnia, thickening of tracheobronchial secretions, labored breathing, and fatigue of respiratory musculature.

Patients with lung disease probably have a less than normal reserve of oxygen and should be protected against sudden demands for oxygen as in intensive exercise. Evidence for such respiratory failure is weakness, bluing of fingernail beds and lips, and labored breathing. This is confirmed by analysis of arterial CO_2, O_2, and pH during a test exercise. Such testing is done under hospital conditions with resuscitation facilities immediately available (see Chapter 23).

Respiratory training through voluntary control of breathing and special breathing exercises may be of considerable therapeutic value in certain respiratory diseases. Because of improved exercise tolerance, mild physical activities such as walking, slow cycling, and easy swimming are generally beneficial to victims of lung diseases such as asthma and emphysema, but intensive exertion may be contraindicated.

Asthma, from the Greek word meaning "gasping for breath," is a respiratory disease characterized by such symptoms as coughing, shortness of breath, and a wheezing or musical type of rattle in the chest. These difficulties are more pronounced on exhaling. The sputum is usually a gray gelatinous material which is gummy and sticky. During an asthma attack the terminal bronchioles are obstructed because of muscle spasm in their walls. During inspiration air can enter the bronchioles with relative ease because of the opening pull of the expanding chest wall. During expiration the caliber of the bronchioles is narrowed and the resistance to the flow of air is increased. The air that is thus trapped in the bronchioles is expelled only by the exerting of extreme pressure by the chest wall. In the presence of edema of the bronchial mucosa and excessive secretions, there may be considerable resistance to both inspiration and expiration. The respiratory rate during such labored breathing is reduced to 10 to 12 breaths per minute from the usual 16 to 18. Asthma is usually associated with allergies, but may be aggravated by physical exertion. Coffee gives temporary relief because the caffeine acts to dilate the bronchioles and make breathing easier. Asthmatics should avoid heavy exercise in dusty, cold air, or in atmospheres known to contain allergenic substances such as pollens and animal hair.

Emphysema, from the Greek word meaning "inflated," is a respiratory disease in which the lungs are overinflated at all times. Such overdistension of the lung tissue destroys the alveolar septal walls distal to the terminal bronchioles. Emphysema is found most frequently in cigarette smokers, residents of air-polluted environments, and heavy users of antibiotics. Usually there is a history of repeated lung infections, and these inflammatory processes result in a gradual destruction of the alveoli, bronchioles, and pulmonary blood vessels. The alveoli rupture into one another, forming larger sacs called bullae which trap the inhaled air. The lungs lose their capacity to expand as the diaphragm descends in inspiration (because of narrowing of the airways) and to expel air in expiration (because of loss of elastic recoil). Sometimes the lungs become so distended that patients become "barrel-chested." The diaphragm, which normally is responsible for about 65% of the work of pulmonary ventilation, surrenders progressively more of its role in respiration to the thoracic and accessory musculature of the upper chest. The extra work to move air in and out of the lungs adds to the energy cost of breathing. The emphysema patient coughs because of irritation of the bronchi. The right heart is subjected to increased pressure by the necessity to pump blood through a restricted vascular bed, with consequent pulmonary hypertension and resulting right ventricular damage, known as cor pulmonale.

Physical exercise is a therapeutic adjunct to drug and inhalation therapy. The emphysema patient is taught to breathe more efficiently by using intercostal rather than shoulder girdle musculature for inhalation, and by using abdominal musculature to assist in more prolonged and effective exhalation. Starting in a position of maximal muscle relaxation, lying in bed with the head, shoulders, and elbows supported by pillows and the knees and hips flexed, the patient's left hand is placed on his chest to remind him not to expand it while inhaling. His right hand is placed on his abdomen to remind him to make his abdomen protrude when he slowly inhales and to tighten his abdominal muscles when he slowly exhales. The next step for the patient is to do this while sitting, standing, and walking. Walking to the limit of good tolerance develops cardiorespiratory endurance. The training program for the emphysema patient begins at a slow pace. Walking is performed in a relaxed manner. An exercise program can be prescribed, using a treadmill or bicycle ergometer to establish the limit of tolerance (see Chapter 23). The objects of the exercise program are to improve pulmonary ventilation, decrease the energy cost of breathing, and increase tolerance to daily activities.

References

1. Åstrand, P.-O., and Rodahl, K.: Textbook of work physiology, New York, 1970, McGraw-Hill Book Co.
2. Clausen, J. P., and Lassen, N. A.: Evidence that the relative exercise bradycardia induced by training can be caused by extra-cardiac factors. In Larsen, O. A., and Malmborg, R. O., editors: Coronary heart disease and physical fitness, Baltimore, 1971, University Park Press.
3. Cumming, G. R.: Physiological studies on Canadian athletes, Paper presented at 1st Annual Meeting, Canadian Association of Sport Sciences, Toronto, Ontario, 1968.
4. Ekblom, B.: Effect of physical training on oxygen transport system in man, Acta Physiol. Scand. Suppl. 328, 1969.
5. Froelicher, V. F., Jr., and others: A comparison of three maximal treadmill exercise protocols, J. Appl. Physiol. 36:720, 1974.
6. Holmér, X., and Åstrand, P.-O.: Swimming training and maximal oxygen uptake, J. Appl. Physiol. 33: 510, 1972.
7. Oscai, L. B., Mole, P. A., and Holloszy, J. O.: Effects of exercise on cardiac weight and mitochondria in male and female rats, Am. J. Physiol. 220:1944, 1971.
8. Paul, P., Issekutz, B., and Miller, H. I.: Interrelationships of free fatty acids and glucose metabolism in the dog, Am. J. Physiol. 211:1313, 1966.
9. Pechar, G. S., and others: Specificity of cardiorespiratory adaptation to bicycle and treadmill running, J. Appl. Physiol. 36:753, 1974.
10. Rowell, L. B.: Distribution of cardiac output during exercise and the effect of training. In Larsen, O. A., and Malmborg, R. O., editors: Coronary heart disease and physical fitness, Baltimore, 1971, University Park Press.
11. Shephard, R. J.: The heart and circulation under stress of Olympic conditions, J.A.M.A. 205:1905, 1968.

Suggested readings

Banister, E. W., Tomanek, R. J., and Cvorkov, N.: Ultrastructural modifications in rat heart: responses to exercise and training, Am. J. Physiol. 220: 1935, 1971.

Bason, R. E., and others: Maintenance of physical training effects by intermittent exposure to hypoxia, Aerospace Med. 44:1097, 1973.

Caplin, I.: The allergic asthmatic, Springfield, Ill., 1968, Charles C Thomas, Publisher.

Clausen, J. P., and others: Central and peripheral circulatory changes after training of the arms or legs, Am. J. Physiol. 225:675, 1973.

Cooper, K. H.: The new aerobics, New York, 1970, M. Evans & Company.

Costill, D.: The relationship between selected physiological variables and distance running performance, J. Sports Med. Phys. Fitness 7:61, 1967.

Fox, E. L., and Mathews, D. K.: Interval training conditioning for sports and general fitness, Philadelphia, 1974, W. B. Saunders Co.

Gleser, M. A., and Vogel, J. A.: Endurance exercise: effect of work-rest schedules and repeated testing, J. Appl. Physiol. 31:735, 1971.

Hartley, L. H., and others: Multiple hormonal responses to graded exercise in relation to physical training, J. Appl. Physiol. 33:602, 1972.

Judd, W. T., and Poland, J. L.: Myocardial glycogen changes with exercise, Proc. Soc. Exp. Biol. Med. 140:955, 1972.

Karvonen, M. J., and Barry, A. J., editors: Physical activity and the heart, Springfield, Ill., 1967, Charles C Thomas, Publisher.

Rodman, T., and Sterling, F. H.: Pulmonary emphysema and related lung diseases, St. Louis, 1969, The C. V. Mosby Co.

Shappell, S. D., and others: Adaptation to exercise: role of hemoglobin affinity for oxygen and 2,3-diphosphoglycerate, J. Appl. Physiol. 30:827, 1971.

Shephard, R. J., editor: Frontiers of fitness, Springfield, Ill., 1971, Charles C Thomas, Publisher.

Williams, C. G., and others: The capacity for endurance work in highly trained men, Int. Z. angew, Physiol. 26:141, 1968 .

Wyndham, C. H., and others: Physiological requirements for world-class performances in endurance running, Human Sciences Laboratory, Chamber of Mines of South Africa, Johannesburg, S. A., Medical Journal, 43:996, 1969.

21 SKILL DEVELOPMENT

We do not yet know whether the learning of a new motor skill results from morphological changes in presynaptic terminals, chemical changes in the neurons, or other subcellular phenomena. We do know from electromyographic studies (see Chapter 4 in the *Laboratory Manual*) and cinematographic observations that the process of skill development involves a simplification of neuromuscular activity. Contractions that are extraneous to an efficient movement are somehow inhibited.

The urgency of movement is decided at a conscious level, according to the way the person perceives his environment. The decision of whether to walk or run is made at higher levels of the central nervous system. The detailed act of movement is controlled at lower subconscious levels of the nervous system. Once the motion is started it is self-regulating, with several subsystems controlling the length and tension of muscles acting on joints. As discussed in earlier chapters, length control of muscles is based on excitation or inhibition of the alpha and gamma neurons and inhibitory afferent fibers from muscle spindles. Tension control is also inhibitory and is generated by Golgi tendon organs. These control systems apparently have a high degree of plasticity and can be altered to adapt to imposed demands. The major change as conditioning occurs seems to be in the inhibitory mechanisms. It is essentially through the inhibition of extraneous contractions and excessive tension that improved coordination and simplification of movement are achieved.

The practical results of such motor simplification are improvement in the force, speed, accuracy and economy of movement, and reduction in excess muscular tension.

Elucidation of skill development from the point of view of a simplification of movement involves the consideration of several mechanisms. In this chapter we shall see how biological, environmental, cultural, behavioral, and psychological factors interact with physiological ones in the process of skill development.

In the execution of a skilled movement, thinking about it during the action is undesirable. Concentration is centered on the wholeness of the act, not upon the parts or upon the consequence of the outcome. An athlete whose performance has been destroyed by the suggestions of others regarding his style of movement is said to be suffering from "paralysis by analysis."

Military combat teams are drilled to respond "by the numbers" in order to prevent delays in time and errors in judgment that are the inevitable consequences of intermixtures of thought and action. In industry, production is higher and waste is reduced when the workers do not have the responsibility of planning and laying out the work and the foremen who do the planning do not perform the work. Thought and action are kept separate.

The shift in attention from the elements of a task to the signal that is the stimulus for the action to take place is the essence of motor learning. During the training process the action becomes automatic, and the performer ultimately can block out the function of the symbolic system. In this way he gains the quickness and positiveness of a nonhuman animal. From the point of view of maximal performance and efficiency, the symbolic system is an element to be opposed.

RESPONSE TO NEW MOVEMENT EXPERIENCES

A person interacting with his environment modifies his patterns of movement to meet the demands of new situations. Such modification, however, is much more than the simple process of adding or subtracting motor skills. Each new experience requires some reorganization of the person's whole pattern of movement—termed *movement gestalt*.

The success with which a person moves to meet the demands of a new situation depends upon how well the required movement fits in with established patterns. In some situations in which the movement requirement is not clearly indicated and the movement vocabulary is narrow in this area of experience, a person may make no response whatsoever at the level of function of movement.

In learning new skills it is necessary for a person to assimilate new motor experiences into his movement gestalt. Failure to learn may reflect his inability to assimilate conflicting motor habits.

PERSISTENCE OF MOVEMENT HABITS

Habits of movement can be either rigidly or less firmly established. Rigid patterns of movement may facilitate the rapid learning of some skills but may interfere with the acquisition of others. If rigidly established habits of movement persist for a long period of time, they may alter the physical structure and thus effect a permanent change in the movement characteristics of a person.

Weak patterns of movement can be altered at will and exist only as long as conditions favoring them are in operation. A person whose movement gestalt is characterized by a high degree of variability may also have difficulty in acquiring and perfecting new skills.

NEGATIVE FEEDBACK THEORY OF SKILL IMPROVEMENT

Human response to new tasks tends to be characterized by oversensitivity and overactivity. With practice there appears to be developed an active inhibitory force that serves to control the movements, making them more direct and efficient. The mechanism of this improvement may be an alteration of the whole system of receptor and effector interaction.

Receptor and effector processes in the nervous system are coordinated in such a way that information fed back to the receptors during performance acts to determine effector function. When a new movement is performed, the feedback tends to be predominantly positive in that the taking of the action encourages its own continuation. The behavior resulting from positive feedback is erratic and clumsy.

After practice the feedback becomes predominantly negative; the taking of action tends to reduce the continuation of the action, and the system becomes self-regulatory. With the onset of negative feedback dominance, the performance takes on two beneficial characteristics.

1. The action is related more to the requirements of the situation than to momentary variations in the individual.
2. The performance tends to remain constant in the face of disturbing elements in the environment so that the achievement is only slightly affected by outside influences.

FACTORS THAT LIMIT SKILL

The maximal skill that can be achieved may be limited by the following factors: (1) body weight, (2) body height, (3) timing, (4) accuracy of movement, which includes eye-muscle coordination, kinesthesis, balance, reaction time, speed of movement, precision, and visual aim, and (5) muscular tension.

Body weight. The heavier a person in relation to his musculature, the greater the limitation of his physical skill. Added weight in the form of fat increases the effort needed to perform a movement. The fatty tissue may also be considered to have a hobbling effect on movement. A reduction of this inactive tissue will aid in improving performance of a skill exercise.

Body height. A tall person displaces his center of gravity through a greater distance than does a short person when the same movement is performed by each. The taller person's center of gravity is always farther from his base of support. When the exercise requires displacement of the center of gravity in any direction except along a horizontal plane, the taller person having the greater displacement requires more muscle activity to achieve the positions and maintain posture during the exercise. The shorter athlete has the advantage in many skill exercises. Errors in diving form are magnified in the tall diver and are less noticeable in the short diver. The same is true in gymnastics. The taller basketball player or baseball pitcher, however, may have better control by being able to guide the ball through a larger range of movement. Tall tennis players have an advantage in covering the court and in placing the serve and the return.

Timing. A skill exercise requires a fine coordination in the timing of the muscular contractions. As the movements of an exercise proceed, each muscle involved must contract or relax at the proper instant or the movement will be interfered with or misdirected entirely. As learning of a skill exercise progresses, there is an improvement in the timing of the muscular contractions and relaxations that control the various movements. The limiting factor in developing the highest degree of muscle timing is the capacity of the central nervous system. A person with a damaged or an underdeveloped central nervous system cannot, even by improved muscular development, attain a high degree of skill in any exercise that requires precise neuromuscular coordination.

Eye-muscle coordination. Accuracy of movement is essential in all skill exercises. Accuracy involves coordination of eye and muscle, proprioceptive sensibility, and integration of the touch receptors, the inner ear, and other organs of balance and positioning. *Eye-muscle coordination* establishes the relationship of the target object to the body so as to guide the movements directly to the target. Eye-muscle coordination is the dominant feature in learning a skill exercise. During the learning period the background of distance relationships is combined with movement-in-space experiences under the guidance of visual observation. As skill is improved the eye-muscle factor becomes less dominant. When the skill is perfected, it can be performed with the eyes closed.

Kinesthesis. The proprioceptors are located in the muscles, tendons, and joints. These receptors are stimulated by stretching. The response to the proprioceptor stimulus is a *kinesthetic impression,* or awareness of a change in the position of the body or of some part of the body.

277

This mechanism enables the tennis player to watch the ball and the court position of his opponents without also having constantly to check the position of his stroking arm and racket in order to contact the ball at the proper time and at the proper place on the racket. The golfer is able, through kinesthetic impressions, to gauge the extent of his backswing and the position of his wrists and hands without looking away from the ball during the backswing. The gross movements of the stroke that involve a coordination of the movements of the legs, hips, waist, shoulders, arms, and wrists become so accurate in practice that the face of the club strikes the ball with force and accuracy, and the ball is sent to a small target 200 yards away. With further practice the timing, accuracy, and force of the stroke are improved and as a result the ball travels farther and lands closer to the target with no greater expenditure of energy.

Balance. Many types of skilled exercise require an accurate *sense of balance* and a rapid restoration of the body to its normal position when balance has been disturbed. This ability depends on nerve impulses originating in the labyrinth of the inner ear (the otolith organs and the semicircular canals).

There are two main groups of labyrinthine reactions: (1) the acceleratory reflexes and (2) the positional reflexes. Acceleratory reflexes are evoked by movements of the head, and the effective stimulus is acceleration (a change in velocity). The response to linear acceleration is useful to the jumper in effecting a landing on the feet. Upon angular acceleration the responses are evoked in the muscles of the eyes, neck, limbs, and trunk. Rotary acceleration produces eye movements known as nystagmus, which is a quick swing of the eyes in the direction of the rotation, alternating with a slow deviation in the opposite direction. If the rotation continues at a constant rate, the nystagmus gradually dies away, an example of the fact that this type of reaction depends upon acceleration, not velocity. Cessation of the rotation may cause turning of the head, body, and arms in the direction of the previously experienced movement, with the result that the individual tends to fall to that side. An example of the positional reflex is the righting reaction that acts upon the neck muscles to keep the head in a normal position regardless of the position of the body. Another example of a positional reflex is the compensatory deviations of the eyes that are evoked by changes in the position of the head. When the body is placed in an abnormal position, there is an immediate effort to restore it to its normal position. A normal, blindfolded person standing on a platform readily adjusts the position of his body when the platform is gradually tilted, but deaf mutes (in whom the inner ear is defective) immediately fall. Impressions

278

from the labyrinth together with the visual and proprioceptive impressions from the muscles control the process by which physical equilibrium is gained or maintained. Impressions from the labyrinth are especially concerned with maintaining the normal position of the head.

Overstimulation of the labyrinthine receptors, as in whirling or rapid tumbling, may produce dizziness and even nausea. Seasickness results from a certain type of overstimulation of these receptors. Dizziness reduces skill and accuracy of movement. A common practice of dancers and figure skaters whose routines include rapid spins is to fix the eyes on a distant point and to watch that point until the head has turned as far as is compatible with comfort. The head is then shifted quickly in the direction of the spin until another point is sighted. The eyes rest on this object until the limit of the turn of the head is reached and the shift is repeated. This momentary pause in the rotation of the head, referred to as "spotting," provides a brief resting period that reduces the dizziness of overstimulation. The susceptibility to dizziness upon continued turning is diminished during training so that skill and accuracy during spinning or tumbling movements are increased.

PATTERNS OF MOVEMENT

Certain reflex actions, originally patterns of movement necessary for survival and now outmoded, still linger at the lower level of nervous system response. The tonic neck reflex is one example of a pattern of movement with an evolutionary background. The tonic neck reflex consists of turning the head and eyes in a given direction, thereby activating and influencing certain responses of the upper and lower extremities. If the person is face down and the oral cavity is turned to one side, there is a lateral movement of the eyes and extensor movement of both extremities on the same side. This is the *homolateral* movement seen typically in the crawling salamander and other amphibians and is often observed in convulsive seizures in man.

Another type of evolutionary movement is the *homologous* pattern in which both upper extremities and both lower extremities are used simultaneously. This produces the hop of the frog, the jump of the rabbit, and the gallop of the horse. It is noted in man when he leaps at a foe or jumps with fright. Both the homolateral and the homologous patterns are observable in an infant placed prone in shallow water.

Babinski's reflex consists of dorsiflexion of the big toe upon stimulation of the sole of the foot. It occurs in lesions of the pyramidal tract and is one of the signs that distinguishes between organic and hysteric hemiplegia. This has been related to the amphibian stage in which the toes are spread to give the frog more surface for the take off on his jump.

A higher type of movement is that found in the turtle in which the lower extremity advances in coordination with the opposite upper extremity. This is known as the *crossed extensor* pattern and is present in walking as one arm swings in time with the opposite leg.

RIGHTING REFLEXES

Posture, both static and dynamic, is the result of the coordination of a great number of reflexes, many of which have a tonic character. Magnus found that in an animal the righting function is carried out by five groups of different reflexes: labyrinthine-righting reflexes, body-righting reflexes acting upon the head, neck-righting reflexes, body-righting reflexes acting on the body, and optical-righting reflexes. Little is known about the way these reflexes react to produce erect posture in man, but it has been shown that whiplash injuries are likely to affect these reflexes and thus injure a person's coordination and balance.

Labyrinthine-righting reflexes. Labyrinthine-righting reflexes originate in the labyrinths and disappear after removal of the labyrinth or after detachment of the otoliths. Labyrinthine-righting reflexes are controlled by gravity. These reflexes act primarily on the neck muscles to provide for orientation of the head in space. One of the problems of manned space flight lies in the fact that the postural-righting reflex seems to cease to function after a few seconds of weightlessness.

Body-righting reflexes acting upon the head. Asymmetrical stimulation of pressure sense organs in the surface of the trunk evokes righting reflexes. The head becomes oriented in relation to the surface with which the body is in contact.

Neck-righting reflexes. When the head is turned, the neck is twisted. This evokes a reflex by which the thorax is moved and brought into symmetry with the head. In skilled athletic events such as springboard diving and gymnastic tumbling the effect of a slight turn of the head in altering body movements is well known.

Body-righting reflexes acting on the body. Sensory nerve endings of the body surface that are stimulated asymmetrically by pressure cause the body to move to secure symmetrical stimulation.

Optical-righting reflexes. Visual impressions contribute to the orientation of the head. In the off-balance position there is a minute dilation of the pupil, which returns to the normal size when balance is recovered.

MASS MOVEMENT PATTERNS

Stimulation of the motor cortex in man and other primates results in combinations of motion termed mass movement patterns. These are all diagonal movements, suggesting that straight movements such as flexion, extension, abduction, and adduction are derived from the synergistic action of contracting diagonal movements. A mass movement pattern will give a greater response against maximal resistance than will a straight pattern. Mass movements of this type result from natural pathways in the central nervous system and are not learned. They appear in normal activities, such as throwing and striking. To a large extent the way in which a person moves to accomplish a task is instinctive. Automatic movements are carried out with a rather high degree of efficiency; others must be learned, and the time taken to acquire efficiency in their use may be prolonged.

PRINCIPLE OF LEAST RESISTANCE

The nervous system functions on the principle of utilizing the path of least resistance. Thus, if a person attempts to make a given motion that requires him to use weak muscles, he will soon learn to substitute stronger ones to accomplish the act. If the hip flexors are very weak, for example, he may substitute the quadratus lumborum and develop a pattern of pelvic elevation when walking. As this abnormal pattern becomes habitual the weakened hip flexors are atrophied because of disuse and finally may become completely paralyzed. Even if innervation of the flexors should be recovered, the abnormal pattern of movement may be so embedded that the flexors continue to be excluded from the pattern of movement. Abnormal patterns of this kind may result in muscle imbalance, and the deformity may become progressively worse.

PRACTICE

Quickness of response to a stimulus such as a starting gunshot is determined by (1) the time taken to recognize the stimulus, (2) the time taken to decide what action to take in response to the stimulus, and (3) the time required to act.

Under simple reflex reaction conditions such as stepping on a tack, touching a hot iron, or tapping the patellar tendon, the quickness of the response is not slowed by recognition or decision processes. This reflex reaction time is established by (1) the length of the neurons activated (eye-blink reaction is faster than finger prick reactions) and (2) the speed of the impulse along the nerve (some nerves conduct impulses faster than other nerves). Neither of these anatomical features can be affected by training.

281

The processes of recognition and decision making can be simplified by proper practice, thereby shortening the time of execution. Proper practice consists of repetitions of the stimulus and correct response to the point that brain involvement is reduced to a minimum and the reaction approaches that of a simple reflex. Practice does not "make perfect" unless each response is a correct one. Practice of erroneous responses—those which result in imperfect performance—delay the development in speed and skill of a movement. If at first you don't succeed, don't try the same thing again. Instead, try doing the task correctly each time. When the movement is perfected, then repeat it until it is "overlearned," that is, the action is unconscious.

CONCENTRATION

Cerebration after the movement is perfected at the unconscious level only slows the response and spoils the neuromuscular coordination. If you think about your leg action as you hurry downstairs, you are apt to fall. A javelin thrower who concentrates on his elbow position and wrist action will shorten the distance of the throw. This is the phenomenon described earlier as "paralysis by analysis." A golfer can unfairly destroy his opponent's performance by giving him a little coaching tip such as "Straighten your left arm" just before he swings. Champions, after their record-breaking performances, often report that they were in a state of concentration in which the details of the event were being registered without any conscious attention or reaction to them. They started without knowing quite what took place, their action was well within maximal capacity ("I felt as if I could have done much better"), and they were surprised to find that they had finished so well ("It was all over before I knew what had happened"). The best performances are those that are executed below the level of consciousness. When higher centers are brought into play, physical performance deteriorates. Complex mental performances, on the other hand, as in chess, require long periods of time for deliberation. Play cannot be speeded without reducing performance because some possible choices must be eliminated from consideration.

PERFORMANCE

Reaction time. The time required to react to a single stimulus is greatly affected by the nature of the stimulus. Response to a sound or a touch is quicker than to a light signal. The time to respond to all types of stimuli is lengthened if the stimuli are complicated. Sound signals that continually vary in pitch and loudness are very difficult to react to. Intermittent distracting noises slow a reaction, but a continuous noise does not seem to affect reaction time.

Reaction is usually faster to easily perceived stimuli. If the sound signal is very faint or the light signal is short, small, dim, or hazy, the reaction is slowed. There is probably a maximal limit of strength of stimuli beyond which increases in loudness, size, and brightness do not speed a reaction and may even slow it down.

Men react faster than women and shortest reaction times in both sexes are during the age period between 21 and 30 years. There are great differences in reaction time among persons. Champion athletes have better than average response times, and sprinters react faster than distance runners. Practice has little effect on shortening reaction time, but can shorten the time required for a total body response to complex stimuli.

Speed of movement. Work is accomplished at a faster rate if component movements are in a continuous curved motion than if movements involve abrupt changes in direction. Maximal velocity of movement is inversely related to weight handled. Also the time required to attain maximal velocity is correlated with weight. Horizontal motions are more rapid than similar motions in a vertical plane.

Urging a person to move more rapidly will increase his speed of movement, but his accuracy may be decreased. Reaction time is unaffected.

Precision. Manual tasks in which movement is away from the body are performed with less error than those in which movement is toward the body. Movement in a downward plane is inaccurate because of a tendency to overshoot. Under stress of speed muscle tension is increased, which in turn decreases motor coordination and results in more errors. Some workers tend to preserve stability of performance under stress and thereby maintain efficiency.

Movements are made most quickly and accurately with the right hand if performed in a counterclockwise direction and more quickly with the left hand if in a clockwise direction. Accuracy and speed of manipulation are best when both hands are used. One hand, either right or left, is 90% as effective as when both are used together.

Positions demanding muscular distortion, such as reaching backward or above shoulder level, are made with difficulty. Motions directly forward or to right or left are made more quickly and accurately. Estimations of displacements of limbs and parts of the body depend somewhat on the physical effort involved during the judgment; more effort leads to greater accuracy.

Visual aim. The accuracy of aim in directing an object toward a distant target is enhanced if a closer object is used as a reference point. The spot system in bowling utilizes this principle. Instead of taking aim on the pins, aim is taken on or near a spot on the alley about 16 feet ahead of the foul line. Because of the defects in the optical system of the eye, visual acuity is greatest when the pupil is fairly constricted. In the act of accommodation the pupil is constricted for near vision and dilated for far vision. For objects near at hand the visual acuity is remarkable. Most persons can see the width of the finest hair at arm's length. The width of the retinal image of the hair is 0.0049 mm., and this is practically the diameter of a single cone in the fovea. The lens is flattened when viewing objects more than 20 feet away and must bulge for clear vision of objects closer than 20 feet (in the normal eye). Associated with the accommodation reflex when an object is viewed at close range is the convergence reflex by which the two eyes are turned in toward the nose through contraction of the internal recti and simultaneous relaxation of the external recti of each eye. The kinesthetic impressions from the converging eye muscles provide an estimate of the distance, the convergence becoming greater as the distance is shortened. Near objects (within 20 feet) viewed with the eyes naturally converged are seen with stereoscopic vision, which allows an estimate of the length, width, and thickness of the object. This spatial discrimination is diminished when the object is viewed from afar. When near objects are viewed with only one eye, spatial discrimination is also lost. The appreciation of the size and shape in three dimensions improves the accuracy of aim and the judgment of distance.

Muscular tension. The degree of muscular tension during the performance of an activity affects the energy requirement of the task, the rate of movement of body parts, and the onset of fatigue. Muscular tension during manual work can be measured by recording grip pressure of the idle hand and of the used hand, by recording the pressure of the point of the pencil in writing, and by recording muscular action potentials.

The level of muscular tension habitually exhibited by a person during muscular activity characterizes him as a tense or relaxed person. Too much tension makes movement jerky, awkward, and often painful. Too little tension makes movement weak and unsteady.

The level of muscular tension is determined by the intensity of the activity of the central nervous system, particularly the cortical and subcortical centers. Impulses from the sensory nervous system received by these centers elicit a discharge of motor impulses that stimulate skeletal muscles, causing a general increase in tension. Mental and emotional experiences affect tension. States of sadness and depression diminish tension and result in slouched posture and "halfhearted" movements. States of happiness and confidence elevate tension and result in more erect posture, alertness, and movements that are more direct and less fatiguing. Fear and intense excitement can increase tension to the point of incapacitating contracture ("scared stiff") and resultant muscular fatigue. Such spasticity during excitement interferes with coordination and often results in fumbles and inaccurate performances during an athletic event. Thinking about muscular performance has been shown to produce an increase in the tension of the muscles that would participate in actual performance. This phenomenon suggests that learning and perfection of skills can proceed by reading and thinking about the technique of the event. Thus a golfer during the winter season may improve his swing by studying texts written on the subject. Divers commonly repeat in their imagination the movements of a new dive before attempting to perform it off the springboard or platform.

Just as thinking about muscular performance increases muscular tension, increased muscular tension during activity also increases the activity of the central nervous system. Clenching the fist exaggerates the knee jerk reflex response. Muscular relaxation reduces the amplitude of the knee jerk response. In one experiment the rate of learning was improved by induced tension achieved by gripping a hand dynamometer. Restlessness and incidental activity such as clenching a fist while writing an examination may conceivably contribute sufficiently to the stimulation of cortical activity to improve the student's score.

READINESS

There is apparently an optimal degree of readiness for physical activity which yields the best performance. This optimal degree is somewhere between a state of relaxation and a state of high tension.

In a relaxed state too much time is required to bring the active muscles into play. If the muscles are too slack, force is dissipated. In the tense state, a certain degree of relaxation must be initiated before movement can occur. Tense muscles act as brakes; they reduce the speed and force of motion, and induce fatigue.

Anticipation of action excites the entire organism. Adrenaline is secreted (test pilots call these secretions "adrenalburgers"), circulation to the splanchnic area slows down and heart rate speeds up ("butterflies in the stomach"), and a vasovagal stimulation causes nausea and sometimes vomiting. The experienced performer welcomes these disagreeable signs as potential benefits to his performance. Once the action is started these signs disappear because the adjustments are in harmony with the demands of exertion. The veteran actor or athlete who does not feel "up" for his performance knows that the results that day will not be the best.

HYPERTONUS AND RELAXATION

Tension is good when it leads to action, but mounting tension without action leads to stress reactions and fatigue. Too much tension, hypertonus, causes restriction of movement. Hypertonic individuals do not move with freedom and grace. They often hold themselves still, thereby increasing their tension. The diaphragm and auxiliary muscles of breathing are held partially contracted during states of excess tension. After a while they spasmodically contract powerfully and then relax completely in a deep sigh. Hypertonus disturbs circulation, digestion, and excretion in individually different ways, the mechanism of which is not clear. Inability to sleep is a common sign of hypertonus. Specific exercises to release tension have been developed by Jacobson and Rathbone. These consist of a deliberate contraction of muscles in a certain region in order to feel the tension and then a conscious relaxation of that tension.

BODY-SENSE AREA OF THE BRAIN

The proprioceptive impressions from the muscles, tendons, and joints and the senses of touch and pressure are represented in the contralateral postcentral convolution of the cerebral cortex. This area is known as the body-sense or somesthetic area. Impulses arriving at the body-sense area result in an awareness of the following:

1. The position of the parts of the body that are being moved
2. The location and extent of the body area that is being touched
3. The weight of an object
4. The size and shape of the object in three dimensions

Combining these sensations we are able to perceive the size, shape, weight, and texture of the stimulating object and also to recognize the position of the parts of the body that are moving to handle the object.

LEARNING

Learning of skills involves a familiarity with the objects to be used and a coordination of the body movements that are required in handling the object. Skills that are unnatural and highly complex are learned more easily if the various elements in the movements can be separated and learned singly. The simplest skill elements are taken up first, and as these are learned there is a progression to the more complex elements. The elements may then be combined and the various skill elements added gradually until the whole skill is performed. Natural activities in simple forms can be learned by practicing the whole skill with attention given to improving the form.

SPECIFICITY

The central nervous system adapts to physical activity of the type that makes demands on it. Repeated attempts at perfecting a skill during such activities as baseball or piano playing undoubtedly involve a re-programming process. Repeated performance of the movement pattern induces conditioned reflexes which enable the physical activity to be performed more precisely and without conscious control.

There is specificity in learning skills just as there is specificity in muscular training. Although two activities may be similar in that like movements are involved, a difference in the objects employed may impede a transfer of the skills learned in the one activity to those used in the other. Badminton practice does not necessarily improve tennis skill. Baseball batting does not necessarily improve golf skill. Also the practice of one skill using an object does not necessarily improve another skill using the same object. For example, passing a football will not necessarily improve the ability to kick a football. Thus during practice those objects and movements that will be employed in the final performance should be used.

The method of training to perform a skill event should be related to the dominant feature of the event. If speed is the dominant feature, as in fencing or tennis, the skills should be practiced at a rapid rate. Practice of such events at a slow speed will produce high initial accuracy, but as speed is increased, further increases in accuracy will be very slight. Race horses are ridden in early training by lightweight jockeys to accustom the horses to the greatest possible speed under the small weight. After this the horses will tend to retain the same speed even while carrying heavier jockeys. When accuracy is the dominant feature, such as in the operation of a telephone switchboard, the new operator should first strive for accuracy at a slow rate and then gradually increase speed.

Suggested readings

Bell, V.: Visual and verbal feedback and its effect upon acquisition and retention of a projectile skill, Res. Quart. **41**:15, 1970.

Bernstein, N.: The coordination and regulation of movement, Elmsford, New York, 1967, Pergamon Press, Inc.

Bilodeau, E., editor: Principles of skill acquisition, New York, 1969, Academic Press, Inc.

Denslow, J., and Gutensohn, R.: Neuromuscular reflexes in response to gravity, J. Appl. Physiol. **23**:243, 1967.

Jacobson, E., and others: Tension in medicine, Springfield, Ill., 1967, Charles C Thomas, Publisher.

Johnson, L. V.: Effects of 5-day-a-week vs. 2- and 3-day-a-week physical education class on fitness, skill, adipose tissue and growth, Res. Quart. **40**:93, 1969.

Lloyd, A.: Muscle activity and kinesthetic position responses, J. Appl. Physiol. **25**:659, 1958.

Oxendine, J.: Effect of mental and physical practice on the learning of three motor skills, Res. Quart. **40**:755, 1969.

Petajan, J., and Eagan, C.: Effect of temperature, exercise and physical fitness on the triceps surae reflex, J. Appl. Physiol. **25**:16, 1968.

Phipps, S., and Morehouse, C.: Effects of mental practice on the acquisition of motor skills of varied difficulty, Res. Quart. **40**:773, 1969.

Rathbone, J.: Relaxation, Philadelphia, 1969, Lea & Febiger.

Roberts, T.: Neurophysiology of postural mechanisms, New York, 1967, Plenum Publishing Corp.

Shick, J.: Effects of mental practice on selected volleyball skills for college women, Res. Quart. **41**:88, 1970.

Singer, R.: Motor learning and human performance, New York, 1968, The Macmillan Co.

Thompson, D.: Immediate external feedback in the learning of golf skills, Res. Quart. **40**:589, 1969.

Wickstrom, R.: Fundamental motor patterns, Philadelphia, 1970, Lea & Febiger.

Yahr, M., and Purpura, D., editors: Neurophysiological basis of normal and abnormal motor activities, New York, 1967, Raven Press.

PART SEVEN

THERAPEUTIC EXERCISE

22 EXERCISE IN RELATION TO OBESITY AND DIABETES

OBESITY

Lack of physical exercise often leads to an excess storage of fat in the body. When this occurs it is because there has not been a proportional decrease in food intake. This relationship is described by the simple equation expressing the conservation of matter: input = output + storage. When body fat exceeds the upper limits of normal values by 10%, the individual is considered to be obese.[6]

Normal values of fat as a percentage of total body weight are different in men and women. The upper limit of normal for men is 18% and for women 28%. Thus any male is considered obese if his body fat is over 28% of his total body weight, and a female is obese if her body fat is over 38%. There are no established minimal values for body fat; in general, leanness is considered an advantage to health. If a person receives adequate nutrition it is not possible to be too lean.

Obesity endangers health because it alters body functions, predisposes the individual to disease, has detrimental effects in established diseases, and engenders adverse psychological reactions.

Mortality rates from "all causes" are 50% greater than normal in obese people. Obesity increases the individual's risk of hypertension, atherosclerosis, and coronary heart disease. It disturbs endocrine function and impairs carbohydrate metabolism. The onset of adult diabetes mellitus and its complications is frequently coincident with the beginning of obesity. Increased adipose tissue distributed throughout the body creates a demand for extra blood. Excess fat stored in the abdominal area makes

291

breathing more difficult by interfering with movements of the chest wall and diaphragm. Obese women may have hirsutism (presence of excessive hair), menstrual abnormalities, and complications in pregnancy. Obese men may become infertile if rolls of fat surround the scrotum.

These cardiovascular, respiratory, metabolic, and endocrine disorders usually disappear when body fat is reduced to normal.

Since in the United States fat people are regarded as unattractive, many such individuals develop an obsessive concern for body image. Because they expect rejection they tend to withdraw and become passive. Under this self-induced confinement they eat more and move less. Instead of responding to internal cues signifying hunger, these obese individuals eat whether they are hungry or not. They are hyperresponsive to food-related tastes and smells and cannot resist bakeries and candy stores.[14]

Inactivity and food intake. In a reasonably active person or animal, food intake is increased in proportion to an increase in activity. However, in sedentary humans and animals slight increases in activity do not stimulate the appetite. Mayer found that unexercised individuals eat more than those who take short walks.[7] Stockmen have been aware of this and they pen their cattle to fatten them for the market. Beef muscles thus larded weigh more and are more tender and juicy because of their higher fat content. Farmers all over the world agree that the first step in the production of lard is to prevent the animals from increasing their energy expenditure by unhampered wandering. It is not until exercise is increased above approximately 300 kilocalories per day (walking 3 to 4 miles during the day) that food intake increases to balance energy output. At higher levels of activity the appetite for food continues to match the utilization of energy.

Appetite and food intake are reduced in humans and animals following periods of severe exercise of short duration but light exercise of long duration does not depress appetite or food intake. Oscai, in his review of the mechanisms of exercise in weight control, suggests that appetite suppression induced by exercise is mediated by the increased levels of catecholamines associated with the stress of exercise.[11] Epinephrine and norepinephrine remain close to resting levels in the blood during light and moderate exercise and increase markedly during severe exercise stress.

Exercise in weight reduction. Individuals who lose weight by severe caloric restriction alone risk malnutrition because their bodies may not get all of the essential substances. As a result these semistarved individuals become lethargic and further avoid physical activity.

Studies of food-deprived populations show that physical working capacity and industrial productivity fall in proportion to the caloric deficiency. Malnutrition also leads to reduced immunity to disease. Therefore, one value of exercise in a weight reduction program is that the reduction of food intake need not be so drastic. The individual has a better chance of meeting the essential food needs of the body and conserving body proteins.

Pollock found that if 300 kilocalories or more are expended in each of four or more 45-minute exercise sessions per week, fat loss occurred without attention to food intake.[13] Twice weekly sessions of similar intensity and duration without dietary control produced no change in fat storage. If the intensity of exercise is increased to 600 kilocalories per exercise period more significant fat loss is achieved, but it is difficult to motivate subjects to expend this much energy in a single session.

After 15 to 20 weeks of exercise it is difficult to obtain further fat loss, perhaps because of an increase in work efficiency which leads to a saving in caloric requirement. At this point it is probably necessary to change the form of exercise, from jogging to stationary cycling or rowing, for example, or to institute dietary control. Fat loss continues after 20 weeks when food input is reduced.[15] The following summary of studies demonstrates the importance of combining diet control with exercise in a fat reduction program.

Study	Weight loss in kg.		
	Exercise, no diet control	Diet control, no exercise	Exercise, diet control
Boileau[3]	−3.2	−17.5	−17
Moody[8]	−2.4	−13	−18
Moody[9]	−1.08	−21	−26
Pollock[13]	−1.3	−24	−30
Pollock[12]	−2.9	−24	−30

Exercise in obese persons. In cases of gross obesity, in which the body has more than 20% above the normal limit of fat, exercise must not be so strenuous as to overstress the individual's cardiovascular system. The cost to that system of supporting the extra blood flow to adipose tissue, and the physical work required to carry the heavy load of fat, are high. Walking up stairs is strenuous work for a grossly obese person; the work required to move the extra body weight increases the total energy cost. An overweight person uses more body reserves than does a slimmer person when both climb the stairs together. If a person's body fat is 20% above the normal limit the energy cost of physical work will be increased by about 20%.

Because of this higher energy cost, an active obese person can occasionally increase food intake above the caloric balance level without much change in body weight. An inactive obese person, however, gains weight to a much greater extent if food intake is increased by the same amount.

Until body weight is reduced it is prudent for the grossly obese person to limit his extra activity to walking, swimming, or cycling. Swimming and cycling are especially indicated because the body weight is supported during these movements.

Physiological bases for weight-reducing exercise. If one desires to lose weight by exercise, the distance traversed should be the guide, not the speed of the movement.[2] The subject can walk at a comfortable speed and not feel the need to exercise strenuously to use calories. A heavy person will use more calories to walk a mile than will a lighter person. In walking a mile, a person will use practically the same number of calories whether he walks it in 25, 20, or 15 minutes.

One does not get the same cardiovascular conditioning effect at slow and fast speeds (see Chapters 20 and 23), but when the fundamental purpose of exercise is to assist in fat reduction it is preferable to walk at the rate at which the most miles can be traversed in comfort. Short bursts of high energy expenditure will fatigue the individual before large numbers of calories have been used, and thus are relatively ineffective in weight reduction.

Fat loss by diet and exercise is a slow process, especially when the individual maintains an otherwise usual daily life-style. The process is slow because one pound of body fat has the energy equivalent of 3,500 kilocalories. To produce this energy expenditure in 7 days by exercise alone would require an extra daily expenditure of 500 kilocalories. For one unused to heavy exercise regimens this is hard work—an extra 5 miles every day. Fat loss by food restriction alone would also be a severe stress. One would have to reduce the daily food intake by 500 kilocalories; an austere regimen, especially for the person who is eating less than 2,500 kilocalories a day.

By combining increased exercise with reduced caloric intake, both regimens are more easily tolerated. Being slightly more active during the day, standing to make telephone calls, and walking instead of driving a few blocks, can add 250 kilocalories of energy utilization. Reducing slightly the quantity of all foods eaten may lessen the caloric intake by 250 kilocalories. In this regimen an eighth of a pound (visualize half a cube of a quarter of a pound of butter) of one's own excess body fat becomes a part of the daily diet.

A further advantage in combining dietary restriction with exercise has been observed by Oscai.[11] When the weight of an individual is reduced by means of caloric restriction alone, lean tissues are lost along with the fat. Exercise during caloric restriction provides considerable protection against the loss of protein; it has a lipid mobilizing effect which may play a role in the conservation of lean tissue by making available more of the energy stored as fat.[4] Increased fat utilization occurs when muscle glycogen is reduced by prior exercise, indicating the advantage of exercise sessions of long duration.

Estimation of fat reduction. Reduction in skinfold thickness or reduction in body circumferences such as waist and hips are more valid guides to fat reduction than are weight scales. Weight scales do not measure separately the weight gain due to increase in muscle mass resulting from extra exercise, and the weight loss in catabolism of body fat. Football players and other heavily muscled athletes appear as overweight on population charts of normal weight, while they may actually be leaner than individuals of the same age, height, and frame size who are considered to be of normal weight or even underweight. These heavy athletes have accumulated excess muscle tissue instead of fat.

Changes in body weight due to factors other than loss of body fat, such as water retention which may initially replace fat lost from adipose cells may obscure the true reduction of fat which occurs in the early stages of a weight reduction program.

Because of these factors, if weight scales are used to monitor a fat reduction regimen the weekly trends in weight change are more valid than daily changes.

The true loss of fat may be noted by using the thumb and forefinger to pinch a doubled thickness of folded skin which contains the attached subcutaneous adipose tissue, and pulling it away from the underlying muscle. Since about 50% of total body fat is situated immediately under the skin, fat loss is readily apparent in skinfold observations. Certain sites, the triceps skinfold in particular, are fairly representative of the fatness of the entire body. An "inch of pinch" in this area is considered to border on obesity. The skinfold thickness of the forehead is also a standard for comparison. If all body skinfolds are no thicker than forehead skinfold there is no excess body fat. Special calipers are available for skinfold measurements. These exert a constant pressure, no matter how wide open the jaws are.

Regimens which induce rapid weight reduction without exercise or caloric restriction commonly rely on dehydration induced by water restriction, diuresis, or induced sweating. Water loss is weight loss and even "dress size" loss, but it is not fat loss—and it is temporary. The body needs fluids in copious amounts and the dehydrated individual usually rehydrates within a few days.

Since the *Laboratory Manual* does not include procedures for measurement of body fat, simple forms will now be described. A direct chemical analysis of the living human body cannot be performed, so

295

indirect measures are employed. Using Archimedes' principle, the body can be weighed in water and body density determined by comparing body weight in air and body weight in water after making appropriate corrections for lung and intestinal gases. Fat content is inversely related to body density, since fat is lighter than water. A simpler method is to use the measurement of skinfold thicknesses at a number of sites on the body for deriving estimates of body density and body fat.[20]

The simplest screening method for obesity employs circumferential measures. In men, body fat is usually uniformly distributed over the body, so that a single waistline measurement compared with body weight gives a useful estimation of body fat. In women, however, fat is distributed differently; some accumulate more fat on their waists, some on their thighs, and others on their upper arms. Therefore in women the approach is to estimate lean body mass by measuring several circumferences and then to calculate body fat percentage from whole body mass measurements by means of scales.

Percent body fat in men is most simply calculated from the formula of Wilmore and Behnke, which employs only two variables, nude body weight (BW), in pounds, and waistline girth (WG), in inches, in a horizontal plane at the level of the umbilicus.[18] Their equation is: lean body weight (LBW) = 98.42 + [1.082 (BW) − 4.15 (WG)]. Percent

fat is then determined from the formula: $\% \text{ fat} = \dfrac{\text{BW} - \text{LBW}}{\text{BW}} \times 100.$

A formula for the estimation of body fat in women which requires only tape and weight measurements was developed by Wilmore and Behnke.[19] Lean body weight (LBW) is first computed from measurements of nude weight, wrist diameter at the level of the styloid process, abdominal circumference in a horizontal plane (subject standing) at the maximal abdominal protrusion inferior to the umbilicus, hip circumference in a horizontal plane at the maximum protrusion of the gluteal muscles, and forearm circumference at the maximum girth just below the elbow with the elbow extended and the forearm supinated. The equation is: LBW in kg. = 8.987 + 0.732 (weight, kg.) + 3.786 (wrist diameter, cm.) − 0.157 (max., abdominal circ., cm.) − 0.249 (hip circ., cm.) + 0.434 (forearm circ., cm.). LBW in kg. is converted to pounds by multiplying by 2.2. The amount of fat, in pounds, is determined by subtracting LBW from weight (weight − LBW = fat). Fat percentage is then computed by dividing fat by weight (fat/weight = % fat).

DIABETES

In diabetes mellitus insufficient insulin is secreted by the pancreas. The function of insulin is to facilitate the entry of glucose into cells for use as an energy source. When insulin is not available a chain of events occurs:

1. Glucose entry and oxidation decrease
2. Glycogen breakdown increases and liver glycogen storage is impaired
3. Protein catabolism liberates amino acids which stimulate gluconeogenesis
4. Triglycerides break down to liberate free fatty acids as an energy source

The glucose which cannot enter the cells is eventually voided in the urine. Ketone bodies resulting from increased fat utilization accumulate and increase hydrogen ion concentration. There may be an odor of acetone on the breath.

In mild cases diabetes mellitus is treated by diet or noninsulin chemicals which stimulate pancreatic insulin secretion. In more severe cases insulin is injected in dosages adjusted to the needs of the individual. Exercise seems to potentiate the hypoglycemic effect of insulin and the patient can maintain control of carbohydrate metabolism with a smaller dose of insulin. This may be the result of some unknown factor independent of insulin which is released during exercise and which promotes transport. Exercise probably does not cause an increase in the pancreatic secretion of insulin.[5] Exercise is most valuable when it is controlled in proportion to the diet and the dosage of insulin. The type of exercise recommended for the diabetic is rhythmic prolonged light effort, which employs large muscle groups and is without emotional stress. Examples are walking, bicycling, rowing or paddling, and swimming. Team sports are usually too demanding and difficult to control. Exhaustion is contraindicated as it complicates existing insulin imbalance. Studies of summer camps in which activities are specially selected for diabetic children show that these children require less insulin at camp than when at school in the winter.[1]

Since the diabetic's diet and insulin dosage are balanced to give the energy for a certain amount of physical activity, this activity should be consistent from day to day. If a sedentary worker who sits at his desk all week works strenuously around the house over the weekend, the unaccustomed activity uses up more than the usual amount of glucose and he may get an insulin-like reaction. By keeping physical activity consistent, diet and insulin dosage are more easily controlled.

References

1. Akerblom, H.: The control of diabetes in summer camps, Diabetologia 5:233, 1969.

2. Åstrand, P.-O., and Rodahl, K.: Textbook of work physiology, New York, 1970, McGraw-Hill Book Co.

3. Boileau, R., and others: Body com-

position changes in obese and lean men during physical conditioning, Med. Sci. Sports 3:183, 1971.

4. Gollnick, P. D., and others: Diet, exercise, and glycogen changes in human muscle fibers, J. Appl. Physiol. 33:421, 1972.

5. Joslin, E. P.: Diabetic manual, ed. 10, Philadelphia, 1959, Lea & Febiger.

6. Kenrich, M., Ball, M. F., and Canary, J. J.: Exercise and weight reduction in obesity, Arch. Phys. Med. Rehab. 323:328, 1972.

7. Mayer, J.: Overweight, Englewood Cliffs, N. J., 1968, Prentice-Hall, Inc.

8. Moody, D. L., Kollias, J., and Buskirk, E. R.: The effects of a moderate exercise program on body weight and skin-fold thickness in overweight college women, Med. Sci. Sports 1:75, 1969.

9. Moody, D. L., and others: The effect of a jogging program on the body composition of normal and obese high school girls, Med. Sci. Sports 4:210, 1972.

10. Moody, D. L., and others: Obesity and health, Washington, D.C., 1966, U.S. Department of Health, Education, and Welfare, Public Health Service.

11. Oscai, L. B.: The role of exercise in weight control. In Wilmore, J. H., editor: Exercise and sports sciences reviews, New York, 1973, Academic Press, Inc.

12. Pollock, M. L., Cureton, T. K., and Greninger, L.: Effects of frequency of training on working capacity, cardiovascular function, and body composition of adult men, Med. Sci. Sports 1:70, 1969.

13. Pollock, M. C., and others: Effects of walking on body composition and cardiovascular function of middle aged men, J. Appl. Physiol. 30:126, 1971.

14. Reichsman, F., editor: Advances in psychosomatic medicine: hunger and satiety in health and disease, Basel, Switzerland, 1972, Karger.

15. Seltzer, C.: An effective weight control program in a public school system, Am. J. Physiol. 60:679, 1970.

16. Whipp, B. J., and Ruff, W. K.: The effect of caloric restriction and physical training on the responses of obese adolescents to graded exercise, J. Sports Med. Phys. 11:3, 1971.

17. Williams, R. H.: Textbook of endocrinology. Philadelphia, 1968, W. B. Saunders Co.

18. Wilmore, J. H., and Behnke, A. R.: Anthropometric estimation of bone density and lean body weight in young men, J. Appl. Physiol. 27:25, 1969.

19. Wilmore, J. H., and Behnke, A. R.: An anthropometric estimation of body density and lean weight in young women, Am. J. Clin. Nutr. 23:267, 1970.

20. Wilmore, J. H., Girandola, R. M., and Moody, D. L.: Validity of skinfold and girth assessment for predicting alterations in body composition, J. Appl. Physiol. 29:313, 1970.

23 MOTOR REHABILITATION

Anatomic perfection was once considered to be a primary component of physical fitness. If one was not anatomically whole, he was classified as unfit. Under the current concept of specificity of fitness, the physically handicapped person may not be vocationally handicapped if he is placed in the right type of job. Permanently disabled individuals can be trained to live and work within the limits of their disabilities "but to the hilt of their capabilities," as Rusk has observed.[9]

According to this dynamic concept the individual is rehabilitated through an active program which maximizes his potentials, rather than mere convalescence in which he is left alone to rest to let time and nature take their course—the word rehabilitation means "to restore."

WHEELCHAIR ATHLETES

The physiological principles of training apply to the physical rehabilitation of disabled persons as well as to the development of athletic fitness. In fact, some severely disabled individuals carry their training to advanced levels and become wheelchair athletes. In the ParaOlympic games these so-called handicapped men and women confined to wheelchairs compete in basketball, archery, fencing, javelin throw, discus throw, wheelchair dash and relay, table tennis, and swimming (ParaOlympic Pamphlet, 1964).

Motor rehabilitation is the application of physical exercise to the restoration of function when body movement has been impaired by injuries or diseases of the neuromuscular or musculoskeletal systems. As students of the physiology of exercise, we will deal here with the physiological phenomena which underlie the restoration of movement functions. More detailed studies of the specific disorders and diseases, and the exercises which can be employed in their treatment, are found in special texts.[6-9]

There are many kinetic dysfunctions that are caused by injury or athetosis, ataxia, and tremor. The differentiating characteristics of these disorders can be corrected to some extent by exercise therapy. These will be discussed in the following sections.

CEREBRAL PALSY

Cerebral palsy is a disorder of movement and posture due to a lesion of the immature brain which affects the motor control of the trunk, arms, and legs and can also cause speech, hearing, visual, and mental deficiencies and emotional disturbances. About half of cerebral palsy victims have some mental retardation or perceptual or learning difficulties.[3]

Cerebral palsy usually occurs before or during birth. In earlier days it was termed "spastic paralysis," but that name was dropped when it was observed that spasticity was found to be only one of several types of deformity in cerebral palsy. Other types of deformity include rigidity, athetosis, ataxia, and tremor. The differentiating characteristics of these deformities are discussed in the following paragraphs.

Spasticity. Spastic muscles are continually in a state of contraction and are hypertonic. Stiffness is the most significant feature, and voluntary control is limited. It involves chiefly the antigravity muscles. As an example, when an arm is severely spastic, it usually goes into flexion deformity and is held in a hooked position by the side. Muscle groups react strongly to a stimulus rather than acting in accordance with it. Spastic muscles do not relax as do normal muscles when an opposite muscle contracts. Instead they contract, with the result that motion is slowed or prevented. Tendon reflexes are exaggerated and the limb resists passive manipulation. The excessive contractility seems to be the result of damage to the basal ganglia. Over 50% of people afflicted with cerebral palsy have some degree of spasticity.

Rigidity. Rigid muscles are also hypertonic, but unlike spasticity there is no "kick-back" stretch reflex, no clonus, and no involuntary motion. Rigidity is caused by a disturbance of the agonist-antagonist relationship which interferes with slow passive motion in both muscle groups. Movements are jerky and sometimes impossible. Rigidity is often due to basal ganglia lesions which may be so extensive that learning is affected.

Athetosis and chorea. Athetosis victims suffer from constantly recurring movements which have no purposeful pattern. Aimless motions which are whip-like and are not possible to control are choreiform. Athetosis is a result of lesions of the basal ganglia. All the impulses from the motor cortex pass through unmodified, causing involuntary wormlike movements of the limbs and trunk which are slow, writhing, and monotonously repetitive. There is also a basic lack of muscle tonus, or hypotonia.

Ataxia. The ataxic person is unable to maintain balance due to faulty equilibrium, hypotonia, and a failure of muscular coordination. Ataxia has many causes, including injury or developmental defects in the cerebellum. Control in walking, sitting, and standing is difficult. The ataxic patient walks with a reeling, unsteady gait and has a tendency to fall toward the side of the cerebellar lesion. He has difficulty in controlling the direction and force of the motion he has started. There is a failure of the kinesthetic or balance sense, or both, which causes a lack of orientation in space, lack of depth perception, and constant stumbling. Exercise therapy is often successful in this disturbance.

Tremor. Tremor is an involuntary and uncontrolled shaking motion that has a regular alternating rhythmic pattern. It is also caused by injury to the cerebellum or basal ganglia and affects the reciprocal action of the flexor and extensor muscles. In lesions of the basal ganglia, tremor may be present at rest and disappear during movement, while the reverse is true in cerebellar lesions.

The victims of cerebral palsy may suffer more than one type of deformity, depending on the area of the brain damaged. The structural damage is irreversible, but it is not progressive. There is no cure. Life expectancy is shortened by a low resistance to infection. Improvement in function is possible to some extent but is very gradual, the rate being dependent on the intellectual level of the individual and the help given by the parents and therapists. The family and the patient must be reconciled and adjusted to the fact of a long-term disability.

The terminology of affliction ordinarily used with spinal cord lesions is often applied to cerebral palsy disorders. If only one extremity is affected, the condition is called monoplegia. If only one side of the body is affected, it is called hemiplegia. Diplegia is paralysis on both sides of either upper or lower limbs. When the lower part of the body is affected it is called paraplegia. Quadriplegia describes an affliction of all four limbs. If an arm and both legs are involved it is termed triplegia. Both motion and sensation are affected, and extent of the deformity may be mild, moderate, or severe.

The therapeutic goal is to bring out the maximal remaining potential of the individual. Surgery increases the physical potential of some patients, and appliances such as braces, splints, and standing tables are helpful in some cases. Drugs have only short-term success. Exercise training improves the functioning of the patient by teaching the undamaged parts of the brain to consciously perform the actions of the damaged parts. Maximum improvement occurs when the patient does as much as he can for himself.

The Bobath approach to treatment is through the suppression of abnormal patterns of movement so that normal patterns can be released.[2]

301

Treatment is started early, before contractures set in and make movement almost impossible. At first the therapist holds the patient and positions various parts of the body in such a way as to inhibit abnormal reflex patterns. Gradually, active automatic and voluntary movements are introduced and visual, tactile, and kinesthetic cues are given so that the patient learns to gain control and develop normal movement patterns. Reduction of overactivity and extension of range of movement are also taught. Resistance exercise is not used because it reinforces existing abnormal patterns of movement.

POLIOMYELITIS

Poliomyelitis is a contagious viral disease.[4] The viruses are transmitted through droplets formed in sneezing and coughing, and in excreta or contaminated articles, and enter the body through the nasopharynx or the gastrointestinal tract. Vaccines are effective in preventing poliomyelitis. There may be an individual difference in the degree of resistance to poliomyelitis viruses, since some families seem to be more prone than others to the disease.

Once contracted the course of the disease is irreversible. In the *flaccid* form of poliomyelitis lesions occur mainly in the anterior horn cells of the spinal cord and the motor nuclei of the cranial nerves. In the *spastic* form of poliomyelitis inhibitory functions are affected by extrapyramidal lesions. There is overactivity of the antigravity muscles of the side contralateral to the lesion. This loss of fixation of parts which set the stage for refined movements makes the control of movement difficult or impossible. With stance the muscles go into a hypertonic state. Proprioceptive ability in the hand is usually preserved, which gives a great advantage in regaining skilled motor use of the affected arm. For some reason the cerebral cortex and the cerebellar cortex escape severe damage. Sensory nerve cells are usually unaffected, so the victim feels pain. Loss of motor nerve impulses to skeletal muscles causes a loss of contractile activity. The nerves and their muscles degenerate. Paralysis, the loss of control of voluntary and reflex movement, causes muscular atrophy and deformities. After the lesion has healed the degree of further recovery depends to a large extent upon physical exercise. Exercise restores function to some degree, depending upon the amount of damage.

Paralysis of the right arm and leg indicates that the lesion is in the left hemisphere of the brain. The terms "hemiplegia," "paraplegia," and so on, as defined in the above section on cerebral palsy, apply to the description of poliomyelitis. In flaccid poliomyelitis the muscles are weak, limp, and flabby. Flaccid paralysis occurs in the absence of motor nerve stimuli. To preserve the muscle it must be stimulated directly, for example, by an electrical current.

During convalescence exercise is effective in restoring the power and tone of the weakened muscles that have some intact motor innervation. Massage and heat relieve muscular discomfort and promote relaxation. Passive forceful stretching helps to prevent contracture, and braces are used to keep the affected joints out of positions of deformity.

As in cerebral palsy, the goal of therapeutic exercise is to use the affected parts in the normal manner as far as possible so that the various coordinating muscles and neurons will begin to interact with each other in new patterns to produce the motions that have been lost. Such motor reeducation is continued indefinitely to maintain function in the afflicted area.[6]

STROKE

Strokes, "cerebral vascular accidents," are commonly caused by cerebral hemorrhage. The resulting damage in one hemisphere of the brain causes paralysis of the opposite side of the body.

The paralysis varies from a mild paresis (incomplete paralysis) or weakness to the complete loss of function of the affected limbs. The degree of paralysis is in direct relation to the size and location of the lesion in the brain.

Following a stroke there is usually some local edema which may reduce with time, resulting in an improvement in function of the affected limbs. The limbs on the hemiplegic side are usually initially flaccid, but after a time they become spastic.

The first task of rehabilitation is to prevent over-stretching of the leg muscles and flexion contractures in the arm region. The patient is encouraged to try supported walking as soon as possible to make the legs capable of ambulation. The leg shows activity before the arm, and often the arm never regains activity. Progressive resistance exercise follows in the final stages of therapy. Emphasis is given to the development of extensor muscles in the arms to overcome the common tendency toward flexion. In the legs, it is important to develop the quadriceps to permit standing and prevent buckling of the knees.

Paraplegic rehabilitation. If a lesion results in permanent paralysis of both legs (paraplegia), the main problem is to enable the patient to adjust himself to his disability state. It is important to put the paraplegic in a standing position with hips and knees extended and ankles at 90 degrees as soon as possible, so that the wearing of braces is feasible. The emphasis of exercise is to develop the shoulder depressor musculature, the triceps, and the latissimus dorsi, because these muscles must be used in order to walk with crutches.

The physiological principles of neuromuscular development which apply to motor rehabilitation have been presented in Chapter 19. Later in this chapter we will outline the general principles of exercise as applied to rehabilitation. It is appropriate now to examine the phenomenon of residual neuromuscular tension which is so often seen in the disabled patient, and is occasionally a problem also in the normal, healthy person.

RELAXATION OF EXCESS TENSION

Muscular tension increases involuntarily during disturbing situations. When this tension becomes excessive it causes fatigue from the incessant contraction which interferes with circulation and prevents the removal of metabolites. The sensory discharges from tense muscles feed back to the central nervous system and interfere with intellectual processes. Such agitation feeds forward to cause a further increase in residual neuromuscular tension. Signs of excessive residual tension are:

1. Grasping a pencil or pen too tightly while writing
2. Talking too loudly or too long
3. Eyes always looking, or staring
4. Eyes squinting, or eyebrows furrowed
5. Fidgeting, foot tapping, or doodling
6. Thighs contracted
7. Excessive eating or smoking
8. Biting fingernails, cheeks, or tongue
9. Jaws clenched
10. Grinding teeth
11. Shoulders elevated
12. Sighing or yawning

Excessive tension can be reduced by a voluntary release of the residual contractions using a relaxation technique developed by Jacobson.[5] The Jacobson technique consists of first sensing the tension by deliberately and forcibly contracting a group of muscles, then discontinuing the contraction and sensing the release of tension. This process of alternate tensing and letting go is performed gradually. During a slow count from 1 to 10 the subject is instructed to feel the increasing tension while "making your muscles as hard as you can." Then, while counting backward from 10 to 1 the instructions are to let the increased tension go back to normal or below while "making your muscles as soft as you can." Each time this process is repeated the subject attempts to let go further to feel complete relaxation.

When the resting pulse rate is counted before and after a session of relaxation, the tense person will find the rate reduced 5 beats per minute or more, indicating a diminished level of metabolic activity due to relaxed musculature.

Excess tension during movement, as in running, impairs motion and induces early fatigue because of the extra energy cost of the muscular resistance. If the runner uses the same Jacobson technique of deliberately increasing tension and then letting it go, a more relaxed running state can be achieved. With excess tension shut off, the runner feels as if movement is continuing on its own momentum, as in coasting out-of-gear. At the point that the speed of running would become slower, the runner can apply just the degree of exertion needed to maintain the desired speed. Experienced runners describe this sensation of easy motion as "floating." This deliberate adjustment of tension to minimal level during action might be termed "dynamic relaxation." This technique can be applied to any continuous activity such as walking, cycling, or swimming.

Motoneuron feedback training. Conscious control over spinal motoneuron activity can be developed by means of audio and visual electromyographic displays, as described in Chapter 4 in the *Laboratory Manual*. These displays provide subjects with an awareness of the involuntary twitching of individual motor units. In a few minutes subjects discover that they can control this twitching somewhat, either increasing or reducing the signals displayed. As conscious control is improved, the volume of the audio and visual electromyograph is gradually reduced and eventually the subject is able to voluntarily reduce undesirable twitching without the aid of the electromyograph.[1]

The general principles of exercise in the motor rehabilitation of the disabled patient are presented below in outline form. Further details are found in the previously mentioned special texts.[6-9]

I. *Types of therapeutic exercise.* There are five categories of movement in therapeutic exercise.

   A. Passive—The patient plays a passive role and the therapist plays an aggressive role. While the patient relaxes, the therapist carries a limb through the full range of motion. This is used to prevent or reduce contracture in spastic muscle.

   B. Passive assistive—The patient plays a partially passive role, but tries to work his paralyzed limb to assist the therapist in carrying the limb through a full range of motion. This is the starting point for muscle reeducation. The patient is made to believe that he is capable of helping himself through the exercises.

   C. Assistive—The patient performs the exercise with the assistance of the therapist. The patient helps himself, using his unaffected limbs to assist his affected ones. Aids such as pulleys or chairs are used. Assistive exercises are prescribed for neuromuscular retraining and mild muscle strengthening.

   D. Active—The patient performs the exercises without any assistance or devices. Active exercises are prescribed for general conditioning, coordination, mobilization, general strengthening, or endurance development.

E. Resistive—The patient performs movements against progressively increased resistance, scaled from the force of gravity to heavy loads. Resistive exercises are prescribed for the development of muscular strength and muscular endurance.

II. *Exercise goals.* The goals of therapeutic exercise, listed in the approximate order of achievement during a course of treatment, are the following.

A. Relaxation of excess tension—The patient first learns the technique of voluntary relaxation (described earlier in this chapter) while lying down. He then applies this technique to the voluntary reduction of excess tension during sitting, standing, and moving.

B. Increase or retention of range of motion—Passive exercise to prevent permanent muscle and joint tightness.

C. Neuromuscular redevelopment—Passive-assistive exercise to restore the strength of weakened muscles which have intact motor innervation, and to educate muscles to perform unaccustomed tasks.

D. Repression of undesired contractions—Assistive and active rhythmic movements to make motion smooth. Exercises may be done in a warm swimming pool or bathtub to relieve the pull of gravity and to make the movements more relaxed.

E. Development of balance and equilibrium—Weight-bearing movement as in walking a straight line or kicking a ball helps to train kinesthetic and vestibular balance mechanisms.

F. Increased muscular endurance—Submaximal resistive efforts for progressively prolonged periods to improve chemical and circulatory systems in muscles.

G. Reversal of the atrophy of disuse—Near-maximal resistive efforts repeated many times to increase the mass of muscular tissue.

H. Increased muscular strength—Maximal resistive effort repeated a few times to increase contractile power.

I. Increased cardiovascular endurance—Prolonged continuous rhythmic movement such as cycling, swimming, and walking to improve the quality of the myocardium and to increase vascularization of cardiac and muscular tissues.

J. Restoration of physical capacity for self-care, employment, and recreational activities—Development of specific coordination and power to perform required motions through repeated attempts to perfect the performances. Not careless practice, but concentrated training to improve accuracy and efficiency of movements.

III. *Therapeutic principles.* The following principles of exercise therapy are applicable to all forms of motor rehabilitation.

    A. The exercise must be so simple that it can be understood by the patient.

    B. The patient should be in a comfortable position.

    C. Proximal joints should be stabilized to eliminate undesired movement.

    D. The number of exercises taught should be few. Three new exercises in one session appear to be optimal.

    E. As a standard form of presentation, start in a preparatory position, initiate the movement, perform the central action, return to the preparatory position, and rest.

    F. The patient should perform a movement immediately after the therapist has demonstrated it.

    G. Short bouts of exercise repeated during the day are preferable to a prolonged session once a day.

    H. Make use of the patient's preexisting habits.

    I. The patient should understand the object of the exercise and the reason why it is performed in a certain manner.

    J. The patient should realize the importance of doing the exercises regularly.

    K. Incentives should be made clear to the patient by the therapist.

IV. *Program planning.* Five considerations are given in the planning of an exercise program.

    A. Indications and contraindications—Will exercise help? What types of exercise should be avoided?

    B. Evaluation—What is the patient's present level of exercise training? What tests and measurements should be made (strength, range of motion, etc.)?

    C. Goal setting—What degree of development can be expected? What gains will give the patient maximal independent function within his limits?

    D. Prescription—What specific exercises should the patient perform? At what intervals should the exercises be increased in intensity and complexity?

    E. Reevaluation—When should tests and measurements be repeated to assess the effectiveness of the prescribed exercises? What adjustments in the exercise prescription are needed?

The therapist incorporates these principles of exercise in planning rehabilitation programs for patients with motor disabilities. Most of these principles apply also in the rehabilitation of cardiac patients, as discussed in Chapter 24.

References

1. Basmajian, J. V.: Muscles alive: their functions revealed by electromyography, ed. 2, Baltimore, 1967, The Williams & Wilkins Co.
2. Bobath, B.: Treatment principles and planning in cerebral palsy, Springfield, Ill., 1966, Charles C Thomas, Publisher.
3. Cruikshank, W. M., editor: Cerebral palsy: its individual and community problems, Syracuse, N.Y., 1966, Syracuse University Press.
4. Ford, F. R.: Diseases of the nervous system in infancy, childhood and adolescence, Springfield, Ill., 1960, Charles C Thomas, Publisher.
5. Jacobson, E.: Progressive relaxation, Chicago, 1944, University of Chicago Press.
6. Kraus, H.: Therapeutic exercise, ed. 2, Springfield, Ill., 1963, Charles C Thomas, Publisher.
7. Krusen, F., Kottke, F. J., and Ellwood, P. M., editors: Handbook of physical medicine and rehabilitation, Philadelphia, 1971, W. B. Saunders Co.
8. Pearson, P., and Williams, C. E., editors: Physical therapy services in developmental disabilities, Springfield, Ill., 1972, Charles C Thomas, Publisher.
9. Rusk, H. A.: Rehabilitation medicine, ed. 3, St. Louis, 1971, The C. V. Mosby Co.

Suggested reading

Brodal, A.: Neurological anatomy in relation to clinical medicine, ed. 2, New York, 1969, Oxford University Press.

24 EXERCISE AND HEART DISEASE

Persistent exercise training may reduce the risk of heart disease. Evidence from epidemiological studies which relate exercise to death from heart disease is inconclusive, perhaps because exercise is only one of many factors, such as smoking, high blood pressure, and elevated serum cholesterol levels, which are associated with a high incidence of heart attacks. The assumption that exercise has a prophylactic effect on the heart has generated a number of theories as to the physiological mechanisms by which this is accomplished. It is in the light of these tentative hypotheses that this chapter treats the subject of exercise and heart disease.

In considering the relation of exercise to heart disease, we must first understand that exercise takes many forms and so does heart disease. The standard parameters of exercise (type, intensity, duration, and frequency) are difficult to define in epidemiological studies of occupations such as mailmen and bus drivers. Unless physiological data such as oxygen consumption or heart rate are provided it is impossible to derive answers to such pertinent questions as "How much exercise is needed to protect against heart disease?"

Heart disease is a catch-all phrase and can include such specific disorders as coronary artery disease and congestive heart failure. We need to know which specific disorder is affected by exercise—or the lack of exercise—before attempting to elucidate physiological phenomena.

At present the effect of an endurance type of exercise training on the prevention of cardiovascular disease is an active area of investigation. Such study is important because 53% of American deaths each year result from cardiovascular disease, according to 1972 estimates by the American Heart Association.

CORONARY HEART DISEASE

A relationship between exercise and the risk of coronary heart disease has not been definitely established. However, since coronary heart disease occurs in epidemic proportions, it is prudent for the student of exercise physiology to explore the possible mechanisms in a search for guidelines to the formulation of submaximal exercise regimens for cardiac conditioning in preventive cardiology and cardiac rehabilitation. Such formulation should always be done in association with a physician.

It has not yet been established that exercise induces coronary collateral vascularization or that exercise increases vessel size in healthy human hearts. Exercise does improve peripheral vascular systems, increasing the efficiency of blood distribution and venous return.[10]

Increased physical activity can be an effective adjunct in controlling some of the risk factors in coronary heart disease. Reduction of obesity (Chapter 22) is aided by increased physical activity. Serum cholesterol levels are lowered when exercise is carried out for 45 minutes per day, 5 days a week, and triglycerides are reduced in less extensive exercise regimens.[13]

Physical training can also lower the resting and exercise blood pressures in coronary heart disease patients, particularly those who are hypertensive.[2] This effect is not often observed in normotensive subjects, especially young ones. Improvement in cardiac function (stroke volume, cardiac output, and myocardial oxygen consumption) can be produced by training in coronary heart disease patients, unless the damage is too severe. Training appears to increase the contractile ability of the myocardium. The bradycardia of training and the concomitant increased stroke volume improve myocardial efficiency.[8] These improvements increase the ability of the heart to perform its pumping duty.

Adaptations in the peripheral circulation occur in coronary heart disease patients after exercise training. Arteriovenous oxygen difference during exercise may be increased in coronary heart disease patients.[5] Furthermore, there is a lessened shift in blood flow from viscera to skeletal muscles.[4] This adaptation may be explained by the morphological and biochemical changes in skeletal muscle (see Chapters 2 and 14).

MYOCARDIAL INFARCTION

Patients with myocardial infarction respond favorably to exercise training after complete healing of the infarct has occurred. A progressive program which included calisthenics, walking, running, and physical recreation produced the following effects in the majority of myocardial infarct patients[6]:

1. Improvement of subjective well-being and decrease of psychological depression

2. Marked improvement of aerobic power and cardiovascular hemo-dynamics (increased stroke volume, decreased tension time index, and increased vigor of heartbeat)
3. Decreased lactate production for the same workload
4. Reduction of hypertensive blood pressure values during exercise
5. Reduction of the heart rate at rest and during exercise
6. Decreased S-T segment displacement during exercise, signifying a reduction of myocardial ischemia
7. Lowering of serum lipid levels
8. Reduction of fat storage in adipose tissue cells
9. Enhanced oxygen extraction by the peripheral tissues
10. Suggestive reduction in mortality from subsequent heart attacks
11. Enhancement of intercoronary collaterals rarely demonstrated by coronary angiograms
12. Partial or complete normalization of pretraining pathological ballistocardiograms

ANGINA PECTORIS

Physical training augments the exercise capacity of patients with angina pectoris. Myocardial oxygen requirement is reduced in the trained state because of a slower heart rate, lower intramyocardial systolic tension, and perhaps an improvement in myocardial contrac-tility.[12] An improved efficiency of the neuromuscular and cardiovascular systems due to training also reduces the demand of the heart for oxygen. If training is carried to an advanced degree, such as daily slow long-distance running, some augmentation of oxygen supply to the heart may be achieved through increased coronary capillarization. As a result, higher levels of physical work can be performed before the onset of myocardial ischemia and anginal pain.

In addition to these specific values, there may be a general feeling of increased well-being and such psychological benefits as an improved self-image and feeling of self-confidence. For some there may be in-creased tolerance to stress and a reduction of tension and agitation.

These benefits may occur in even the most sedentary individuals at any age if the exercise is adjusted to the condition of the person. Sudden lifestyle changes from inactivity to vigorous exertion can be harmful. Rapid transition from sedentary life to heavy exercise can result in dangerous myocardial ischemia, extreme elevation in blood pressure, and injury to musculoskeletal elements.

CARDIAC EXERCISE PRESCRIPTION

In order to prescribe exercise it is necessary first to know the degree of impairment and to understand the mechanism of impairment. This

311

information is gained by a study of the person's responses to a graded exercise test (GXT), using a bicycle ergometer, treadmill, or stepping bench for exercise as described in Chapter 7 in the *Laboratory Manual.*

The exercise can be graded in terms of the *physical work* performed by progressively increasing the resistance of the ergometer pedals, increasing the slope or speed of the treadmill, or increasing the rate or height of stepping. A safer and more meaningful approach is to grade the exercise in terms of the *physiological effort* exerted.

Physiological effort is graded in terms of the response to exercise such as heart rate or oxygen uptake. Heart rate is preferred as a controller of exertion in graded exercise tests because it is easily and accurately measured, it is a direct index of the stress on the heart, and under usual nonemotional test conditions it correlates well with oxygen uptake, ventilation rate, cardiac output, and other indices of physiological effort.

In a typical graded exercise test the subject exercises for about 4 minutes at a heart rate of 100 per minute while his blood pressure, electrocardiogram, oxygen uptake, respiratory rate, and other physiological responses are measured and signs of intolerance such as pain and shortness of breath are observed.

If the subject tolerates that grade well, the effort is increased by raising the exercise heart rate to 120 per minute. Responses are evaluated continuously and the test is terminated at the onset of the first sign of poor tolerance. Such signs or end-points are defined fully later in this chapter (p. 314).

If the subject tolerates the 120 heart rate grade well, the effort is again increased by raising the heart rate to 140. The next grade would be at a 160 heart rate, unless the subject is over 35 years of age. If he is over 35 an age-adjusted limit is set according to the following procedure.

In testing exercise tolerance for the purpose of setting a prescribed level of therapeutic or prophylactic exercise, a limit of 85% of the individual's maximal heart rate limit need not be exceeded. A convenient formula for estimating an individual's maximal heart rate is to subtract the age from 220. The maximal heart rate in populations of 20-year-olds is about 200 beats per minute, the rate decreases about 1 beat per year of age after that. To compute the 85% target heart rate for the fourth grade of the exercise test the formula thus becomes $(220 - age) \times 0.85$. In a 43-year-old person the target heart rate at grade four is 150 per minute. Persons 55 and older do not advance beyond grade three, the 140 target heart rate.

The grade well tolerated by the subject for the complete 4-minute period becomes the upper limit of that person's training heart rate zone.

The lower limit of the training heart rate zone is 10 beats per minute less. Thus, if exercise was stopped during the 140 heart rate grade, the upper limit of this training heart rate zone is 120, the grade he tolerated well. The lower limit is 10 beats per minute less, or 110. This means that the individual should start his training at an exercise heart rate of between 110 and 120 per minute.

CARDIAC EXERCISE TRAINING

The initial duration of the training exercise should not exceed that of the test, namely 4 minutes. The duration of exercise can be extended as the condition improves.

The total length of the initial exercise session would be at least 10 minutes, allowing 4 minutes for warm up and gradually increasing the heart rate to the training level and 2 minutes for cooling down after the 4-minute training exercise.

An essential objective of exercise training in patients with heart disease is to increase work capacity. The physical limitations imposed on these patients by the disease process reduces their quality of life.

Equally important objectives of exercise are to reduce the risk of a heart attack and to diminish its severity should one occur. In line with these objectives, exercise is included as a part of a medical regimen of preventive cardiology. The total regimen would include: (1) controlled exercise, (2) hypolipogenic diet, (3) reduction of obesity, (4) control of diabetes, (5) reduction of stress and excess tension, (6) reduction of high blood pressure, (7) lowering of high heart rate, and (8) elimination of cigarette smoking.

Exercise is not a desirable mode of therapy if it accelerates cardiac deterioration or threatens to shorten the patient's life. It is thus necessary for the physician first to qualify each patient as a candidate for exercise, and then to monitor those who do qualify to treat complications such as cardiac arrest and to assure that their response to exercise and training is good enough to warrant continued exercise therapy.

EXERCISE STRESS ELECTROCARDIOGRAPHY

Symptom-limited exercise stress testing. The purposes of a submaximal symptom-limited exercise test are to: (1) define the degree of exertion at which the patient reaches his limit of good tolerance for exercise, (2) identify the type of impairment, and (3) establish the intensity of exercise to be prescribed.

Procedure. The patient is tested no earlier than 2 hours after a light meal. His history, including the drugs he is taking, is recorded, and a cardiovascular examination, including a 12-lead resting electrocardiogram, is completed immediately before the test.

Proscriptions. Patients with coronary heart disease need to take un-usual precautions while exercising. Conditions which affect exercising heart rate such as large meals, caffeine beverages, cold or hot fluids, and tobacco must be avoided so that the heart rate can be used reliably to control the intensity of exercise. The demands on the heart during exercise must not be made to compete with demands for digestion or body cooling. Extremes of heat or cold exposure such as experienced when wearing sweat clothes during endurance exercise, or when shower-ing after exercise, or when passing from a warm room into chilling outdoor weather while still sweating evoke considerable cardiac strain. The combined effects of chilling and sudden exertion during snow shoveling are believed to cause acute coronary insufficiency and ar-rhythmias in unconditioned subjects.

The electrocardiogram is displayed continuously during the exercise test on an oscilloscope and recordings are made periodically with an electrocardiograph. The patient performs a trial exercise at a low level as a warm up. At the end of the test the patient recovers in a reclining position until the heart rate returns to near the resting level. A hot or cold shower is not permitted for at least an hour after the test, for it may precipitate cardiac arrest.[3]

End points. The end point of a symptom-limited exercise test is de-termined either by the subject or by the operator. Exercise is halted at the onset of the first sign of poor tolerance or the attainment of an age-predicted level of near-maximal heart rate as follows:

1. Subjective
   a. Exhaustion
   b. Inability to maintain the preset pace of work
2. Symptomatic
   a. Chest pain
   b. Labored breathing
   c. Palpitation
   d. Signs such as pallor, ataxia, or cold sweat
   e. Central nervous system symptoms such as confusion and incoordination
3. Objective
   a. Reaching a predetermined heart rate level, such as 85% of the patient's estimated maximal heart rate (220-age $\times$ 0.85)
   b. Abnormal ECG changes such as ischemic S-T segment changes or arrhyth-mias
   c. Conduction defects which appear as wave form changes in the ECG
   d. Blood pressure decrease or lack of increase with increasing work intensity, or disproportionate increase (more than 10 mm. Hg increase per 10 beats/min. heart rate increase)
   e. If oxygen uptake is measured the test is halted when the patient reaches his maximal oxygen uptake (when additional increase in workload does not result in further increase in oxygen uptake)

The following postexercise responses are signs of cardiac stress: (1) breathlessness, rapid pounding heart, or extreme weakness or shakiness that lasts for more than 10 minutes after exercise; (2) broken sleep or unusual restlessness during the night following strenuous exercise; and (3) a definite sense of fatigue that persists through the next day.

Exercise response evaluation. In evaluating the severity of heart disease, oxygen uptake is measured during the graded exercise test because it defines the pumping capacity of the heart. Under hospital conditions this test is carried to maximal effort in order to obtain the maximal oxygen uptake. Maximal oxygen uptake is equal to the product of maximal cardiac output and maximal arterial-mixed venous oxygen difference. Since the maximal arterial-venous oxygen difference is usually not affected in heart disease, the maximal oxygen uptake is a reliable index of cardiac output.[11]

Change in heart rate from rest to maximal exercise is a crude index of cardiac output, since in upright exercise there is little change in stroke volume.[7] Myocardial oxygen requirement is also influenced more by changes in heart rate than in stroke volume.[9] Change in systolic blood pressure from rest to maximal exercise is a crude index of the contractile force of the heart, but the magnitude of the increase is underestimated because of the concomitant decrease in peripheral resistance during exercise.[1]

Coronary arteriography. Exercise electrocardiography provides indirect physiological data regarding coronary heart disease. These data are confirmed by coronary arteriography, which involves x-rays of the heart to visualize the course of an opaque fluid that has been injected in the bloodstream. The arteriograms show the anatomic site of coronary arterial obstruction and the extent of the obstructive lesions. At the same time the movement of the left ventricle is studied to determine the functional state of the myocardium. Arteriography is not infallible and it is possible that some patients whose electrocardiographic responses to exercise are abnormal have vascular disease that is not detectable by current arteriographic methods.

CARDIAC PHYSICAL ACTIVITIES

Type of exercise. In order to develop the heart and its coronary arteries the exercise should be of the type which makes the greatest demands on the cardiovascular system. This system functions in exercise mainly for oxygen transport, and thus the training exercise must impose a great demand for oxygen. Physical activities of the type which call into play large masses of skeletal muscles for sustained periods impose the greatest demand for oxygen.

The fundamental prerequisite of exercise for cardiac reconditioning is that the activities involve rhythmical isotonic contraction of large groups of muscles. A wide variety of activities meet this specification: vigorous walking, jogging, running, stationary and mobile cycling, swimming, bench stepping, rope jumping, and rhythmic calisthenics.

Jogging or running may be poorly tolerated by patients with arthritic changes in the feet, ankles, knees, hips, or spine. Running on grass or wearing shoes with flexible ribbed soles may increase tolerance.

The bicycle seat may be uncomfortable for patients with sparse gluteal adipose tissue, varicocele, or prostatic difficulties. An extra pad on the seat may improve comfort.

Referring to Tables 11 through 14 in the *Laboratory Manual*, the effort may be classified approximately as follows:

Classification	Heart rate	Total kcal./hr.
Very light	Under 110	Under 150
Light	110-120	150-200
Moderate	120-130	250-300
Heavy	130-140	300-400
Very heavy	Over 140	Over 400

The propriety of the exercise is determined by monitoring the heart rate or other function, and by noting the symptoms. With practice the patient can perceive the level of exertion without checking his heart rate.

Physical reconditioning is a part of a comprehensive treatment program consisting of diet designed to improve nutrition and attain normal weight and serum lipids, abstinence from the use of tobacco, medication, and psychological and social adjustment which includes continuation of gainful employment and customary mode of social life.

To have a beneficial effect the physical activity must be pleasurable and gratifying. Compulsive dedication to a dull routine may induce tension, which would tend to negate the benefits of exercise training. A variety of activities can increase the functional capacity of the whole individual, including his heart.

References

1. Åstrand, P.-O.: Experimental studies of physical working capacity in relation to sex and age, Copenhagen, 1952, Munksgaard.
2. Boyer, J. L., and Kasch, F. W.: Exercise therapy in hypertensive men, J.A.M.A. **211**:1668, 1970.
3. Bruce, R. A., and Kluge, W.: Defibrillatory treatment of exertional cardiac arrest in coronary disease, J.A.M.A. **216**:653-658, 1971.
4. Clausen, J. P., and Trap-Jensen, J.: Effects of training on the distribution of cardiac output in patients with coronary heart disease, Circulation **42**:611, 1970.
5. Detry, J. R., and others: Increased arteriovenous oxygen difference after physical training in coronary heart disease, Circulation **44**:109, 1971.
6. Hellerstein, H. K.: Exercise therapy in coronary disease, Bull. N.Y. Acad. Med. **44**:1028, 1968.
7. Kassar, I. S., and Bruce, R. A.: Comparative effects of aging and coronary heart disease on submaxi-

mal and maximal exercise, Circulation 39:759, 1969.

8. Katz, L. N.: Physical fitness and coronary heart disease: Some basic views, Circulation 35:405, 1967.

9. Kitamura, K., and others: Hemodynamic correlates of coronary blood flow and myocardial oxygen consumption during upright exercise, Am. J. Cardiol. 26:643, 1970.

10. Larson, O. A., and Malmborg, R. O., editors: Coronary heart disease and physical fitness, Baltimore, 1971, University Park Press.

11. Mitchell, J. J., Sproule, B. J., and Chapman, C. B.: The physiological meaning of the maximal oxygen intake test, J. Clin. Invest. 37:538, 1938.

12. Redwood, D. R., Rosing, D. R., and Epstein, S. E.: Circulatory and symptomatic effects of physical training in patients with coronary-artery disease and angina pectoris, N. Eng. J. Med. 286:959, 1972.

13. Tooshi, A.: Effects of three different durations of endurance exercises upon serum cholesterol (abstract), Med. Sci. Sports 3:1, 1971.

Suggested readings

Andersen, K. L., and others: Fundamentals of exercise testing, Geneva, 1971, World Health Organization.

Committee on Exercise: Exercise testing and training of apparently healthy individuals: a handbook for physicians, New York, 1972, American Heart Association.

De Haas, J. H., and others: Ischaemic heart disease, Baltimore, 1970, The Williams & Wilkins Co.

Holloszy, J. O.: Biochemical adaptations in muscle: effects of exercise on mitochondrial oxygen uptake and respiratory enzyme activity in skeletal muscle, J. Biol. Chem. 242:2278, 1967.

Morse, R. L., editor: Exercise and the heart: guidelines for exercise programs, Springfield, Ill., 1972, Charles C Thomas, Publisher.

Naughton, J. P., Hellerstein, H. K., and Mohler, I. C., editors: Exercise testing and exercise training in coronary heart disease, New York, 1973, Academic Press, Inc.

Physical Exercise Committee: Physician's handbook for evaluation of cardiovascular and physical fitness, Nashville, 1971, Tennessee Heart Association.

Rosing, D. R., and others: Blood fibrinolytic activity in man: diurnal variation and the response to varying intensities of exercise, Circ. Res. 27:171, 1970.

Russek, H., and Zohman, B. L., editors: Changing concepts in cardiovascular disease, Baltimore, 1972, The Willams & Wilkins Co.

Tibblin, G., editor: Preventive cardiology, New York, 1972, John Wiley & Sons, Inc.

Zohman, L. R., and Tobis, J. S.: Cardiac rehabilitation, New York, 1970, Grune & Stratton, Inc.

25 CONNECTIVE TISSUE

Connective tissue, which comprises a large portion of the total body mass, limits not only the range but also the speed of movement. The condition of the connective tissue is affected by exercise, and it is believed that the aches and pains commonly associated with aging are associated with connective tissue changes due to inactivity. It is also postulated that the fatigue of sedentary work is in large measure a connective tissue phenomenon.

It is, of course, difficult to study the functions of connective tissue in the living body, and thus there are many aspects that are as yet little understood. This subject needs more attention because of its importance to physical performance and well-being.

Connective tissue consists of a fine, interlaced network of fibers lying within a *ground substance* of varying consistency, thickness, and other characteristics. Some of the body components that are entirely or largely composed of connective tissue are bones, cartilage, joints, aponeuroses, tendons, ligaments, fasciae, the corium of the skin, the dura mater, the various tubes that must be kept open (such as the trachea and the bronchi), the fibrous neurilemma that sheaths the peripheral nerve fibers, and the sarcolemma, endomysium, and perimysium, that surround the units of the muscular system.

The mucoid intercellular material comprising the ground substance is relatively inert chemically, but it is postulated that it is consumed in physiological function and removed through absorption of smaller molecular aggregates into the blood and lymph. It is renewed by the secretion of the fibroblastic cells. Blood is a form of connective tissue in which the ground substance has become completely fluid.

FIBERS

There are three types of connective tissue fibers—*collagenous, reticular,* and *elastic.* The nature of the three types is not well understood. Collagen tends to form large bundles of fine fibers. These are practically inextensible; excessive strains cause them to break rather than to stretch. Their great tensile strength makes them ideal for tendons, ligaments, aponeuroses, and fasciae. The pericardium surrounding the heart and the adventitia surrounding the large blood vessels contain collagen fibers that serve to prevent overdistention of these organs. A prolonged steady tension may, however, result in a weakening and stretching of these fibers. Collagen fibers are able to withstand great tensional stress but only comparatively small compressional stress.

It has proved difficult to separate reticulin from collagen, but it appears to consist of very fine protein fibers combined with a carbohydrate component. These fibers form an important constituent of lymph nodes and blood-forming organs.

Elastic connective tissue is composed of threads of sulfate polysaccharides in combination with protein embedded in an amorphous matrix.

MECHANICAL STRUCTURE

The stresses to which articulations are subjected must be absorbed by a relatively small area of cartilage. The mechanical problem involved necessitates that the fibers be arranged in such a way that a sufficient number will always be at right angle to the imposed stresses. All articulating cartilages are fibrocartilages, and the density of the fibrous material is normally proportional to the customary pressures that it must withstand.

STRENGTH AND ELASTICITY

In animal tissues *hyaluronic acid,* a polysaccharide, binds water in the interstitial spaces and holds the connective tissue cells together in a jelly-like matrix. Certain functions of the skin, the ocular fluids, synovial fluid, and connective tissue in general appear to depend at least in part on the quantity and degree of aggregation of hyaluronic acid. The long-chain structures of chondroitin sulfuric acid and hyaluronic acid, together with the fiber proteins, may be the basis of the tensile strength and elasticity of connective tissue.

Synovial fluid consists of tissue fluids with a high hyaluronic acid content and appears to function as a lubricant and shock absorber. The synovial cavity of a joint normally contains only enough fluid to moisten and lubricate the synovial surfaces, but it may accumulate in painful amounts in an injured or inflamed joint. Other types of

319

ground substances have different functions, but these are almost unexplored.

AGING

There is a difference in the consistency and distribution of newly formed and adult connective tissue. Ground substance is abundant in an infant, less plentiful in an adult, and scanty in an elderly person. This reduction in ground substance in elderly persons may be correlated with their greater vulnerability to physical shock since diminution of ground substance results in a smaller space within which to meet changes in vascular volume. This makes it difficult for them to compensate for the rapid changes that occur in disease, injury, and surgery. Furthermore, as one grows older the distensibility of connective tissue decreases. The tendency of fascia to contract under certain conditions (to be discussed later) remains, and as distensibility decreases with advancing age, the range of movement of joint is likely to become restricted.

However, during the aging process the hyaline covering of bone surfaces remains remarkably intact although localized areas of cartilage softening due to specific trauma or disease or to the wear and tear of abnormal joint mechanics may develop. These are usually found in the weight-bearing surfaces of the lower extremities.

STRETCHING

Exercises to stretch ligamentous connective tissue have been used for at least 2,000 years for the relief of the discomforts associated with the menstrual period. These have proved of definite value, and a rather extensive literature has accumulated on this subject.

Other conditions of malfunction of connective tissue are common to both men and women, especially those leading a sedentary life. The most common of these is *fascial contraction*. Contracture of the fibrous elements of a muscle may result in shortening of the contractile muscle fibers and prevent them from extending to their normal relaxed length, hence limiting their power and placing them under tension. Afferent and efferent nerve fibers pass through various fascial and ligamentous planes in the muscle. If the fascia tightens abnormally (as may result from age, chilling, poor posture, inactivity, strain, and other causes), it constricts these nerve fibers, thus causing a pressure irritation of the nerves, resulting in neuralgia and other ailments. If the fasciae are stretched by gradual, repetitive, forcible, and progressive exercises, part of the elongation thus achieved remains after the exercise is completed. This affords an opportunity for the correction of bad mechanical alignment and for the elimination of compressions of peripheral nerves. Fascia displays a tendency to contract during rest, and this is especially in evidence during inactivity following a period of activity. Thus after a night's rest a person awakens feeling stiff and with a natural tendency to stretch. Athletes, dancers, contortionists, and other performers of this type find it necessary to limber up carefully before engaging in their activities.

CARTILAGE

Cartilage withstands compressional stress very well and tensional stress to a considerable extent. *Hyaline cartilage* consists of groups of cells lying in a structureless or faintly granular, pale blue matrix. It is found on the articular surfaces of bone joints and in the costal and laryngeal cartilages. The cartilage that ultimately becomes bone is of this type. *White fibrous cartilage* is made up of a mixture of white fibrous tissue and cartilaginous tissue. This is found in the attachment of ligaments and tendons to bone, at the symphysis pubis and certain other joints, and in the intervertebral disks. *Yellow fibrous cartilage* is composed of a mixture of yellow elastic fibers and cartilaginous tissue and is found in the external ear, the auditory tube, and in some of the cartilages of the larynx.

Cartilage probably is always in a state of greater or lesser deformation during periods of activity, resuming its shape during rest.

Articular cartilage in growing animals that have been exercised is thicker than in animals that have been kept at rest. During exercise articular cartilage increases in thickness, and during the rest period following exercise the thickness of the cartilage diminishes about 10%.

Stiffness after heavy exercise may have its basis in the viscosity and amount of synovial fluid, as demonstrated by the following experiment. When one leg of an experimental animal was exercised and the other leg was left undisturbed, the exercised joint contained a larger amount of synovial fluid than did the unexercised joint. The longer the exercise, the greater was the amount of fluid present. The viscosity of the synovial fluid tended to increase, the hyaluronic acid concentration dropped to about 70% of that of the rested muscle, the total protein decreased to about 65%, and microscopically visible cellular elements were present in greater numbers. From this it was concluded that the increase in synovial volume was chiefly the result of the inflow of water. The larger number of particles probably resulted from abrasion of the surrounding tissues.

EXERCISE AND BONE

When bones are not used they undergo resorption. This degenerative process, known as disuse osteoporosis, is related to the withdrawal of mechanical stress. It is speculated that bones and collagen have piezo-

321

electric properties by which mechanical force can be transduced into electrical potential, which may somehow influence membrane transport and cell metabolism.

Withdrawal of mechanical stress does not reduce osteoblastic activity. Bone formation continues, but resorptive activity is elevated. The four minerals that constitute most of the inorganic material of bone (calcium, phosphorus, magnesium, and sodium) are mobilized from bone and excreted.

Means of maintaining bone stability are important problems of prolonged space flight, bed rest, immobilization by casts or bandages, and paralysis. The minimal strain stimulus necessary to maintain normal bone structure is not yet known, but it is well established that simple muscle exercise that provides muscle strain on bones prevents bone resorption.

The stresses and strains of physical activity act on bones as they do on soft tissue. A mild degree of trauma stimulates the development of new supportive trabeculae and the readjustment of osseous struts without an increase in bone size. Training does not increase stature. In addition to these alterations in structure exercise increases the diameter of bones. The mechanism by which bone development is stimulated by exercise is not well defined. Without stimulation the primitive mesenchymal cells are quiescent and bone is resorbed instead of renewed.

A severe or prolonged strain resulting from excessive or repetitive stresses to bone can cause fracture or inflammation (osteochondritis). Rest results in healing and compensatory new bone formation.

A line has not yet been established between the mild degree of trauma needed to stimulate the development of bone and the severe degree of trauma which causes bone necrosis. Until this line is drawn it is prudent to avoid exercise programs that place excessive or repetitive stress on the skeletal framework of growing children and older adults. If long or high jumping, long-distance running, or similar severely stressful activities are contemplated, a long period of very gradual conditioning should be provided in order to develop supporting trabeculae and to strengthen the epiphyseal plates.

Whether heavy physical activities alter the normal ossification processes in young children is not clearly demonstrated, due to individual variation in growth. There is apprehension that the "microtrauma" of severe and repetitive mechanical pressures on the growth plate, particularly in the zone of proliferating cells, may overstimulate cellular ossification and eventually limit growth potentials.

Repetitive stress to a single epiphysis can cause injury, especially in children under age 14 in whom the epiphysis is still open. An example is "Little Leaguer's elbow," properly termed "traumatic epiphysitis of the medial epicondylar epiphysis of the humerus." This condition is initiated in pitchers at the site of origin of the tendon of the flexor-pronator group of muscles in the forearm. Throwing a baseball with maximal effort exerts considerable traction tension on this tendon, especially when curve balls are thrown. Adams observed epiphysitis in roentgenograms of every one of the eighty Little League pitchers he studied.[1] Nonpitching players and nonplayers generally were free of these changes. Young pitchers should avoid long practice sessions and should probably pitch a limit of two innings per game, with a rest period of one day between games or throwing practice.

Vigorous throwing also causes traumatic epiphysitis of the proximal humeral epiphysis. At the completion of a maximal throw the head of the humerus is strongly pulled away from the glenoid, which subjects the proximal humeral epiphysis to considerable strain. The tibial tubercle of the knee is another common site of traumatic epiphysitis, as it is strained by jumping and running, especially downhill running.

References

1. Adams, J. E.: Injury to the throwing arm—a study of the traumatic changes in elbow joints of boy baseball players, Calif. Med. **102**:127, 1965.
2. Larson, R. L.: Physical activity and the growth and development of bone and joint structures. In Rarick, G. L., editor: Physical activity: human growth and development, New York, 1973, Academic Press, Inc.

Suggested readings

Adams, A.: Effect of exercise upon ligament strength, Res. Quart. **37**:163, 1966.

Bootzin, D., and Muffey, H., editors: Biomechanics, New York, 1969, Plenum Press.

Bruce, D., and Wiebers, J.: Mineral dynamics during hibernation and chronic immobility: a review, Aerospace Med. **40**:855, 1969.

Brunnstrom, S.: Clinical kinesiology, ed. 2, Philadelphia, 1966, F. A. Davis Co.

Cooper, J., and Glassow, R.: Kinesiology, ed. 3, St. Louis, 1972, The C. V. Mosby Co.

Harris, M.: A factor analytic study of flexibility, Res. Quart. **40**:62, 1969.

Mack, P., and LaChance, P.: Effects of recumbency and space flight on bone density, Am. J. Clin. Nutr. **20**:1194, 1967.

Rathbone, J., and Hunt, V.: Corrective physical education, ed. 7, Philadelphia, 1965, W. B. Saunders, Co.

Steindler, A.: Kinesiology of the human body under normal and pathological conditions, Springfield, Ill., 1964, Charles C Thomas, Publisher.

Wells, K.: Kinesiology, ed. 4, Philadelphia, 1966, W. B. Saunders Co.

PART EIGHT

AGE AND SEX FACTORS

26 AGE AND SEX

Throughout this text we have occasionally made reference to individual differences in physiological responses to physical exercise. Racial, body type, and body size differences were discussed in Chapter 15. In this final chapter an attempt will be made to examine the relation of exercise to growth and aging, and to consider differences in human male and female responses to exercise.

Such examination of individual differences is obscured by the influence of training. It is not uncommon to see a 70-year-old man whose aerobic capacity matches that of a 30-year-old, or a woman athlete whose muscular strength is greater than that of a sedentary man. It can be argued that the major cause of the differences seen between young and old, and male and female, is their degree of activity—or state of training. Indeed, when activity is taken into account, age and sex differences in strength and endurance are nearly obliterated.[16] Thus cross-sectional studies of age groupings of male and female populations must be interpreted with caution. Longitudinal studies in which activity habits, nutrition, and other factors in exercise response are either carefully controlled or accurately documented are necessary to analyze the influence of growth and aging. Sex differences can be elucidated only when activity habits and other factors are likewise controlled.

Do functional and structural changes as a result of training during youth persist into the adult years? For the most part, exercise training induces only temporary changes in the organism; they disappear when training is terminated. There may, however, remain some slight residual changes which should enhance physical capacity in later years. This is suggested by a comparison[15] of the aerobic capacity of sedentary men aged 50 to 59, some of whom were nonathletes during youth and others who had been athletes but had given up all sports 20 years before. The maximal oxygen uptake of the nonathletes was 30 ml./min./kg., while that of the ex-athletes was 38 ml./min./kg. A third group, former athletes who had kept up regular activities in adult years, had a maximal oxygen uptake of 53 ml./min./kg. It is possible, of course, that the differences between athletes and nonathletes was due to superior original endowment of the ex-athletes and not to any remaining training effects.

The ages when children appear to be more susceptible to factors which can influence growth and strength are from 5½ to 7 years for both sexes, and again from 11 to 13 for girls and 13 to 15 for boys.[4]

GROWTH, DEVELOPMENT, AND AGING

Growth, which is the increase in size and mass of body tissues, is essentially completed during the first 20 years of life. Growth stops at about the time maximal height is reached. Further enlargement of cell size can occur after that, as a result of increased activity, but such hypertrophy remains only as long as the changed activity status exists.

Development, in which the body is brought to a more complete or useful state, can continue into advanced years. For nearly as long as a person lives, there is some potential for further development.

Aging consists of the progressive changes which take place in the organism with the passage of time. One view is that aging begins at conception and continues throughout life; others argue that it begins after maturation has been completed. Cells are generated, they grow and develop, and they die. New cellular units in skin, blood, liver, bone marrow, and the mucous lining of the gastrointestinal tract replace those which are continuously or occasionally destroyed, but with increasing age the rate of destruction may exceed the rate of replacement. Other kinds of cells, such as those in brain and muscle do not have the capacity for cell division, so those that are destroyed are not replaced.

Effects of exercise on growth. The effects of exercise training on the development of the various organs and systems of the body has been treated in previous chapters. Now we shall examine the few studies available on the effects of exercise habits on growth.

Adams' comparative study of 100 women 17 to 21 years of age who had undergone hard manual labor from early childhood and 100 women of similar age who had engaged in no heavy manual labor showed that the working girls were taller and heavier, and their muscle girth, chest dimensions, knee width, and hip width were larger.[1]

The growth of children is affected by nutrition and disease. Whether or not excess or lack of exercise affects growth is uncertain. There are shreds of evidence that exercise may stimulate prepubertal growth. Relying on the assumption that the amount of DNA per cell nucleus is constant, Bailey concluded from a study of the ratio of protein to DNA in an exercise and a control group of young rats that exercise has a positive effect on growth.[5]

Responses of youths and adults to exercise. The highest continuous work loads of which males are capable increase from 90 watts for 8-year-olds to over 270 watts for 20-year-olds. During growth spurts at about 12 years of age maximal working capacity continues to increase.

The heart rate response to moderate exercise (walking on a treadmill at 3.5 miles per hour up a grade of 8.6%) declines progressively with advancing age. At age 6 the heart rate response is 170 beats per minute; at age 26 the rate is only 143 per minute. Apparently the greater increase in heart rate in the younger subjects is due to a more pronounced influence of the sympathetic nervous system. Robinson[13] postulated that the high heart rates among boys reflect the prodigality of youth as contrasted with the conservatism of age.

Oxygen consumption during moderate activity shows no significant variation with age, but the maximal oxygen uptake during strenuous exertion declines slowly with advancing age. A subject who is able to use 5 liters of oxygen per minute at the age of 20 years will probably be able to use not more than 4 liters per minute at age 40 years. At the same time, the maximal heart rate he can attain during exercise decreases; it is likely to be between 160 and 170 at the age of 50 years and may not exceed 150 at the age of 70 years. These measurements indicate that man's best performance during strenuous activity is attained between the ages of 18 and 25 years. His maximal heart rate then lies between 190 and 210, and he can reach higher levels of oxygen consumption during this time than at any period either earlier or later.

Responses of young children to exercise. The physiological systems of younger children are apparently not as well developed to meet the demands of strenuous exercise as they become when puberty is reached. Children under 12 years of age possess a highly active sympathetic nervous system that predisposes to a high heart rate and an easily depleted capacity for endurance activities such as running. They do not have the capacity to utilize oxygen that older boys do because of a relatively smaller stroke volume of the heart and a consequent smaller capacity for increased circulation of blood through the muscles. The younger boys also possess a smaller carbohydrate store.

The net mechanical efficiency (work done divided by excess oxygen used above the basal level) in cycling is observed to be greatest in boys between 9 and 11 years of age. Similar previous studies are not in agreement with this observation; according to the earlier studies prepubertal boys required more oxygen than 13-year-old boys for a

329

given output of energy of the muscles and also had a lower mechanical efficiency in grade walking.

The physiological processes involving the brain, nerves, heart, lungs, and kidneys, which are coordinated to maintain normal constancy of the internal environment of the body (homeostasis), are weak during infancy and early childhood, are strengthened at puberty, continue to improve during early adulthood, and then decline. This strengthening at puberty may be a result of the hormonal factors associated with puberty.

Before puberty maximal physical output is directly proportional to age, circumference of the chest and thigh, and vital capacity. From puberty upward to 19 years of age physical fitness for maximal exercise is related more to body size than to age.

The ability of the body to respond to and recover from exercise and other stresses of the homeostatic mechanisms improve markedly at about 14 years of age. This vitality declines in boys with the onset of adolescence, showing a significant decrease at the age of 17 years; it then rises slightly between the ages of 21 to 25 years, and thereafter declines gradually. In girls there is a temporary increase in fitness for strenuous exercise at 17 years of age and possibly again at 20 years of age.

The ability of boys to perform athletic activities requiring strength, speed, endurance, and skill increases steadily between 5 and 20 years of age, adolescence retarding but not interrupting the progress. Athletic ability in girls reaches a maximum at the age of 13 or 14 years and then tends to decline so that a 9-year-old girl usually has a better performance than a girl 18 years of age.

Physical capacity of adults. After 25 years of age the ability of men to perform maximal work declines about 1% each year. It decreases slightly more rapidly in women. A decrease in aerobic capacity is accompanied by a similar decline in functional capacity of the musculoskeletal, the respiratory, and the cardiovascular systems. The ability to perform moderate work in extreme heat, at least for brief exposures, does not appear to decline with age.

On the whole, the evidence, although far from complete, indicates that after the age of 25 to 30 years, the capacity for intense effort slowly decreases, while the capacity for exercise of endurance may suffer little impairment *provided some degree of training is maintained.* The greatest danger in participation in athletics or sports in middle age (assuming that a subject is otherwise in good health) is the interspersing of spasmodic bouts of strenuous exercise in a sedentary life. This usually results in more harm than good, even though the heart and blood vessels are sound, and it may have serious effects if disease or degenerative changes of the cardiovascular system are present. The following principles should be observed:

1. If possible, a regular though necessarily curtailed program of exercise should be maintained after the school years.
2. If exercise is to be commenced again after a long period of sedentary life, it should be begun in moderation and gradually increased to the desired level of intensity.
3. There should be a thorough physical examination at regular intervals, preferably once each year.

When working within the limit of their ability, many men well advanced in years can carry on long-continued work with a lower heart rate and less evidence of fatigue than that exhibited by young men. The capacity for anaerobic work appears to be maximal in the early twenties and to be small in young boys and old men. The highest blood lactate levels are reached in the twenties, and there is only a slight lactate increase in the hardest work attempted by young boys or old men. Work or sport activities with the emphasis on speed and strength are best suited to young men. Older men are best fitted for jobs or sports requiring skill, coordination, and endurance.

SEX

The working capacity of young untrained boys and girls of similar age and size is about the same. The young female and the young male respond physiologically to physical training in the same way, but most males develop a higher working capacity than most females. Increase in functional capacity as expressed by maximal oxygen uptake is largely a function of training. When women train intensively in swimming and running, positive adaptive changes in heart volume and functional capacity occur without adverse effects.[8]

Differences in exercise capacity of men and women exist only when population samples are compared.[7] Females with the highest exercise capacity are superior to males of similar age with low exercise capacity. When averaged, males have a higher exercise capacity than females.

A study of Table 13 leads to many inferences, one being the need for a truly feminine competitive sport with the following characteristics: The new female sport would be geared to ages 8 through 14, which includes the peak period of aerobic capacity and endurance. Girls would start training for this sport at age 6 and be expected to retire from championship competition at age 16 or shortly thereafter. The event would be of short duration. The intensity of effort would be submaximal. Movements would not demand great strength of the arms and shoulders, or risk shocks or blows to the arms and shoulder girdles. The environment would be cool. The motions of the body would feature high

Table 13. Characteristic differences between males' and females' exercise capacities

Factor	Females	Males
Center of gravity (% of height above ground)	Lower	Higher
Body agility (change directions)	Lesser	Greater
Pelvic width	Broader	Narrower
Susceptibility to hip fracture	Greater	Lesser
Obliquity of femurs	Greater	Lesser
Hip sway in running	Greater	Lesser
Leg length	Shorter	Longer
Running speed	Slower	Faster
Jumping distance	Shorter	Longer
Injury in sprinting and jumping	Greater	Lesser
Arm length, upper	Shorter	Longer
Arm length, forearm	Shorter	Longer
Bone size	Smaller	Larger
Bone strength	Lesser	Greater
Ligament and tendon size and strength	Lesser	Greater
Connective tissue/body weight	Lesser	Greater
Injuries in running and jumping	More	Less
Upper vs. lower body development	Lower	Upper
Arm and shoulder injuries	More	Less
Digestion affected by exercise	Greater	Lesser
Muscle size/weight	Lower	Higher
Strength/height	Lower	Higher
Strength	Lower	Higher
Endurance	Lower	Higher
Fat/body weight	Greater	Lesser
Anaerobic capacity	Lower	Higher
Aerobic capacity	Lower	Higher
Age of peak aerobic capacity	Younger	Older
Age of peak physical endurance	Younger	Older
Metabolic rate level (due to fat)	Lower	Higher
Metabolic rate variability	More (due to menstruation)	Less
Core-skin temperature gradient	Lesser	Greater
Sweating threshold	Higher	Lower
Heat tolerance	Poorer	Better
Cold tolerance	Better	Poorer
Endurance for swimming in cold water	Better	Poorer
Breathing capacity	Lesser	Greater
Thoracic vs. abdominal respiration	Thoracic	Abdominal
Hemoglobin	Less	More
Erythrocytes	Less	More
Oxygen carrying capacity	Lesser	Greater
Heart size	Smaller	Larger
Heart rate, resting	Faster	Slower
Heart rate increase in exercise	Greater	Lesser
Heart rate recovery after exercise	Slower	Faster
Exercise blood pressure	Lower	Higher
Susceptibility to bruising	Greater	Lesser

stability and low agility, and would require no fast running, jumping, body contact, or explosive effort. The activity which meets these criteria most closely at present is swimming. This selection is verified by a comparison of male and female swimming records. Every record set by the all-time great men swimmers Johnnie Weismuller and Buster Crabbe has been broken by young girls.

Is there a "maleness" and "femaleness" in response to exercise? Aside from the differences in physical training, body build, and body fat content, are there "maleness" and "femaleness" factors which differentiate the physiological responses of boys and girls and men and women? When Davies calculated the maximal oxygen uptake of boys and girls working on a bicycle ergometer and expressed the uptake in terms of the volume of the leg muscles or active tissue involved in the exercise instead of using the standard total body weight constant, the sex difference disappeared.[6] This study suggests that there may be no "maleness" or "femaleness" in human muscle tissue metabolism or circulorespiratory functions. Women may have a lesser ability to perform exhausting work because of their adiposity, rather than because of differences in physiological functions. When working at a given submaximal load the strain on their circulorespiratory systems is greater in most women and girls than in men and boys, but the difference is small or nonexistent between thin boys and girls.[12]

Women have smaller hearts and smaller blood volumes than men, so they obviously carry less total hemoglobin and oxygen in their blood.[3] During light to moderate effort cardiac output and oxygen uptake are about the same in men and women. The women's smaller hearts must beat faster to compensate for their lower stroke volume, but their lower body weight makes a lower stroke volume adequate. These differences are related to body size and do not constitute a "maleness" or "femaleness" of physiological response to exercise.

The effects of training on women's physiological responses to exercise has not been thoroughly investigated, but a study by Kilbom showed no differences from the changes commonly observed in men.[11]

The energy expenditure during walking[9] and cycling[2] is about the same for men and women when the cost is expressed in relation to body weight.

Women have a larger number of active sweat glands than men do, yet for some reason they have a lower total body sweat rate when they work in a hot environment.[17] Adjustment to heat is more efficient in women, but men are able to acclimatize to work in hot environments as well as women.

There does not seem to be any effect of the menstrual cycle on the physiological effects of exercise, except that core temperatures are higher during the postovulatory phase when work is performed in a hot environment.[10] Olympic female athletes compete successfully during all phases of the menstrual cycle. Most of these sportswomen do not interrupt their training regimen, but may reduce the intensity of training if flow is excessive during menstruation. Trained girl athletes experience less pain during menstruation and have a more regular cycle than do untrained girls. If there is a "femaleness" factor, it is not manifested during the menstrual cycle.

After puberty, males are about 40% stronger, on the average, than women.[14] Taken as a ratio of strength to body weight the difference is even greater, due to the adiposity of women. Men also have a mechanically advantageous bony structure, more so in the shoulders than in the legs. The adult male has about 29% more skeletal muscle fibers than the adult female. It is not known, however, whether there is a difference in the individual fiber strength of untrained men's and women's skeletal muscles.

Since no real "femaleness" or "maleness" physiological differences in response to exercise have yet been identified, it is futile to speculate on hormonal or muscular metabolic factors which may play some role. "Femaleness" and "maleness" in relation to exercise seem to be more a matter of morphology than physiology, at least at the present stage of incomplete knowledge.

References

1. Adams, E. H.: A comparative anthropometric study of hard labor during youth as a stimulus of physical growth of young colored women, Res. Quart. 9:102, 1938.
2. Adams, W. C.: Influence of age, sex, and body weight on the energy, J. Appl. Physiol. 22:539, 1967.
3. Åstrand, P.-O., and others: Cardiac output during work submaximal and maximal, J. Appl. Physiol. 19:268, 1964.
4. Asmussen, E.: Growth in muscular strength and power. In Rarick, G. L., editor: Physical activity—human growth and development, New York, 1973, Academic Press, Inc.
5. Bailey, D. A., Bell, R. D., and Howarth, R. E.: The effect of exercise on DNA and protein synthesis in skeletal muscle of growing rats, Growth 37:323, 1973.
6. Davies, C. T. M.: Body composition in children: a reference standard for maximum aerobic power output on a stationary bicycle ergometer. In Thoren, C., editor: Pediatric work physiology, Acta Paediat. Scand. Suppl. 217, 1971.
7. Drinkwater, B. L.: Physiological responses of women to exercise. In Wilmore, J. H., editor: Exercise and sport sciences reviews, Vol. 1, New York, 1973, Academic Press, Inc.
8. Drinkwater, B. L., and Horvath, S. M.: Response of young female track athletes to exercise, Med. Sci. Sports 3:56, 1971.
9. Durnin, J. V. G. A., and Passmore, R.: Energy, work and leisure, London, 1967, Heineman Educational Books, Ltd.
10. Haslag, W. M., and Hertzman, A. R.: Temperature regulation in young women, J. Appl. Physiol. 20:1283, 1965.
11. Kilbom, A.: Physical training of women, Scand. J. Clin. Lab. Invest. 119:1, 1971.
12. Macek, M., and Vavra, J.: Cardio-

pulmonary and metabolic changes during exercise in children 6-14 years old, J. Appl. Physiol. **30**:200, 1971.

13. Robinson, S.: Experimental studies of physical fitness in relation to age, Arbeitsphysiol. **10**:18, 1938.

14. Rodahl, K., and Horvath, S. M., editors: Muscle as a tissue, New York, 1962, McGraw-Hill Book Co.

15. Saltin, B., and others: Response to exercise after bed rest and training, Circulation, Supp. 7, 37/38:1, 1968.

16. Wessel, J. A., and Van Huss, W. D.: The influence of physical activity and age on exercise adaptation of women, 20-69 years, J. Sports Med. **9**:173, 1969.

17. Wyndham, C. H., Morrison, F. F., and Williams, C. G.: Heat reaction of male and female Caucasians, J. Appl. Physiol. **20**:357, 1965.

Suggested readings

Asmussen, E., and Mathiasen, P.: Some physiological functions in physical education students re-investigated after 20 years, J. Am. Geriat. Soc. **10**:379, 1962.

Brozek, J., editor: Human body composition—approaches and applications, New York, 1966, Pergamon Press.

Cureton, T.: The physiological effects of exercise programs on adults, Springfield, Ill., 1969, Charles C Thomas, Publisher.

Dill, D., and Consolazio, F.: Responses to exercise as related to age and environmental temperature, J. Appl. Physiol. **17**:645, 1962.

Ekblom, B.: Effect of physical training in adolescent boys, J. Appl. Physiol. **27**:350, 1969.

Ismail, A.: Body composition and relationships to physical activity. In Fall, H., editor: Exercise physiology, New York, 1968, Academic Press, Inc.

Jokl, E., and Brunner, D.: Physical activity and aging, vol. 4, Medicine and Sports Series, Baltimore, 1969, University Park Press.

Jokl, E., and Jokl, P.: The physiological basis of athletic records, Springfield, Ill., 1968, Charles C Thomas, Publisher.

Ricci, B.: Physiological basis of human performance, Philadelphia, 1967, Lea & Febiger.

GLOSSARY

acid-base balance The factors involved in the maintenance of a slightly alkaline state of the blood and tissues.

acidosis A shift of the acid-base balance toward the acid side. In uncompensated acidosis, both the pH and the buffer capacity are lowered; in compensated acidosis, the pH has been restored nearly to normal but the buffer capacity remains lowered.

action potential The voltage change across a cell membrane that results in excitation of the cell in response to a stimulus.

acute Of brief duration; disappearing on removal or cessation of the immediate stimulus, for example, the increase in heart rate during exercise.

adrenaline (epinephrine) A hormone secreted by the medulla of the adrenal glands, especially under conditions of emotional stress. The physiological effects of adrenaline include increase in heart rate and arterial blood pressure and increase in the blood sugar concentration.

aerobic Requiring the presence of oxygen.

alkalosis A shift of the acid-base balance toward the alkaline side.

alveolar air Literally, the air present in the pulmonary alveoli that participates in gas exchange with the blood in the pulmonary capillaries. This air cannot be obtained for analysis, so that for practical purposes the last portion of air expelled in a deep expiration, which probably comes from the respiratory bronchioles and alveolar ducts, is assumed to be approximately equivalent in composition.

anaerobic Occurring in the absence of oxygen.

angina Spasmodic attacks of intense suffocative pain usually referred to the chest.

antigravity muscles The muscles (predominantly extensors) that maintain the body in an upright posture against the force of gravity.

aortic body A small mass of tissue located between the aorta and the pulmonary artery and having a function similar to that of the carotid body.

aortic sinus A dilatation of the aortic arch having a function similar to that of the carotid sinus.

arterioles The small terminal arteries that regulate the flow of blood into the capillaries.

asthenia Weakness. Loss of strength or energy.

athlete's heart The large, strong heart of an endurance athlete. Returns to prior size and power after cessation of training.

atrophy A wasting of tissues. Muscular atrophy is usually the result of disuse, as in poliomyelitis.

autonomic nervous system The division of the nervous system that controls the activity of smooth muscle, heart muscle, and glands.

basal metabolism The energy expenditure of the body under conditions of complete rest.

blood pressure The force with which the blood distends the walls of the blood vessels.

bradycardia Slowing of heart rate; resting heart rate less than 50 per minute.

buffer A compound that minimizes the change in pH of a fluid when acids or bases are added.

callus Horny patches of epidermis caused by chronic physical trauma in areas of friction.

Calorie The amount of heat required to raise the temperature of 1 kilogram of water 1° C. Also called kilocalorie.

capillaries The tiny, thin-walled blood vessels interposed between the arteries and the veins in which occurs the exchange of materials between blood and tissues or in the lung between blood and alveolar air.

cardiac Pertaining to the heart.

cardiac arrest Cessation of cardiac function.

cardiac cycle The sequence of events in the heart—volume and pressure changes and valve actions—during one complete period of contraction and relaxation.

cardiac impulse The impulse that originates in the pacemaker of the heart and stimulates the heart muscle, producing systolic contraction.

cardiac output The volume of blood pumped by each ventricle of the heart in 1 minute.

cardiac reserve The ability of the heart to increase its output of blood by increasing the heart rate, the stroke volume, or both.

cardiotachometer An instrument that makes a continuous record of the heart rate.

carotid body A small mass of tissue located near the bifurcation of the carotid artery at the angle of the jaw.

carotid body reflex Reflex increase in the minute volume of breathing due to stimulation of receptors in the carotid body by chemical changes in the blood (decreased oxygen tension, increased carbon dioxide, or increased acidity).

carotid sinus A small dilatation of the internal carotid artery at the bifurcation of the artery near the angle of the jaw.

carotid sinus reflex A reflex decrease in heart rate and blood pressure resulting from stimulation of stretch receptors in the wall of the carotid sinus by a rise in arterial blood pressure.

cerebellum A portion of the brain concerned with the adjustment of the strength, range, and smoothness of muscle contractions.

chronic Continuing for a long time; persisting after cessation of the immediate stimulus, for example, the increase in muscle size resulting from training.

chronotropic Affecting rate (of heartbeat).

concentric contraction Muscle shortens.

coronary blood vessels The blood vessels that supply blood to the heart muscle.

crest load The largest work load for which the oxygen intake of the body is adequate to meet the oxygen requirement.

cyanosis A bluish discoloration of the skin and mucous membranes caused by deficient oxygenation of the blood.

dead space The combined volume of all the air passages in which no gas exchange occurs. It includes the trachea, bronchi, and bronchioles down to, but not including, the respiratory bronchioles.

diastole The period during which the heart is relaxing after a previous contraction.

diastolic pressure The lowest level to which the arterial blood pressure falls in the interval between successive heartbeats.

dissociation curve The oxygen dissociation curve expresses the relation between the percentage saturation of hemoglobin and the oxygen tension of the blood.

distensibility The capacity of a body for being stretched.

dynamic contractions Contractions alternating with relaxations, as in alternate flexion and extension of an extremity in running.

dynamometer An apparatus for testing muscular strength.

dyspnea Labored breathing associated

with unpleasant sensations of breathlessness.

eccentric contraction Muscle lengthens.

elasticity The capacity of a body for recovering its original shape after having been distended or otherwise deformed.

electrocardiogram A graphic record of the spread of the cardiac impulse through the heart.

electrocardiograph An instrument that amplifies and records the electrical changes resulting from the spread of the cardiac impulse in the heart.

ergogenic Tending to increase work output.

ergograph An instrument for recording the work done by contracting muscles. In the instrument designed by Mosso a record is made of the contractions of the finger lifting a weight.

ergometer An apparatus for measuring the amount of work performed by a subject. The bicycle ergometer is a stationary bicycle in which the rear wheel is replaced by a heavy flywheel or electric brake against which the subject performs work.

exercise One occasion of physical activity.

exercise conditioning Exercise repeated with sufficient intensity and duration to increase strength and endurance.

exercise training Exercise repeated with improved economy of movement to increase performance.

expiratory reserve volume The volume of air that can be expelled by the strongest possible expiratory effort after a normal expiration.

extension The straightening out of two parts of the body bent upon one another by a previous flexion.

fatigue A diminished capacity for work caused by previous work. The term is also frequently applied to accompanying subjective sensations.

flexion The bending of one part of the body upon another part.

functional residual capacity The volume of air left in the lungs at the end of a natural, unforced expiration.

glycogenesis The formation of glycogen from glucose or its breakdown products.

glycolysis The breakdown of glucose or glycogen to pyruvic acid or lactic acid.

heart sounds Sounds produced by the closure and vibration of the valves of the heart.

hematocrit The percentage of the volume of a sample of blood that is occupied by the blood cells.

hemoglobin A pigment present in the red blood cells that combines reversibly with oxygen.

homeodynamics Maintenance of steady state in the organism at elevated levels of metabolism.

homeostasis The normal constancy of the internal environment of the body.

hormone A chemical agent produced in one of the endocrine glands and transported in the blood to other tissues or organs where it produces a specific alteration of function.

hydrogen ion The positively charged ion (proton) that results from the dissociation of acids; the concentration (or "activity") of hydrogen ions determines the acidity of a solution.

hyperglycemia An increased concentration of glucose in the blood.

hyperpnea Increased minute volume of breathing.

hypertension A pathological increase in the resting arterial blood pressure.

hypertrophy An increase in the size of a tissue or organ independent of the general growth of the body. There is no increase in the number of cells, but each cell becomes larger.

hyperventilation Pulmonary ventilation increased out of proportion to metabolic requirements.

hypocapnia A decreased arterial carbon dioxide tension.

hypoglycemia A subnormal blood sugar concentration.

hypoxemia A deficiency of oxygen in the blood.

hypoxia A deficiency of oxygen in the tissues.

inotropic Affecting the force of muscular contractions.

inspiratory reserve volume The volume of air that can be taken in by a maximal inspiratory effort over and above the tidal volume.

internal environment The tissue fluid that bathes the cells of the body and through which occurs the exchange of materials between the blood and tissue cells.

intraperitoneal Within the abdominal (peritoneal) cavity.

intrapleural Within the pleural cavity (the fluid-filled space between the outer surface of the lungs and the inner surface of the chest wall).

intrapulmonary Within the lungs.

intrathoracic Within the chest (thoracic) cavity.

in vitro Occurring outside the body, for example, in a test tube.

in vivo Occurring in the body.

ischemia Deficiency of blood flow, often localized and temporary.

isoelectric Having the same electric potential throughout and therefore producing no current.

isometric contraction A contraction in which a muscle is unable to shorten, the total tension developed eventually being dissipated as heat. No movement is produced and no work is performed.

isotonic contraction A contraction in which a muscle shortens against a load, resulting in movement and the performance of work.

lactic acid An organic acid having the formula $C_3H_6O_3$; the end product of the anaerobic metabolism of glucose or glycogen.

leukocytosis An increase in the number of leukocytes per unit volume of blood.

mechanical advantage The ratio of load to effort or ratio of power arm to weight arm.

mechanical efficiency The proportion of the energy requirement of an act that is converted into mechanical work. The mechanical efficiency of the human body ranges from 10 to 30%, according to the type of activity.

metabolism The chemical reactions that occur in living tissues; the term is often confined to the oxidations that are the ultimate source of biological energy.

metabolite One of the intermediate or final products in the metabolic breakdown of foodstuffs in the body.

mitochondria Filamentous or globular structures occurring in cytoplasm of cells; they contain the respiratory enzyme systems responsible for the formation of ATP.

motor area The area of the cerebral cortex that controls the contractions of individual skeletal muscles in voluntary movements.

motor nerve A nerve that transmits excitation to a muscle.

motor pool The group of motor nerve cells in the spinal cord or brain stem that give rise to the nerve fibers that comprise the motor nerve to a muscle.

motor unit The unit of neuromuscular function, including a ventral horn cell, its motor nerve fiber, and the group of muscle fibers supplied by branches of the nerve fiber.

muscle spindle A type of receptor, located among the fibers of a skeletal muscle, that is stimulated by changes in tension in the muscle.

muscle tone See *tonus.*

myocardium Heart muscle.

myofibrils The longitudinally arranged contractile elements embedded in the sarcoplasm of a muscle fiber.

myogram A graphic record of muscle contractions.

myograph An instrument for recording muscle contractions.

neuromuscular Pertaining to the relation between nerve and muscle.

neuromuscular coordination The nervous control of muscle contractions in the performance of motor acts.

normal load A light or moderate load of work in which the oxygen intake is adequate to supply the needs of the body.

normotensive Having normal blood pressure.

optimum The most favorable condition (as of temperature) for a particular function or process.

overload A heavy work load in which the oxygen intake is inadequate to meet the requirement.

oxidation The removal of hydrogen or electrons from a compound. In biological oxidations, oxygen does not directly combine with the substance being "oxidized," but ultimately combines with the hydrogen to form water.

oxygen deficit The difference between the oxygen requirement of a task and the oxygen intake during performance of the task.

oxygen uptake The rate of oxygen consumption.

oxygenation The loose, reversible combi-

339

nation of oxygen with hemoglobin; not a true chemical oxidation.

oxyhemoglobin Hemoglobin loosely combined with oxygen.

pericardium The fibrous sac that encloses the heart.

pH A convenient notation for expressing the degree of acidity or alkalinity of a solution. At neutrality, pH = 7; values above 7 indicate alkalinity; those below 7, acidity.

phasic contraction A contraction of a muscle or group of muscles that results in movement.

placebo Inactive chemical resembling experimental drug in appearance and taste, given to a control group.

plasma The liquid part of the blood in which the blood cells are suspended.

plethysmograph An instrument that measures volume changes in an organ or other part of the body.

postural contraction A contraction of a muscle or group of muscles that results in no movement but serves to maintain a posture or attitude.

postural tone The slight sustained contraction of muscles engaged in maintaining a posture or attitude; especially pronounced in the extensor muscles, which maintain the body in an upright posture against the force of gravity.

posture A position or attitude of the body as a whole or of parts of the body with respect to one another.

prestart Conditioned response to exercise resulting in elevation of body processes prior to activity.

proprioceptor A receptor located within the body and stimulated by mechanical deformation (pressure, stretching, tension, etc.), for example, muscle spindles, stretch receptors in the carotid sinus.

psychic Pertaining to or originating in the higher centers of the brain (cerebral cortex).

pulmonary ventilation The periodic partial renewal of the air in the lung alveoli.

pulse The distention of the arterial walls (by the systolic ejection of blood) which travels down the arteries as a wave.

pulse pressure The difference between the systolic and the diastolic blood pressures.

receptor A specialized sensory organ in which the sensory nerve fibers originate peripherally and which is stimulated by some specific type of environmental disturbance (heat, cold, light, sound, etc.). See also proprioceptor.

reflex An involuntary motor response resulting from stimulation of sensory receptors.

reflex arc The nervous pathway that forms the anatomical basis of a reflex, consisting of a receptor, a sensory nerve fiber, a synapse, a motor nerve fiber, and an effector (muscle, gland, etc.).

relative humidity The ratio of the amount of moisture in the air to the amount that would be present if the air were completely saturated with moisture at the same temperature—usually expressed in percent of complete saturation.

residual volume The volume of air (about 1,500 ml.) that remains in the lungs after the deepest possible expiration.

respiration The sum total of the processes involved in the exchange of gases between an organism and its environment.

respiratory center A group of nerve cells in the medulla that controls contraction of the respiratory muscles and thus regulates the rate and depth of breathing.

respiratory quotient (R.Q.) The ratio of the volume of carbon dioxide expired to the volume of oxygen absorbed during a given period of time.

smooth muscle Involuntary muscle occurring in the walls of the hollow viscera (blood vessels, gastrointestinal tract, etc.).

spasm A sudden involuntary muscular contraction, attended by pain and interference with function.

sphygmomanometer An instrument that is used to measure indirectly the arterial blood pressure in man.

spirometer An apparatus for the collection, measurement, or storage of gases. It consists of a movable bell inverted in a cylinder filled with water; the bell rises when gas enters and falls when gas leaves, so that a record of the rate and depth of breathing may be made with a suitable recording device.

splanchnic Pertaining to the abdominal organs.

sprain A joint injury in which some of the fibers of a supporting ligament are ruptured, but the continuity of the ligament remains intact.

Starling's law The stroke volume of the heart is proportional to its diastolic volume. This results from the fact that the force of muscle contraction is increased by stretching of the muscle fibers.

static contractions Contractions in which muscle tension is sustained throughout the period of activity, as in weight lifting.

strain Excessive stretching or overextension of a musculotendinous unit.

stretch reflex A reflex contraction of a muscle resulting from stretching of the muscle.

striated muscle Skeletal muscle; voluntary muscle whose contraction produces movement of parts of the skeleton with reference to other parts.

stroke volume The volume of blood ejected by each ventricle of the heart during a single systole.

synapse The points of contact between the terminal branches of a nerve fiber and the cell body and dendrites of the next neuron in the chain.

systole The contraction phase of the heart.

systolic pressure The highest level to which the arterial blood pressure rises during the systolic ejection of blood from the ventricle.

tachycardia Rapid heart rate; resting pulse rate above 100 per minute.

tendon organ A receptor located in muscle tendon that is stimulated by stretching, with a resulting reflex contraction of the muscle.

tension (gas) The pressure exerted by a gas dissolved in a liquid.

tension (muscular) The force exerted by a contracting muscle.

tetanus A smooth sustained contraction of skeletal muscle caused by fusion of individual muscle twitches.

tidal volume The volume of air exchanged in each inspiration and expiration.

tonus A slight, sustained contraction of muscle; in skeletal muscle, tonus is the result of incomplete tetanus in a small fraction of the fibers.

total lung volume The volume of air in the lungs after a maximal inspiration; the sum of the vital capacity and the residual volume.

treadmill An apparatus with a continuous moving belt that can be made to run at various speeds and inclinations.

treppe A progressive increase in the tension developed by a muscle in the first few contractions following a period of inactivity.

Valsalva maneuver Attempted forced expiration against a closed glottis resulting in an increase in intrathoracic pressure, which reduces venous return to the heart and decreases arterial pressure.

vascular Pertaining to blood vessels.

vasoconstriction Decrease in the caliber of arterioles produced by contraction of the circular rings of smooth muscle in the vessel walls.

vasoconstrictor center A group of nerve cells in the medulla that discharges impulses over the vasoconstrictor nerves and that regulates the amount and distribution of constriction of the arterioles in various parts of the body.

vasoconstrictor nerve A nerve that stimulates the smooth muscle in the arterioles, causing narrowing of the lumen of the vessels.

vasodilatation An increase in the caliber of a blood vessel.

vasodilator nerve A nerve that produces an increase in the caliber of a blood vessel (usually an arteriole) by inhibiting the tone of the smooth muscle in the wall of the vessel.

viscosity Resistance to flow (in fluids) or to change in shape (in solids).

vital capacity The greatest volume of air that can be forcibly exhaled after a maximal inspiration.

work The product of a force and the

distance through which the force is applied; for example, if a 1-pound weight is lifted a distance of 1 foot, the work performed is 1 foot-pound.

work load The intensity of work, usually expressed in terms of foot-pounds or kilogram-meters of work per minute; sometimes the work load is expressed in terms of the oxygen requirement per minute.

WEIGHTS AND MEASURES

Conversion factors

To change	to	Multiply by
millimeters	inches	0.03937
meters	inches	39.37
meters	feet	3.2808
meters	yards	1.0936
kilometers	miles	0.62137
cubic meters	cubic yards	1.3079
liters	cubic inches	61.025
liters	liquid quarts	1.0567
liters	gallons (U.S.)	0.2642
liters	pounds of water	2.205
liters	kilograms of water	1.0
kilograms	pounds avdp.	2.2046
kilograms	ounces	35.274
inches	millimeters	25.4
inches	centimeters	2.54
feet	meters	0.3048
yards	meters	0.9144
cubic yards	cubic meters	0.7646
pounds avdp.	ounces	16.0
pounds avdp.	grams	453.6
pounds avdp.	kilograms	0.4536
ounces	grams	28.35
liquid quarts	liters	0.9463
centimeters	inches	0.3937
square centimeters	square inches	0.155
cubic centimeters	milliters	1.0
cubic centimeters	cubic inches	0.061
cubic centimeters	grams of water	1.0
cubic centimeters	grains of water	15.432
cubic centimeters	drops	12.0
feet	centimeters	30.48
square feet	square inches	144.0
square feet	square centimeters	929.0

Continued.

Conversion factors—cont'd

To change	to	Multiply by
cubic feet	gallons	7.4805
cubic feet	quarts	29.922
cubic feet	kilogram of water	28.32
cubic feet	liters of water	28.32
cubic feet	pounds of water	62.43
gallons	quarts	4.0
gallons	liters	3.785
gallons	pounds of water	8.345
gallons	kilograms of water	3.785
grams	ounces	0.035274
grams	pounds	0.002205
grams	grains	15.432
inches	centimeters	2.54
square inches	square centimeters	6.4516
cubic inches	cubic centimeters	16.387
cubic inches	pints	0.0346
cubic inches	liters	0.0164
cubic inches	grams of water	16.39
cubic inches	pounds of water	0.0361
cubic inches	grains of water	252.89
square meters	square yards	1.196
square meters	square feet	10.764
square meters	square inches	1,550.0
square meters	square centimeters	10,000.0
cubic meters	liters	1,000.0
cubic meters	quarts	1,056.7
cubic meters	cubic feet	35.31
cubic meters	metric tons of water	1.0
cubic meters	pounds of water	2,204.6
miles	feet	5,280.0
miles	yards	1,760.0
miles	meters	1,609.3
miles	kilometers	1.6093
square miles	acres	640.0
square miles	square kilometers	2.59
ounces	grams	28.3495
ounces	pounds	0.0625
ounces	grains	437.5
pints	quarts	0.5
pints	cubic centimeters	473.18
pints	ounces of water	16.0
pints	pounds of water	1.043
pints	kilograms of water	0.47318
pints	cups	2.0
pints	tablespoons	32.0
pints	teaspoons	96.0
quarts	pints	2.0
quarts	cups	4.0
quarts	cubic centimeters	946.4
quarts	tablespoons	64.0
quarts	teaspoons	192.0
quarts	ounces of water	32.0

Conversion factors—cont'd

To change	to	Multiply by
quarts	pounds of water	2.086
quarts	kilograms of water	0.946
tablespoons	cups	0.0625
tablespoons	cubic centimeters	15.0
tablespoons	dessert spoons	1.5
tablespoons	teaspoons	3.0
tablespoons	drops	180.0
teaspoons	cubic centimeters	5.0
teaspoons	cups	0.02
teaspoons	drops	60.0

1 foot-pound = 0.1382 kilogram meter = 0.000324 Calorie
= 0.001286 B.T.U. = 0.0005 foot-ton
1 foot-pound per minute = 0.02261 watt
1 kilogram-meter = 7.233 foot-pounds = 0.002343 Calorie
= 0.009298 B.T.U. = 0.1635 watts
1 horsepower-hour = 1,980,000 foot-pounds = 641.3 Calories
1 joule = 0.2423 Calorie = 10,000,000 ergs = 10,198 gram centimeters
= 0.00987 liter centimeter
1 horsepower = 33,000 foot-pounds per minute = 550 foot-pounds per second
= 1,980,000 foot-pounds per hour
= 4,564 kilogram meters per minute = 746 watts
= 0.746 kilowatt = 2.1 liters of oxygen/minute
= 642 Calories/hour
1 B.T.U. = 0.252 Calorie at 15° C. = 778 foot-pounds
watt = work at the rate of about ¼ calorie per second
= 0.012 kilogram meter per second = 7 kilogram meters per minute
= 1 joule per second
1 watt-minute = 6.12 kilogram meters per second
= 0.01435 calorie
Kilowatt = 1,000 watts = 0.239 Calorie per second = 15.34 Calories per minute
= 101.9 kilogram meters per second = 737.56 foot-pounds per second
= 1,000 joules per second = 10 billion ergs per second = 1.34 horsepower
1 kilogram meter per second = 9.81 watts
1 watt hour = 0.85968 Calorie
1 kilowatt hour = 3,412 B.T.U.
1 atmosphere of pressure = 760 mm. Hg = 29.92 in. Hg = 10.33 meters water
= 33.9 ft. water = 1,033.3 Gm./sq. in.
= 14.7 lb./sq. in. = 2,116.3 lb./sq. ft.

Temperature conversion:

$$°C. = \frac{°F. - 32}{9} \times 5 \qquad °F. = \frac{°C. \times 9}{5} + 32$$

Heat equivalent of 1 liter of oxygen:
  5.14 Calories for glycogen
  4.4 Calories for oils
  4.6 Calories for fat
  4.6 Calories for protein
  5.06 Calories for starch
  5.08 Calories for sucrose

22.4 liters of oxygen = 30 grams of glycogen

1 liter of oxygen (R.Q. = 1) = 5.047 calories = 15,575 foot-pounds
= 2,153 kilogram meters
= 0.47 horsepower if used in 1 minute

1 gram of oxygen = approximately 3.5 calories

At 0° C., 760 mm. Hg pressure, 1 liter CO_2 = 1.9652 grams
1 liter O_2 = 1.4292 grams
1 liter air = 1.2928 grams
1 liter water vapor = 0.8038 gram
1 gram water vapor = 1.2440 liters

1 Calorie = 1 kilogram calorie = 1,000 gram calories
= 3.968 B.T.U. at 60° F. = 4,185 joules
= 3,087 foot-pounds = 426.7 kilogram meters
= 69.7 watt-minutes

INDEX